# THE CLEVELAND CLINIC GUIDE TO
# Surgical Patient Management

### Editor
### Jeffrey Ponsky, M.D.
Director, Endoscopic and Minimally Invasive Surgery
Department of General Surgery
The Cleveland Clinic Foundation
Cleveland, Ohio

### Co-Editors
### Michael Rosen, M.D.
Research Fellow, Minimally Invasive Surgery Center
The Cleveland Clinic Foundation
Cleveland, Ohio
Resident in Surgery
Massachusetts General Hospital
Boston, Massachusetts

### Jason Brodsky, M.D.
Resident in Surgery
George Washington Medical Center
Washington, D.C.

### Fredrick Brody, M.D.
Staff Surgeon
The Cleveland Clinic Foundation
Cleveland, Ohio

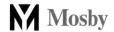

**Mosby**

*A Harcourt Health Sciences Company*

St. Louis   London   Philadelphia   Sydney   Toronto

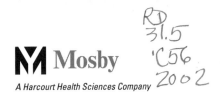

RD
31.5
'C56
2002

*Publishing Director:* Richard Lampert
*Senior Editorial Assistant:* Elizabeth LoGiudice
*Production Manager:* Donna L. Morrissey

Mosby, Inc.
*A Harcourt Health Sciences Company*
11830 Westline Industrial Drive
St. Louis, Missouri 63146

Printed in the United States of America

**Library of Congress Cataloging in Publication Data**

The Cleveland Clinic guide to surgical patient management / [edited by] Jeffrey Ponsky ... [et al.]
      p. ; cm.
   Includes index.
   ISBN 0-323-01709-6
   1. Operations, Surgical. 2. Preoperative care. 3. Postoperative care.
I. Title: Surgical patient management. II. Ponsky, Jeffrey L. III. Cleveland Clinic Foundation.
   [DNLM: 1. Surgical Procedures, Operative. 2. Intraoperative Care.
WO 500 C635 2002]
RD31.5 .C56 2002
617'.9—dc21
                                        2001044503

Last digit is the print number: 9 8 7 6 5 4 3 2 1

To all our colleagues
past, present, and future.

# CONTRIBUTORS

**Hazem Abou El Fettouh, M.D.**
Urologic Transplant Fellow
The Cleveland Clinic Foundation
Cleveland, Ohio

**Lee Akst, M.D.**
Otolaryngology Resident
The Cleveland Clinic Foundation
Cleveland, Ohio

**Justin Albani, M.D.**
Urology Resident
The Cleveland Clinic Foundation
Cleveland, Ohio

**Kevin L. W. Banks, M.D.**
Urology Resident
The Cleveland Clinic Foundation
Cleveland, Ohio

**Hani Baradi, M.D.**
Surgical Resident
The Cleveland Clinic Foundation
Cleveland, Ohio

**Eren Berber, M.D.**
Surgical Resident
The Cleveland Clinic Foundation
Cleveland, Ohio

**Jason Brodsky, M.D.**
Surgical Resident
George Washington University
Washington, D.C.

**Fredrick Brody, M.D.**
Staff Surgeon
The Cleveland Clinic Foundation
Cleveland, Ohio

**Brett Butler, M.D.**
Surgical Resident
The Cleveland Clinic Foundation
Cleveland, Ohio

**Ali Chahlavi, M.D.**
Neurosurgery Resident
The Cleveland Clinic Foundation
Cleveland, Ohio

**Bipand Chand, M.D.**
Surgical Resident
The Cleveland Clinic Foundation
Cleveland, Ohio

**Edward E. Cherullo, M.D.**
Urology Resident
The Cleveland Clinic Foundation
Cleveland, Ohio

**Babak Dadvand, M.D.**
Surgical Resident
The Cleveland Clinic Foundation
Cleveland, Ohio

**Christopher Discolo, M.D.**
Otolaryngology Resident
The Cleveland Clinic Foundation
Cleveland, Ohio

**Martin Goodman, M.D.**
Clinical Fellow, Surgical Oncology
University of Pittsburgh
Pittsburgh, Pennsylvania

**Jeffrey Hazey, M.D.**
Staff Surgeon
Eastern Tennessee State University
Greenville, North Carolina

**Michael J. Henderson, M.D.**
Chairman, Department of General Surgery
The Cleveland Clinic Foundation
Cleveland, Ohio

**Douglas Jones, M.D.**
Surgical Resident
The Cleveland Clinic Foundation
Cleveland, Ohio

**Venkatesh Krishnamuthi, M.D.**
Staff Urology Surgeon
The Cleveland Clinic Foundation
Cleveland, Ohio

**Wayne Kuang, M.D.**
Urology Resident
The Cleveland Clinic Foundation
Cleveland, Ohio

**Walter Lee, M.D.**
Otolaryngology Resident
The Cleveland Clinic Foundation
Cleveland, Ohio

**Abeel A. Mangi, M.D.**
Surgical Resident
Massachusetts General Hospital
Boston, Massachusetts

**Floriano Marchetti, M.D.**
Surgical Resident
The Cleveland Clinic Foundation
Cleveland, Ohio

**Ikenna Okereke, M.D.**
Surgical Resident
The Cleveland Clinic Foundation
Cleveland, Ohio

**Edward Panzeter, M.D.**
Surgical Resident
The Cleveland Clinic Foundation
Cleveland, Ohio

**Jeffrey Ponsky, M.D.**
Staff Surgeon
The Cleveland Clinic Foundation
Cleveland, Ohio

**Lee E. Ponsky, M.D.**
Urology Resident
The Cleveland Clinic Foundation
Cleveland, Ohio

**Todd Ponsky, M.D.**
Surgical Resident
George Washington University
Washington, D.C.

**Eric E. Roselli, M.D.**
Surgical Resident
The Cleveland Clinic Foundation
Cleveland, Ohio

**Michael Rosen, M.D.**
Research Fellow, Minimally Invasive
  Surgery Center
The Cleveland Clinic Foundation
Cleveland, Ohio
Resident in Surgery
Massachusetts General Hospital
Boston, Massachusetts

**Adheesh A. Sabnis, M.D.**
Surgical Resident
George Washington University
Washington, D.C.

**David Sharp, M.D.**
Urology Resident
The Cleveland Clinic Foundation
Cleveland, Ohio

**Conrad Simfendorfer, M.D.**
Surgical Resident
The Cleveland Clinic Foundation
Cleveland, Ohio

**Jitendra V. Singh, M.D.**
Surgical Resident
Nassau Hospital
Long Island, New York

**Michael Tarnoff, M.D.**
Clinical Fellow, Minimally Invasive
  Surgery Center
The Cleveland Clinic Foundation
Cleveland, Ohio

**David P. Vogt, M.D.**
Staff Surgeon
The Cleveland Clinic Foundation
Cleveland, Ohio

**Justin S. Wu, M.D.**
Fellow in Hepatobiliary-Pancreatic
  Surgery
The Cleveland Clinic Foundation
Cleveland, Ohio

**Emad Zakhary, M.D.**
Surgical Resident
The Cleveland Clinic Foundation
Cleveland, Ohio

**Keith Zuccala, M.D.**
Clinical Fellow, Minimally Invasive
  Surgery Center
The Cleveland Clinic Foundation
Cleveland, Ohio

# PREFACE

Fear is a common emotion experienced by young surgical residents as they begin a new and unfamiliar rotation. Each surgical specialty demands precise, unique care of its patients. Although medical school provides a broad overview of pathophysiology and patient care, graduates are hardly prepared to face the rigorous specifics of preoperative and postoperative care in patients with complex surgical problems. Rapid technical and cognitive developments in the surgical specialties have added to the vast knowledge base that residents must acquire when beginning a new rotation. Traditionally residents new to a specialty have relied on more senior colleagues and experienced nursing staff to assist them in writing orders and planning the care of patients.

The purpose of this book is to provide a ready and handy resource for surgical housestaff that will facilitate the daily care of their patients. Each chapter will briefly explain the nature of a disease process, its appropriate workup, operative strategy, and postoperative care. This work is a compilation of the effort of surgical residents, most at the Cleveland Clinic, who have experienced the frustration and anxiety of working on a new surgical rotation and wish to enhance the experience of those to follow. In the end we hope that this is a usable and helpful resource that will effect better care for our patients and a better work experience for surgical housestaff.

**Jeffrey Ponsky, M.D., F.A.C.S.**

# CONTENTS

**PART I**
**FLUIDS, ELECTROLYTES, AND NUTRITION**

1 Fluids and Electrolytes, 3
*Jeffrey Ponsky*

2 Enteral Feeding Access, 9
*Justin Albani*

3 Surgical Enteral Nutrition, 15
*Justin Albani*

**PART II**
**SURGICAL EMERGENCIES**

4 Upper Gastrointestinal Tract Bleeding, 27
*Brett Butler*

5 Lower Gastrointestinal Tract Bleeding, 31
*Todd Ponksy*

6 Intestinal Obstruction, 35
*Douglas Jones*

7 Shock, 41
*Jason Brodsky*

**PART III**
**ESOPHAGUS AND STOMACH**

8 Achalasia, 47
*Michael Rosen*

9 Gastroesophageal Reflux Disease and Paraesophageal Hernia, 53
*Eric E. Roselli*

10 Ulcer Disease, 61
*Edward Panzeter*

11 Gastric Cancer, 67
*Conrad Simfendorfer*

**PART IV**
**SMALL AND LARGE INTESTINE**

12 Appendectomy, 75
*Jason Brodsky*

13 Diverticular Disease, 81
*Hani Baradi*

14 Colon Cancer, 85
*Hani Baradi*

15 Inflammatory Bowel Disease, 91
*Hani Baradi*

## PART V
## ANORECTAL

16  Fistula in Ano, 99
    *Floriano Marchetti*

17  Perirectal Abscess, 105
    *Floriano Marchetti*

18  Hemorrhoids, 111
    *Keith Zuccala*

19  Rectal Cancer, 115
    *Floriano Marchetti*

## PART VI
## HEPATOBILIARY AND PANCREAS

20  Cholecystectomy, 125
    *Michael Rosen*

21  Acute Pancreatitis, 133
    *Michael Tarnoff*

22  Cirrhosis, 143
    *Justin S. Wu*
    *Michael J. Henderson*

23  Liver Cancer and Resection, 151
    *Eren Berber*

24  Pancreatic Cancer, 159
    *Martin Goodman*

25  Endoscopic Retrograde Cholangiopancreatography, 167
    *Jeffrey Hazey*

## PART VII
## HERNIA

26  Inguinal Hernia, 175
    *Keith Zuccala*

27  Umbilical Abdominal Hernia, 183
    *Conrad Simfendorfer*

## PART VIII
## ENDOCRINE

28  Thyroidectomy, 189
    *Jitendra V. Singh*

29  Parathyroidectomy, 197
    *Lee Akst*

30  Neoplasms of the Endocrine Pancreas, 205
    *Eric E. Roselli*

31  Adrenal Disease, 213
    *Lee E. Ponsky*

32 Breast Cancer, 223
*Michael Rosen*
*Emad Zakhary*

**PART IX**
**VASCULAR**

33 Carotid Endarterectomy, 235
*Babak Dadvand*

34 Mesenteric Ischemia, 241
*Jeffrey Hazey*

35 Dialysis Access: Chronic Ambulatory Peritoneal Dialysis, 249
*Jeffrey Hazey*

**PART X**
**SKIN AND SOFT TISSUE**

36 Wound Healing and Management, 257
*Edward E. Cherullo*

37 Skin and Soft Tissue Tumors, 265
*Brett Butler*

38 Melanoma, 269
*Lee Akst*

**PART XI**
**HEMATOLOGY**

39 Splenectomy, 279
*Bipand Chand*

**PART XII**
**CARDIOTHORACIC SURGERY**

40 Coronary Artery Bypass Grafting, 287
*Abeel A. Mangi*

41 Cardiac Valve Disease, 297
*Abeel A. Mangi*

42 Lung Cancer, 307
*Michael Rosen*
*Emad Zakhary*

43 Lung Volume Reduction Surgery, 317
*Ikenna Okereke*

44 Video-assisted Thoracoscopic Surgery, 321
*Eric E. Roselli*

**PART XIII**
**EAR, NOSE, AND THROAT**

45 Nosebleeds (Epistaxis), 327
*Walter Lee*

46 Tracheotomy, 331
   *Lee Akst*

47 Parotidectomy, 337
   *Christopher Discolo*

**PART XIV**
**TRANSPLANT**

48 Renal Transplantation, 345
   *Wayne Kuang*
   *Hazem Abou El Fettouh*

49 Transplantation of the Pancreas, 353
   *Kevin L. W. Banks*
   *Venkatesh Krishnamuthi*

50 Liver Transplantation, 361
   *Justin S. Wu*
   *David P. Vogt*
   *Michael J. Henderson*

51 Pulmonary Transplantation, 371
   *Eric E. Roselli*

52 Cardiac Transplantation, 379
   *Eric E. Roselli*

**PART XV**
**PALM PILOTS**

53 Digital Peripheral Brains, 389
   *Adheesh A. Sabnis*

**PART XVI**
**BEDSIDE PROCEDURES**

54 Chest Tubes, 401
   *Michael Rosen*

55 Thoracentesis, 405
   *David Sharp*

56 Lumbar Puncture, 411
   *Ali Chahlavi*

Index, 417

# ABBREVIATIONS

| | |
|---|---|
| ABGs | Arterial blood gases |
| ACBE | Air-contrast barium enema |
| ACT | Activated clotting time |
| ACTH | Adrenocorticotropic hormone |
| ad lib | As desired |
| AFP | Alpha-fetoprotein |
| ALP | Alkaline phosphatase |
| ALT | Alanine aminotransferase |
| APR | Abdominoperineal resection |
| aPTT | Activated partial thromboplastin time |
| AST | Aspartate aminotransferase |
| ATG | Antithymocyte globulin |
| ATN | Acute tubular necrosis |
| AV | Arteriovenous; atrioventricular |
| AVM | Arteriovenous malformation |
| BAO | Basal acid output |
| BCT | Breast-conserving therapy |
| BEE | Basal energy expenditure |
| BM | Basement membrane |
| BMI | Body mass index |
| BMP | Basic metabolic profile (Na, K, Cl, $HCO_3$, BUN, Cr, glucose) |
| BP | Blood pressure |
| bpm | Beats per minute |
| BUN | Blood urea nitrogen |
| CAA | Coloanal anastomosis |
| CABG | Coronary artery bypass graft |
| CAD | Coronary artery disease |
| CAH | Congenital adrenal hyperplasia |
| CAPD | Continuous ambulatory peritoneal dialysis |
| CBC | Complete blood count |
| CBD | Common bile duct |
| CCK-HIDA | Cholecystokinin-hepatobiliary iminodiacetic acid |
| CCK-PZ | Cholecystokinin-pancreozymin |
| CEA | Carcinoembryonic antigen |
| CFS | Cancer family syndrome |
| CHF | Congestive heart failure |
| CI | Cardiac index |
| CK | Creatine kinase |
| CLM | Conjoined longitudinal muscle |
| CMP | Complete metabolic profile (Na, K, Cl, $HCO_3$, BUN, Cr, glucose, LDH, uric acid, total protein, GGT, LFTs) |
| CMV | Cytomegalovirus |
| CNS | Central nervous system |

| | |
|---|---|
| COPD | Chronic obstructive pulmonary disease |
| CPK | Creatine phosphokinase |
| Cr | Creatinine |
| CRC | Colorectal cancer |
| CRH | Corticotropin-releasing hormone |
| CSF | Cerebrospinal fluid |
| CT | Computed tomography |
| CUSA | Cavitron Ultrasonic Surgical Aspirator |
| CVA | Cerebrovascular accident |
| CVC | Central venous catheter |
| CVP | Central venous pressure |
| CXR | Chest x-ray examination |
| DBP | Diastolic blood pressure |
| D/C | Discontinue |
| DCIS | Ductal carcinoma in situ |
| DDD | Arterial universal pacemaker |
| DHEA | Dehydroepiandrosterone |
| DIC | Disseminated intravascular coagulation |
| DVT | Deep venous thrombosis |
| EAS | External anal sphincter |
| EBV | Epstein-Barr virus |
| ECG | Electrocardiogram |
| ECR | Endocavitary radiation |
| EEA | End-to-end anastomosis |
| EGD | Esophagogastroduodenoscopy |
| ELND | Elective lymph node dissection |
| ER | Estrogen receptor |
| ERCP | Endoscopic retrograde cholangiopancreatography |
| ER-PR | Estrogen receptor-progesterone receptor |
| ESLD | End-stage liver disease |
| ESR | Erythrocyte sedimentation rate |
| ESRD | End-stage renal disease |
| ET | Enterostomal therapy |
| ETT | Endotracheal tube |
| EUA | Examination under anesthesia |
| EUS | Endoscopic ultrasonography |
| F | French |
| FAP | Familial adenomatous polyposis |
| FFP | Fresh-frozen plasma |
| FNA | Fine needle aspiration |
| FNAB | Fine-needle aspiration biopsy |
| FOBT | Fecal occult blood test |
| Foley | Foley urinary catheter |
| GE | Gastroesophageal |
| GERD | Gastroesophageal reflux disease |
| GGT | Gamma glutamyl transferase |

| | |
|---|---|
| GI | Gastrointestinal |
| GIA | Gastrointestinal anastomosis |
| HA | Horseshoe abscesses |
| HAT | Hepatic artery thrombosis |
| Hb | Hemoglobin |
| HBC | Hepatitis C virus |
| HBE | Harris-Benedict equation |
| HBV | Hepatitis B virus |
| HCC | Hepatocellular cancer |
| HCT | Hematocrit |
| H/H | Hematocrit and hemoglobin |
| HIV Ab | Human immunodeficiency virus antibody |
| HIDA | Hepatobiliary iminodiacetic acid |
| HLA | Histocompatibility leukocyte antigen |
| HNPCC | Hereditary nonpolyposis colorectal cancer |
| HONK | Hyperosmotic nonketotic coma |
| HR | Heart rate |
| HSSCC | Hereditary site-specific colon cancer |
| HSV | Herpes simplex virus |
| IAS | Internal anal sphincter |
| I&D | Incision and drainage |
| I&O | Input and output |
| IBC | Inflammatory breast cancer |
| IBD | Inflammatory bowel disease |
| IBW | Ideal body weight |
| ICP | Intracranial pressure |
| ICU | Intensive care unit |
| IM | Intramuscular |
| IMA | Inferior mesenteric artery |
| IMV | Intermittent mandatory ventilation |
| INR | International normalized ratio |
| IPAA | Ileal-pouch anal anastomosis |
| IPF | Idiopathic pulmonary fibrosis |
| IS | Incentive spirometry |
| IV | Intravenous |
| IVPB | Intravenous piggyback |
| KUB | Kidney ureter bladder film |
| KVO | Keep vein open |
| LABC | Locally advanced breast cancer |
| LAR | Low anterior resection |
| LCIS | Lobular carcinoma in situ |
| LCWS | Low continuous wall suction |
| LDH | Lactate dehydrogenase |
| LES | Lower esophageal sphincter |
| LFTs | Liver function tests |
| LIWS | Low intermittent wall suction |

| LR | Lactated Ringer's |
|---|---|
| LV | Left ventricular |
| LVRS | Lung volume reduction surgery |
| MAP | Mean arterial pressure |
| MCT | Medullary carcinoma of the thyroid |
| MR | Mitral regurgitation |
| MRA | Magnetic resonance angiography |
| MRCP | Magnetic resonance cholangiopancreatography |
| MRI | Magnetic resonance imaging |
| NG | Nasogastric |
| NGT | Nasogastric tube |
| NKDA | No known drug allergies |
| NPC/N ratio | Nonprotein calories/nitrogen ratio |
| NPO | Nothing by mouth |
| NS | Normal saline (isotonic sodium chloride solution) |
| NSAID | Nonsteroidal antiinflammatory drug |
| N/V | Nausea/vomiting |
| OGT | Orogastric tube |
| OLT | Orthotopic liver transplantation |
| OOB | Out of bed |
| OR | Operating room |
| PA | Pulmonary artery |
| PAC | Pulmonary artery catheter or Swan-Ganz catheter |
| PACU | Postanesthesia care unit |
| PAP | Pulmonary artery pressure |
| PAS | Pneumatic antiembolism stockings; Pneumoboots |
| PCA | Patient-controlled analgesia |
| PCM | Protein-calorie malnutrition |
| PD | Pancreatic duct |
| PDGF | Platelet-derived growth factor |
| PEEP | Positive end expiratory pressure |
| PEG | Percutaneous endoscopic gastrostomy |
| PEH | Paraesophageal hernia |
| PEJ | Percutaneous endoscopic jejunostomy |
| PET | Positron-emission tomography |
| PFTs | Pulmonary function tests |
| PICC | Peripherally inserted central catheter |
| PO | By mouth |
| POD | Postoperative day |
| PPD | Purified protein derivative test |
| PPI | Proton pump inhibitor |
| PR | By rectum |
| PRBCs | Packed red blood cells |
| PRM | Puborectalis muscle |
| prn | As needed |
| PS | Pressure support |

| PSA | Prostate-specific antigen |
| PT | Prothrombin time; physiotherapy |
| PTCA | Percutaneous transcatheter angioplasty |
| PTH | Parathyroid hormone |
| PTHC | Percutaneous transhepatic cholangiography |
| PTT | Partial thromboplastin time |
| PUD | Peptic ulcer disease |
| PVD | Portal venous drainage |
| PVR | Pulmonary vascular resistance |
| PVS | Peripheral vascular study |
| RBC | Red blood cell |
| REE | Resting energy expenditure |
| RIND | Reversible ischemic neurologic deficit |
| RPR | Rapid plasma reagin |
| RR | Respiratory rate |
| RUQ | Right upper quadrant |
| RV | Residual volume |
| SBP | Systolic blood pressure |
| SC | Subcutaneous |
| SICU | Surgical intensive care unit |
| SMA | Superior mesenteric artery; Sequential Multiple Analyzer |
| SMV | Superior mesenteric vein |
| s/p | Status post |
| SVD | Systemic venous drainage |
| T | Temperature |
| TAPP | Transabdominal preperitoneal approach |
| T&C | Type and crossmatch |
| T&S | Type and screen |
| TEE | Total energy expenditure; transesophageal echocardiography |
| TEM | Transanal endoscopic microsurgery |
| TEPA | Totally extraperitoneal approach |
| TIA | Transient ischemic attack |
| TIPS | Transjugular intrahepatic portosystemic shunt |
| TPN | Total parenteral nutrition |
| UA | Urinalysis |
| UNOS | United Network for Organ Sharing |
| UOP | Urine output |
| US | Ultrasound |
| UUN | Urinary urea nitrogen |
| UW | University of Wisconsin (preservation solution) |
| VATS | Video-assisted thoracoscopic surgery |
| VMA | Vanillylmandelic acid |
| VZV | Varicella zoster virus |
| WBC | White blood cell |
| WSR | Westergren sedimentation rate |
| YAG | Yttrium-aluminum-garnet |

# PART I

## Fluids, Electrolytes, and Nutrition

# FLUIDS AND ELECTROLYTES

*Jeffrey Ponsky*

The subject of fluids and electrolytes can be complicated and intimidating. For the surgical house officer the important issue is the ability to confidently assess the fluid and electrolyte needs of his or her patients and to provide them in an efficient manner. There is usually little time each day to ponder the basic science behind the decisions to be made. However, once a basic understanding of the requirements is in hand, a rapid and systematic approach to the writing of proper intravenous (IV) fluid orders can be attained.

## I. MAINTENANCE FLUIDS AND ELECTROLYTES

Each person uses water daily to excrete waste products. The fluids are lost in urine, sweat, and respiratory losses (insensible losses) and in the stool (fecal losses). For a 70-kg adult, the range of losses is as follows:

| | |
|---|---|
| Urine | 700-1500 ml/d |
| Insensible | 500-1000 ml/d |
| Fecal | 200-500 ml/d |
| TOTAL | 1400-3000 ml/d |

So each day an adult requires in the range of 1400 to 3000 ml of water to excrete wastes. This is called the **maintenance-free water.**

NOTE: In children the maintenance-free water requirement is 100 ml/kg/d up to 10 kg. Then it is an additional 50 ml/kg for the next 10 kg.

Along with the water that is lost each day, there is a small amount of electrolyte lost. This will be lost even in the face of total electrolyte restriction. Every day, therefore, this small amount of electrolyte must, with the maintenance water, be replaced. These are called the **maintenance electrolytes.** For a 70-kg adult these are as follows:

| | |
|---|---|
| Na | 70-150 mEq/d |
| Cl | 70-150 mEq/d |
| K | 40-60 mEq/d |

NOTE: In children the requirements are 1 to 2 mEq/kg/d.

It is important to be aware of the electrolyte composition of various fluids:

| | Na (mmol/L) | K (mmol/L) | Cl (mmol/L) |
|---|---|---|---|
| $D_5W$ | 0 | 0 | 0 |
| Normal saline (0.9%) | 154 | 0 | 154 |
| ½ normal saline (0.45%) | 75 | 0 | 75 |
| ¼ normal saline (0.2%) | 33 | 0 | 33 |
| Lactated Ringer's solution | 130 | 4 | 110 |

To satisfy the requirements for maintenance fluids and electrolytes, we use hypotonic fluid such as 0.3% or 0.2% normal saline (NS; isotonic sodium chloride solution). We add (in adults) 20 mEq of potassium to each bottle. In most adults 2 L of maintenance fluid (2000 ml) is sufficient. Therefore maintenance IV orders might be:

Bottle 1: 1000 ml $D_5$/0.2% NS with 20 mEq KCl
Bottle 2: 1000 ml $D_5$/0.2% NS with 20 mEq KCl

Rate: 80 ml/h

*or*

Bottle 1: 1000 ml $D_5$/0.3% NS with 20 mEq KCl
Bottle 2: 1000 ml $D_5$/0.3% NS with 20 mEq KCl

Rate: 80 ml/h

Each of these sets of orders will provide maintenance fluids and electrolytes. Using 0.3% NS gives the patient a bigger salt load, but with normal kidneys this is not a problem.

NOTE: For every 1 L you wish to run in over 24 hours, increase the rate by 40 ml/h, so 1 L is 40 ml/h; 2 L is 80 ml/h; 3 L is 120 ml/h; and so on.

**Every patient must have maintenance fluids each day!**
Obviously when patients can take fluids by mouth, maintenance fluid is provided in their diet, but when a patient is NPO, it is the physician's responsibility to provide this requirement.

## II. GASTROINTESTINAL LOSSES

Gastrointestinal losses (ie, diarrhea, fistula output, NGT output) must be measured and replaced milliliter for milliliter with the "appropriate" **fluid in addition to maintenance fluids.** The appropriate fluid is determined by measuring a small amount of the fluid in question and determining its electrolyte composition. An appropriate replacement fluid is then chosen. In adults if losses are small, less than 1 L/d, they may be measured and replaced with the maintenance fluids of the following day. If losses are great, however, the replacement can be given every shift or even every hour piggyback into the maintenance fluid line.

Intake and output (I&O) must be carefully recorded.

Following are example IV orders for a patient who has lost 1 L of fistula drainage. The drainage was measured and approximates 0.45% NS with 20 mEq KCl.

Bottle 1: 1000 ml $D_5$/0.2% NS with 20 mEq KCl
Bottle 2: 1000 ml $D_5$/0.2% NS with 20 mEq KCl
**Bottle 3: 1000 ml 0.45% NS with 20 mEq KCl**
Rate: 120 ml/h

NOTE: The first two bottles represent maintenance fluid. The third bottle is replacement for the gastrointestinal loss.

Nasogastric tube drainage contains:

Na: 75 mEq/L
Cl: 110 mEq/L
K: 10-15 mEq/L

This can be replaced with either normal saline with 20 mEq KCl/L or 0.45% normal saline with 40 mEq KCl/L.

So IV orders for a patient who has lost 1 L of NGT output in the past 24 hours would be:

Bottle 1: 1000 ml $D_5$/0.2% NS with 20 mEq KCl
Bottle 2: 1000 ml $D_5$/0.2% NS with 20 mEq KCl
**Bottle 3: 1000 ml NS with 20 mEq KCl**

Rate: 120 ml/h

*or*

Bottle 1: 1000 ml $D_5$/0.2% NS with 20 mEq KCl
Bottle 2: 1000 ml $D_5$/0.2% NS with 20 mEq KCl
**Bottle 3: 1000 ml $D_5$/0.45% NS with 40 mEq KCl**

Rate: 120 ml/h

Again, the first 2 L are maintenance, and the third is replacement of NGT output.

NOTE: You may see some people write 3 L of $D_5$/0.45% NS with 20 mEq KCl for patients who have lost 1 L of NG suction fluid. That is the same as giving $D_5$/NS as the replacement fluid for NGT output.

## III. THIRD SPACE LOSSES

A "third space" is a body compartment where fluid may be sequestered but is not readily available for exchange with the intravascular space. Such compartments include the peritoneal cavity, the soft tissue, the thoracic cavity, and the intestinal lumen. When fluid accumulates in a third space, it is transferred there from the intravacular space and essentially represents a transudate of the plasma. Therefore, the fluid has an electrolyte composition similar to serum electrolytes and should be replaced with lactated Ringer's solution, which approximates serum electrolytes.

Third space losses occur after major abdominal surgery, trauma, and burns. These losses begin immediately and must be replaced immediately **in addition** to maintenance fluids.

The amount of third space fluid to be replaced is essentially a guess, but the goal of replacement is to maintain adequate perfusion. The latter may be assessed by insertion of a urinary catheter and observation of urine output. Output should be noted each hour, with an optimum desired range of 0.5 to 1 ml/kg/h, or 30 to 60 ml/h in an adult.

When IV orders are written after surgery in anticipation of third space loss, a reasonable amount of Ringer's to include, in addition to maintenance fluids, is a volume equal to that of maintenance.

Also, in the immediate postoperative period, potassium is usually omitted until there is assurance that there is satisfactory urine output.

So postoperative IV orders when third space loss is anticipated might be:

Bottle 1: 1000 ml $D_5$/lactated Ringer's solution
Bottle 2: 1000 ml $D_5$/0.2% NS
Bottle 3: 1000 ml $D_5$/0.2% NS
Bottle 4: 1000 ml $D_5$/lactated Ringer's solution
Rate: 160 ml/h

NOTE: **This rate is only a guess, and the urine output will now be used to help guide the titration of the IV rate.**

Three scenarios help explain what may happen.

## Scenario 1

Over the next several hours the patient's urine output is high (ie, 100 ml/h). The IV rate should be cut to perhaps 120 ml/h and the output assessed over the next few hours. When the output remains in the desired range with no further adjustments, then reducing the IV rate has reduced the amount of third space fluid replaced by 1 L.

Third space losses may end after 24 to 36 hours, and replacement on the second day will depend on assessment of urine output.

## Scenario 2

Over the next several hours the patient's urine output is low (ie, 10 ml). After checking the catheter for obstruction, a bolus of third space replacement should be given.

In an adult or child a bolus of up to 20 ml/kg can be rapidly given. In an adult, that can be up to 1500 ml. However, it is best to try smaller boluses first and assess their effect. So in this case a bolus of 500 ml of lactated Ringer's should be given in addition to the ongoing IV fluids. If the urine output responds appropriately, nothing further need be done. If later on the output again drops, an additional bolus (or two) may be given.

## Scenario 3

Over the next several hours the patient's urine output is low. Boluses up to 1500 ml are given, and there is no response.

Several problems may be at play here, and further assessment is required. The patient could still be intravascularly depleted and require more fluids or he or she may have cardiac or renal failure.

After giving the initial boluses up to 1500 ml there is a need for central venous pressure (CVP) monitoring to assess fluid status. This can be done with a CVP line or a pulmonary artery (Swan Ganz) catheter. A normal CVP or wedge pressure can be up to 15 mm Hg.

If the CVP is less than 10, further Ringer's or colloid should be pushed until the CVP rises above 10, or good urine output is achieved. Diuretics should not be used until adequate volume (as indicated by CVPs) is restored and may not be necessary at all if the urine output responds to the rising CVP.

Should the CVP be greater than 15 mm Hg, the IV rate should be reduced and attention turned to assessment of the heart and kidneys. When only a small amount of urine is being excreted, the specific gravity should be high (ie, 1.030). If the specific gravity is low (ie, 1.010), renal damage must be suspected.

FLUIDS AND ELECTROLYTES

# ENTERAL FEEDING ACCESS

*Justin Albani*

## PEG (PERCUTANEOUS ENDOSCOPIC GASTROSTOMY)

Since its initial description by Ponsky and Gauderer in 1980, PEG has had a profound impact on enteral access and techniques of alimentation. Enteral feeding is now the second most common indication for upper gastrointestinal endoscopy in hospitalized patients. The PEG method allows for the creation of a tube gastrostomy without the need for general anesthesia or laparotomy.

**2**

## I. INDICATIONS

1. **Chronic inability to eat orally:** The most common indication for gastrostomy is enteral access in patients with a functional gastrointestinal tract who are unable to take oral nutrition. Candidates for this procedure include those with profound neurologic deficits due to multiple sclerosis, cerebrovascular accidents, dementia, trauma, Parkinson's disease, or anoxic encephalopathy. In addition, patients with extensive facial trauma, tumors of the esophagus or orpharynx, or who are receiving ongoing radiotherapy are also excellent candidates. PEG can provide supplemental nocturnal feeding for children with malabsorptive or inflammatory bowel disease.

2. **Prolonged gastric decompression:** As a palliative procedure in patients with chronic bowel obstruction due to radiation enteritis or carcinomatosis, gastrostomy drainage serves as a gastric vent sufficient to prevent nausea and vomiting and thus preclude prolonged nasogastric intubation. However, gastrostomy drainage typically does not provide drainage volumes comparable to nasogastric suctioning.

3. **Replacement of biliary drainage** either with intended biliary fistulas (percutaneous transhepatic catheter drains) or unintended biliary fistulas due to injury or operative complications. Here the PEG would function as a biliogastric shunt by recycling bile from a biliary fistula back into the stomach.

4. **Reduction of a chronic intermittent gastric volvulus:** The volvulus is reduced either laparoscopically or endoscopically, then anchored with a PEG in the body and a PEG in the distal antrum with removal of the gastrostomy tubes a few weeks later.

5. **A route of administering medications** to pediatric patients unable or unwilling to ingest unpalatable medications or diet because of underlying metabolic deficiencies such as urea cycle deficiencies or glycogen storage diseases.

## II. TYPICAL PRESENTATION

The typical patient who presents for PEG placement possesses a fully functional gastrointestinal tract but is unable to take oral nutrition. This includes patients with profound neurologic impairments due to maladies such as stroke, amyotrophic lateral sclerosis, or pseudobulbar palsy, as well as patients with extensive facial trauma or tumors of the esophagus or orpharynx.

## III. PREOPERATIVE EVALUATION

Obtaining a history ensuring a functional gastrointestinal system is essential. Typical preoperative evaluation includes a coagulation panel ensuring normal prothrombin time (PT) and activated partial thromboplastin time (aPTT). The surgeon must exclude any condition that precludes the passing of the endoscope into the stomach or prevents transillumination of the abdominal wall. These relative contraindications include morbid obesity, significant hepatomegaly, gastric varices, and multiple abdominal surgeries. In addition, patients with massive ascites are poor candidates because adhesion of the stomach to the abdominal wall is not likely. Patients with severe gastroesophageal reflux disease (GERD) or a history of frequent aspiration are poor candidates as well.

Perhaps the most overlooked contraindication to PEG placement is a patient with severe comorbidities that suggest a life expectancy too brief to justify invasive enteral access, such as patients with systemic sepsis or rapidly deteriorating medical conditions with multiple system organ failure.

### PREOPERATIVE ORDERS

**Diet:** NPO 8 hours before the procedure
**Medications:** a single preoperative prophylactic dose of an IV cephalosporin antibiotic; IV sedation available for the procedure

## IV. CONDUCT OF OPERATION

This procedure may be performed in an operative suite or any closely monitored setting such as an intensive care unit or endoscopy suite.

The patient is supine; therefore an assistant is needed to suction the posterior pharynx when secretions accumulate. The patient is given an intravenous sedative, and the mouth and pharynx are swabbed with an antiseptic solution. The abdomen is prepped and draped in the normal sterile fashion.

Room lights are turned down as the gastroscope is passed into the stomach, and the stomach is insufflated. This pushes the colon caudad and the liver and spleen cephalad. Transillumination of the abdominal wall by the endoscope indicates that no intervening structures are present, and allows selection of the optimum site for gastrostomy insertion. A point is chosen on the abdominal wall approximately two thirds the distance along a line drawn from the umbilicus to the midpoint of the left costal margin.

The skin and fascia are then infiltrated with local anesthetic (1 to 3 ml 1% lidocaine [Xylocaine]), and a 5-mm incision is made in the skin and anterior rectus muscle sheath at the site of transillumination. Next, a safe tract technique is used. A 10-cc syringe with saline is placed on a needle and passed directly into the stomach. Simultaneously, the endoscope is directed to the point where the needle will pass through the stomach wall. Under direct vision the needle is passed into the stomach and withdrawn so that at the point air is obtained in the syringe the needle is also seen entering the stomach. This will avoid undetected passage through the lumen of the colon. A smoothly tapered 16-gauge intravenous catheter is then placed through the abdominal wall and stomach under direct visualization by the gastroscope. A wire polypectomy snare is passed through the gastroscope and looped around the catheter. A stout suture or wire is passed through the catheter and grabbed by the snare of the endoscope, and the endoscope and suture are then withdrawn through the mouth.

A lubricated modified mushroom catheter is then attached to this suture through the drainage end of the gastrostomy tube and pulled retrograde through the mouth, esophagus, stomach, and abdominal wall and through the abdominal entry site. This action ensures that the gastrostomy tube moves down the esophagus and out the abdominal wall. The gastroscope is reinserted to check the abdominal wall and the position of the head of the tube and to ensure that excessive tension is not applied to the head of the catheter. The endoscope is removed, and an outer bolster is attached to hold the gastric and abdominal walls together. The total procedure typically takes approximately 15 minutes.

## VARIATIONS OF PEG

**Pull (Ponsky).** The most common PEG technique, it is described in the preceding discussion.

**Push (Sacks-Vine).** This variation is similar to the pull technique except that a long guidewire is placed through the inserted catheter and grasped with the endoscopic snare and pulled from the patient's mouth. A special gastrostomy tube with a tapered dilator end is then *pushed* over the guidewire. The tube is pushed down the esophagus to exit the abdominal wall and then pulled from the abdominal wall once it is visible at the surface.

**Introducer (Russell).** This variation of PEG involves percutaneous gastrostomy without passing the tube through the mouth and with only one insertion of the endoscope. The gastroscope is passed into the stomach, room lights are dimmed, the abdominal wall is transilluminated, and finger pressure at the point of best transillumination is used to note the best location for puncture. The skin is anesthetized, a small incision is made, and a needle is introduced into the gastric lumen. A guidewire is passed through the needle, the needle is removed, and an introducer with an outer peel-away sheath is placed over the guidewire into the stomach. Once the introducer and wire are removed, only the sheath remains in the stomach. A urinary catheter is then placed through the sheath, the balloon is inflated, and the sheath is removed. The catheter is then sutured to the skin to hold the tube in place.

**Radiologic Procedure.** A previously placed feeding or nasogastric tube is used for insufflating the stomach. Ultrasonography is then used to locate the skin entrance site in the left upper quadrant. Local anesthesia is achieved with a subcutaneous lidocaine injection. Under ultrasonographic guidance, a gastric puncture is performed through a small incision at the anesthetized site and a T-bar is placed. A guidewire is then coiled into the stomach, the needle is removed, and a gastrostomy tube is placed. The tube is then secured to the skin with sutures.

**Laparoscopic PEG.** This variation is used in situations requiring laparoscopic visualization of the gastric puncture site because anatomic limitations prevent safe PEG placement.

## POSTOPERATIVE ORDERS

**Admit to:**
**Diagnosis:** s/p PEG
**Condition:** stable
**Vital signs:** per routine
**Activity:** ad lib
**Allergies:**
**Nursing:** strict I&O's, NPO × 24 hours

- Start tube feeds the morning after placement with sterile water at a low rate (50 ml/h for 2 hours) and advancing to formula tube feedings if water is well tolerated to achieve a maximum goal rate over a number of hours. Gastric residuals are checked every 4 to 6 hours to ensure that the patient is tolerating the tube feedings. The tubes are flushed with lukewarm tap water (30 ml each flush) every 4 hours once tube feeding has begun to ensure patency.
- The tube exit site is cleaned with soap and water daily after tube placement, and a split sterile gauze dressing is placed under the external bumper once each day for the first 5 days, and then prn.
- Other orders are specific to the purpose of the gastrostomy tube and include placing the tube to gravity drainage or suction for decompression. The tube is plugged and can be reopened and drained if the patient experiences nausea or vomiting.

## V. POTENTIAL COMPLICATIONS

Results from large series demonstrate that the PEG procedure may be performed safely with minor complications in 4% to 13% of patients, with procedure-related mortality less than 1%.

1. **Peristomal infections:** The most common procedure-related side effect of PEG placement (5%-30%) is infection caused by the escape of gastric or oral flora into tissues of the abdominal wall. This manifests as erythema around the gastrostomy tube days after the procedure with local tenderness, edema of the skin, low-grade fever, and leukocytosis. This can easily be treated with local incision and drainage.
2. **Necrotizing fasciitis:** This rapidly progressive infectious process is characterized by fascial and subcutaneous involvement and systemic toxic manifestations. Signs include crepitance, ecchymosis, erythema, and bullae on the abdominal wall or flank with or without pus. Plain abdominal x-ray films show fluid and gas in the subcutaneous tissues of the abdominal wall. Risk factors include diabetes mellitus, atherosclerosis, alcoholism, malnutrition, immunosuppression, and age older than 50 years.
3. **Leakage of feedings into the peritoneal cavity** usually is due to necrosis of the abdominal wall tissue as a result of excessive tension on the catheter. Patients should have water-soluble contrast instilled into the gastrostomy tube to evaluate for leaks. If a leak is seen, the patient's gastrostomy tube should be pulled, a nasogastric tube should be inserted, and intravenous fluids and antibiotics should be initiated.
4. **Peritonitis** is seen in 0 to 1.2% of patients undergoing PEG. It is potentially fatal and may be due to premature removal of the catheter before the firm adhesions between the stomach and abdominal wall have formed or to the stomach's not having been brought into apposition with the parietal surface of the abdominal wall during the PEG procedure.
5. **Gastrocolocutaneous fistula** may be due to puncture of the colon at the time of gastrostomy placement or entrapment of the colon between the gastric and abdominal walls. Diagnosis can be made by injection of Gastrografin through the PEG to identify the catheter tip in the colon.
6. **Pneumoperitoneum** is due to air escaping around the puncturing needle site. If the patient has abdominal pain, leukocytosis, or fever, he or she should be evaluated with a water-soluble contrast study through the gastrostomy tube.
7. **Bronchopulmonary aspiration** may occur during the PEG procedure or after placement. It is often prevented by administering minimal sedation during the procedure, by placing the PEG to gravity drainage

for 12 to 24 hours after the procedure, and by elevating the head of the bed at least 30 degrees during tube feedings.

8. **Buried bumper syndrome:** Over several weeks the PEG may migrate anteriorly through the stomach wall if excessive traction is applied and ischemic necrosis of the gastric epithelium occurs. Thus, the PEG may lie completely outside the stomach and embed itself in the abdominal wall.

9. **Hemorrhage** commonly is due to gastric ulcers beneath the internal bolster created by frictional abrasion or excessive traction.

## VI. DISCHARGE ORDERS

Discharge orders are the same as those for postoperative care, because many PEGs are placed in an outpatient setting. The patient may keep the gastrostomy tube indefinitely, as long as simple tube care is performed and the tubes are removed when they are no longer needed, are causing complications, or require replacement. Methods of removal typically involve simply applying gentle traction until the tube exits the abdominal wall. The remaining abdominal wall defect can be covered with gauze and will close in a number of days. Older methods of removal included using an endoscope to snare the remaining catheter portion within the stomach after the catheter was cut off at skin level.

## PERCUTANEOUS ENDOSCOPIC JEJUNOSTOMY

Initially described independently by Ponsky and Aszodi and Gottfried and Plumser in 1984, percutaneous endoscopic jejunostomy (PEJ) is a modification of the PEG allowing jejunal feeding with simultaneous gastric decompression for patients with a history of frequent aspiration or gastroesophageal reflux and in patients with functional motility disorders such as diabetes mellitus or postoperative nonfunctioning gastrojejunostomy. The placement technique is similar to that for PEG but with a parallel longer enteric tube placed in the pylorus for feeding solutions.

Complications are similar to that of PEG, with a greater incidence of tube dysfunction, because clogging is the most common problem seen with PEJ feeding and occurs in 13.8% to 45% of cases. Thus, saline flushing every 4 to 6 hours is highly recommended even with continuous drip feedings.

# SURGICAL ENTERAL NUTRITION

*Justin Albani*

Adequate nutrition in the perioperative period is paramount for optimization of the surgical patient. Although a well-nourished, healthy person undergoing an uncomplicated major procedure has enough fuel reserves for 1 week of starvation, studies indicate that 20% to 60% of patients admitted to hospitals in the United States are undernourished. These patients have higher mortality rates and often are two to three times more likely to have postoperative complications. Clinical studies suggest that early enteral feeding reduces postoperative septic complications by maintaining gut integrity and preventing bacterial translocation. Nutritional support aids in wound healing, immune function, and basal metabolic activity to expedite the patient's postoperative recovery.

## I. METABOLIC CHANGES WITH STRESS

### FASTING AND STARVATION

The body's fuel components consist of carbohydrates in the form of glucose, glycogen, proteins, and lipids. The metabolism of these components varies with food availability. After a meal, glucose is driven into cells as blood levels of insulin increase and glucagon decrease. Obligate glycolytic cells in the brain and red and white blood cells consume 180 g/d of glucose in the average man. Two to three hours after a meal, the liver breaks down glycogen by means of glycogenolysis, and the blood levels of glucagon and catecholamines increase. Four to six hours after fasting, gluconeogenesis begins, as lactate produced by red blood cells and muscles is converted to glucose by means of the Cori cycle in the liver. After 30 hours, the 75 g of glycogen stored in the liver is completely depleted, and gluconeogenesis serves as the sole source of energy. An increase in glucagon levels causes adipose tissue to degrade into fatty acids. These are then oxidized by tissues for energy and converted to ketone bodies for use by the brain. Muscle protein also is degraded into amino acids and ketone bodies to prevent protein loss. In prolonged starvation (after 3 to 5 days), adipose tissue becomes the primary source of energy through the oxidation of fatty acids and conversion into ketone bodies.

### TRAUMA, SEPSIS, OR MAJOR OPERATION

Similar to the stress of starvation, the physiologic stress of sepsis, trauma, or surgery induces important metabolic changes that are often described in the following three phases.

**Catabolic Phase (Adrenergic-Corticoid Phase).** After injury, increased levels of glucagon, glucocorticoids, and catecholamines produce a

15

hypercatabolic state characterized by an increase in both energy expenditure and nitrogen excretion. Low insulin concentrations result in an increase of glucose turnover and lipolysis. These changes are thought to be due to proinflammatory cytokines present after major injury.

**Early Anabolic Phase (Corticoid-Withdrawal Phase).** Within 3 to 8 days after an uncomplicated elective surgery or weeks after sepsis or a major operation, the body shifts from catabolism to anabolism, characterized by an abrupt decrease in nitrogen excretion and positive nitrogen balance. Patients experience increased appetite, diuresis of retained water, weight gain, and increased muscle strength, because anabolic factors such as insulinlike growth factor-1 predominate. Although all the nitrogen lost during the catabolic phase is regained during this period, repletion of nitrogen occurs at a much slower rate.

**Late Anabolic Phase.** Weeks to months after the initial injury, nitrogen balance approaches normalcy with the gradual restoration of adipose stores. A slow but consistent weight gain occurs and is attributed to the high energy content of fat (9 kcal/g).

## II. TYPE OF MALNUTRITION

Protein-calorie malnutrition (PCM) is the most prevalent form of malnourishment seen in hospitals today. Properly identifying patients with severe PCM is important to decrease the risk of perioperative complications, including infections, respiratory failure, poor wound healing, and ultimately death.

Two types of PCM span the continuum of disease severity. **Marasmus** (*marasmos,* a dying away) develops from an inavailability of all nutrients, resulting in wasting of muscle and fat stores. This is best evidenced in patients with anorexia nervosa. Other causes of such malnutrition include decreased intake because of malabsorptive processes such as short bowel syndrome or cardiac cachexia. Clinically, patients have a *normal serum albumin* with wasting of subcutaneous fat and muscle and often have normal mentation and appetite. **Kwashiorkor** ("condition of the displaced child" from Ghana), or **hypoalbuminemic PCM,** is characterized by loss of visceral protein stores, edema, and energy. This is often an extension of marasmus and can be seen commonly in intensive care unit patients associated with sepsis, trauma, and surgery.

## III. INDICATIONS

In otherwise healthy patients, intravenous fluids alone with a minimum of 100 g of glucose daily are sufficient to minimize protein catabolism. Indications for nutritional support include:

1. Fasting expected to last longer than 1 week (eg, prolonged ileus)
2. Weight loss over a period 6 months greater than 10% of the patient's ideal body weight (IBW)
3. Hypermetabolic states such as sepsis, trauma, burns, and major surgery
4. Organ system failure, including respiratory, renal, or hepatic failure
5. Neurologic dysfunction including cerebrovascular accidents (CVAs), dementia, or head trauma
6. Gastrointestinal dysfunction including inflammatory bowel disease (IBD), pancreatitis, or esophageal obstruction
7. Oncology patients undergoing chemotherapy and radiotherapy

## IV. ASSESSMENT

Although the physical examination may elicit signs of malnutrition, including muscle wasting, peripheral edema, glossitis, and angular stomatitis or cheilosis, clinically there is no one highly sensitive or specific method for quantifying malnutrition.

**Anthropometric measurements** estimate somatic protein and body fat stores. The most commonly used measurements allow for the calculation of ideal body weight (IBW) and body mass index (BMI).

Ideal Body Weight
Men: IBW = 47.7 kg (106 lb) + (2.7 kg [6 lb] for every 2.5 cm [1 in.] above 1.5 m [5 ft])
Women: IBW = 45 kg (100 lb) + (2.25 kg [5 lb] for every 2.5 cm [1 in.] above 1.5 m [5 ft])
IBW may be adjusted ± 10% based on an individual's frame size
Body Mass Index
Weight (kg)/(height [m])$^2$
Normal BMI in men is 18.5-23.5 and in women is 19.5-24.5.
A BMI of greater than 35 indicates morbid obesity

## LABORATORY TESTS

Laboratory tests are useful in assessing visceral protein status and monitoring the patient's response to nutritional therapy (Table 3-1). Serum levels of albumin, transferrin, and prealbumin serve as indicators of mal-

### TABLE 3-1
**LABORATORY STUDIES**

| Protein (g/dl) | Half-Life | Normal | Mildly Depleted | Severely Depleted |
| --- | --- | --- | --- | --- |
| Albumin | 21 d | 3.5-5.0 | 3.0-3.4 | <2.1 |
| Transferrin | 7-8 d | 176-315 | 134-175 | <117 |
| Prealbumin | 2-3 d | 18-45 | 10-17 | <5 |

nutrition in the absence of other nonnutritional variables (ascites, liver disease, hydration status). The half-life of each protein determines its sensitivity in assessing protein status. Thus prealbumin with the shortest half-life of 2 to 3 days is the most responsive in evaluating the patient's progress.

Nitrogen balance assesses the adequacy of nutritional intake and the extent of catabolism. Positive nitrogen balance indicates adequate nutrition is present for protein synthesis. Generally, the goal is to achieve a nitrogen balance of $+2$ to $+4$ g. Nitrogen balance is calculated after collecting a 24-hour urine nitrogen sample (UUN; urinary urea nitrogen) as follows:

$$N_2 \text{ balance} = N_{in} - N_{out}$$

$$\text{Nitrogen balance (g)} = (\text{Protein intake}/6.25) - (\text{UUN} + 4)$$

(6.25 demonstrates the average of 6 to 7 g of amino acids per gram of nitrogen, and the 4 accounts for fecal and other nonurinary losses.)

Several additional studies including creatinine-height index, various research techniques, and skeletal muscle function tests are also used for assessing nutritional status but are far less common than those mentioned previously.

## V. NUTRITIONAL REQUIREMENTS

**Calories.** Energy demands are based on weight, height, age, and activity level and are commonly calculated based on the Harris-Benedict equation (HBE) for basal energy expenditure (BEE) in kilocalories per day as follows:

$$\text{HBE: } 655 + (9.6 \times \text{WT}) + (1.7 \times \text{HT}) - (4.7 \times \text{A})$$

$$\text{BEE: } 66 + (13.7 \times \text{WT}) + (5 \times \text{HT}) - (6.8 \times \text{A})$$

where WT = weight in kilograms; HT = height in centimeters; A = age in years.

BEE is the amount of energy required for performing only essential body functions such as respiration, thermal regulation, and cardiac function. Resting energy expenditure (REE) includes stress and body temperature variations and is the preferred clinical measurement. This is calculated by multiplying the stress factor by the BEE. Stress factors include:

Minor operation: 1-1.1
Multiple trauma: 1-1.2
Sepsis: 1.2-1.7
Burn 1.5-2

Total energy expenditure (TEE) includes BEE, REE, and activity plus several other usually clinically insignificant factors. Usually 1.5 to 1.75 × BEE estimates TEE adequately in the hospitalized patient.

Alternatively, caloric goals can be estimated for most hospitalized patients and are between 25 and 35 kcal/kg/d or 125% to 175% of calculated BEE.

Thus, calculating the energy goals for a patient in the absence of indirect or direct calorimetry can be done as follows:

1. Estimate basal energy requirements (20-35 kcal/kg/d) or use HBE.
2. Multiply BEE by stress factor.
3. Add 0 to 20% basal energy expenditure.
4. Add for weight gain if necessary: 500-1000 kcal/d

0.45 kg (1 lb) of adipose tissue requires ~3500 kcal; thus 500 kcal/d extra will allow a patient to gain 0.45 kg per week

**Protein.** Protein demands are often based on stress level or body weight. The nonprotein calories/nitrogen ratio (NPC/N ratio) refers to the amount of nonprotein calories per gram of nitrogen. An oral diet typically has a NPC/N ratio of 300:1. Under stress the body may require a 80 to 150:1 ratio for anabolism. Most feeding solutions have a 150:1 NPC/N ratio.

Optimal protein intake ranges from 0.8 to 2 g/kg/d and varies with the stress.

| | |
|---|---|
| No stress | 0.8 g/kg/d |
| Mild stress | 0.8-1 g/kg/d |
| Moderate stress | 1-1.5 g/kg/d |
| Severe stress | 1.5-2 g/kg/d |

**Carbohydrates.** Intravenous dextrose is the most common energy source providing 3.4 kcal/g. Minimum requirements are approximately 1 mg/kg/min or 100 g/d for a 70-kg man. (1 L of $D_5W$ contains 50 g dextrose). The body tolerates a carbohydrate maximum of approximately 5 to 7 mg/kg/min. Because stressed and septic patients have an impaired glucose tolerance, an intake of less than 5 mg/kg/min is recommended for these patients. Excess carbohydrates have been associated with hyperglycemia, hepatic steatosis, and ventilator dependence. Most commercial enteral formulas have 40% to 50% calories from carbohydrates.

**Lipids.** Generally 35% to 45% of all enteral formula calories are from fat. Sources are often from corn, safflower, sunflower, or soybean oil. In the adult, linoleic acid is the only fatty acid considered essential in the diet of humans, because it is needed for making eicosanoids and prostaglandins from arachadonic acid.

## VI. ENTERAL NUTRITION

Delivering nutrients into the gastrointestinal tract by means of a feeding tube is the method of choice for providing nutritional support to patients

SURGICAL ENTERAL NUTRITION

3

with a fully functional digestive tract. Several clinical trials have noted that patients receiving enteral nutrition have fewer septic complications and use nutrients more efficiently than those receiving parenteral or no additional nutritional support.

## INDICATIONS

Enteral feeding is appropriate in patients who are unable to take oral nutrition and have a functional gastrointestinal tract. These include patients with neurologic impairments such as dysphagia or stroke, facial trauma, or tumors of the oropharynx or esophagus, as well as critically ill patients. Tube feeding is contraindicated in patients having a mechanical bowel obstruction, short bowel syndrome, bowel ischemia, active gastrointestinal bleeding, severe malabsorption, severe inflammatory bowel disease, or a high output gastrointestinal fistula (>200 ml/d). Whenever possible, the gut is the preferred method of choice for nutritional therapy.

## ACCESS

*Nasogastric* tubes are the most appropriate method of tube feeding for most hospitalized patients. *Nasoenteral* feeding into or past the third portion of the duodenum is preferred in patients at risk for aspiration because of gastroparesis or gastroesophageal reflux by bypassing the stomach and using the pyloric and gastroesophageal sphincters. The tube position is always confirmed by means of fluoroscopic guidance or abdominal radiograph before use. A 3.3-mm diameter (10 F) feeding tube is most commonly used to maximize patient comfort and to minimize the risk of clogging when administering enteral nutrition.

Surgical or endoscopic (PEG/PEJ) gastrostomy or jejunostomy tubes are appropriate in patients requiring tube feedings for more than 1 month.

## ALIMENTAL FORMULA TYPES

Several formula types are available and often tailored to specific clinical conditions. Standard formulas usually contain 50% to 55% carbohydrates, 15% to 20% protein, and 30% fat. They have a caloric density of 1 kcal/ml or greater, with an osmolality ranging from isotonic (280 mOsm/L) to hypertonic, and most are lactose free to avoid complications of disaccharidase deficiency. Formulas can be divided into three major categories: polymeric, hydrolyzed, and modular. Polymeric and hydrolyzed formulas comprise most commercial products and are nutritionally complete, whereas modular products are used only to supplement existing commercial formulas.

**Polymeric** or **whole protein** formulas are similar to a regular diet with protein derived from casein and soy protein, long- and medium-chain triglycerides and polysaccharides, and glucose polymers. Examples include *Isocal, Osmolite, Jevity,* and *Ultracal.*

High-calorie/concentrated polymeric formulas have a greater caloric density of 1.5 to 2 kcal/ml and are useful when fluid restriction is indicated. These formulas have a higher osmolality (400-600 mOsm/kg) and thus must be monitored to prevent dehydration. Examples include *Magnacal* and *Isocal HN.*

**Hydrolyzed** or **chemically defined elemental** formulas contain products of protein hydrolysis combined with carbohydrate macronutrients to form oligopeptides, short-chain peptides, and oligosaccharides. These chemically simple products are optimal for patients with impaired absorption, because they do not require digestion. They have a low fat content (1%-15% calories) and thus are unpalatable. They are hyperosmolar (450-700 mOsm/kg water) and four to five times more expensive than polymeric formulas. Examples include *Vivonex TEN, Criticare HN.*

**Modular** products like *Casec* and *Moducal* have a single or few macronutrients and are used solely for supplementation with other enteral formulas.

## Disease-Specific Formulas

**Renal failure** formulas like *Amin-Aid, Nepro, Suplena,* and *Renal Cal* are low in protein but enriched in essential amino acids, are hyperosmolar, and contain low or no electrolytes or fat-soluble vitamins. Because of their low protein content, these can only be used safely for a short period.

**Hepatic failure** formulas like *HepaticAid II* and *Nutrihep* are enriched with branched-chain amino acids (valine, isoleucine, leucine) and are low in aromatic amino acids (tyrosine, phenylalanine, methionine). The true efficacy of these products remains controversial.

**Pulmonary** formulas provide the most calories (up to 55%) as fat in an attempt to decrease the carbohydrate caloric load for and thus the levels of $CO_2$ produced in the mechanically ventilated patient.

**Glucose intolerance** formulas like *Choice DM* are low in carbohydrates, high in fat, isotonic, and supplemented with fiber.

**Immunomodulatory** formulas such as *Impact* and *Alitraq* are enriched with immunostimulatory amino acids such as glutamine and arginine and lipids. These may benefit critically ill patients by reducing infections. The true efficacy of these products remains controversial.

## METHODS OF INFUSION

**Continuous infusion** with a mechanical pump is the preferred method, especially if feeding the duodenum or jejunum directly to avoid dumping syndrome. One should initiate feeding with a full-strength product at 20 to 25 ml/h and increase the rate every 6 to 8 hours by 20 to 25 ml increments until the goal rate is reached. See Table 3-2 for sample caclulation for goal rate.

3

SURGICAL ENTERAL NUTRITION

| TABLE 3-2 |
| --- |
| CALCULATING GOAL RATE |
| 70-kg postoperative multiple trauma and malnourished with functioning GI tract |

1. Calculate caloric needs: BEE (35 kcal/kg/d)
   35 kcal/kg/d × 70 kg = 2450 kcal/d
2. Multiply BEE by stress factor:
   2450 kcal/d × 1.0 = 2450 kcal
3. Choose enteral product:
   Isocal ~ 1.06 kcal/ml
   (2450 kcal/d)/1.06 kcal/ml = 2490 ml/d Isocal per day
4. Calculate fluid requirement:
   70 kg needing maintenance fluids = (4,2,1 rule) = 110 ml/h or 2640 ml/d
5. Total fluid and calories = 2640 kcal/d and 2450 ml/d
6. Divide total tube feeding fluid by 24 h = goal rate of 103 ml/h

**Cyclic infusion** over a period of 10 to 12 hours may be used for the patient at risk of nocturnal aspiration or may be given at nighttime to allow patients to eat more during the day.

**Intermittent infusion** is useful for ambulatory patients or those scheduled for daily treatments. These are often administered by a gravity drip, usually for a total of 250 to 750 ml at a maximum of 60 ml/min.

## COMPLICATIONS

**Metabolic:** Abnormalities in potassium, sodium, calcium, phosphorous, glucose intolerance, and dehydration are common if patients are not carefully monitored. Hyperosmolarity is treated with free water administration and, if overlooked, could result in hyperosmotic nonketotic coma (HONK).

**Mechanical:** Placement of the feeding tube must be confirmed with a radiograph, because improper position may result in pleural or esophageal perforation. Clogging of the feeding tube can be prevented with frequent flushing (30 ml lukewarm tap water after each bolus or every 4 hours during continuous infusion). Unclogging is often achieved by inserting carbonated drinks, meat tenderizer (1 tsp papain in 30 ml water), 95% ethyl alcohol, pancreatic enzymes, or cranberry juice. If the tube cannot be unplugged, it should be replaced.

**Infectious:** Aspiration of tube feedings may lead to pneumonia. Highest risk patients are ones who are sedated or neurologically impaired. The risk of aspiration is decreased by feeding at or below the ligament of Treitz. Risks of aspiration may be decreased by elevating the head of the bed 30 degrees during feeding and for the hour afterward and by checking gastric residuals every 8 to 12 hours during continuous feedings. Residuals greater than 100 ml suggest increased risk.

**Gastrointestinal:** Diarrhea occurs as a consequence of tube feeding in up to 30% of patients. Other causes of diarrhea should be ruled out before changing the volume or strength of tube feedings. Other causes include drug-induced diarrhea from antibiotic use (*Clostridium difficile* colitis) or infectious colitis, sorbitol-based medications, hypoalbuminemia, magnesium in the formula, too little fiber, or a hyperosmolar solution. If the cause of the diarrhea cannot be explained or eliminated, the strength or volume of tube feedings can be decreased, the formula changed, or antidiarrheal agents such as loperamide elixir (*Imodium*) or diphenoxylate hydrochloride with atropine (*Lomotil*) may be used. Additional complications include bloating, nausea, vomiting, and abdominal pain. Often these symptoms are due to gastric distention and may be controlled with a slow continuous infusion or the addition of a prokinetic agent such as metoclopramide or cisapride.

# PART II

## Surgical Emergencies

# UPPER GASTROINTESTINAL TRACT BLEEDING

*Brett Butler*

Upper gastrointestinal tract (GI) bleeding is a common clinical problem seen on both medical and surgical services. Upper GI bleeding is defined by bleeding in the GI tract proximal to the ligament of Trietz.

## I. PATHOPHYSIOLOGY

A wide array of disease processes are associated with upper GI bleeding. Specifically, some causes include peptic ulcer disease, gastritis (stress, alcohol, or drug-induced), esophagitis, nosebleed, Mallory-Weiss tear, Dieulafoy's lesion, aortoduodenal fistula, polyps, or pancreatitis-induced pseudoaneurysm. The original assessment and workup are the same for all the preceding, but the definitive treatment plans vary.

## II. TYPICAL PRESENTATION

Both melena and hematemesis can indicate upper GI bleeding. The presence of "coffee-ground" material after insertion of a nasogastric tube is indicative of slower bleeding. Hematochezia (bright red blood per rectum) can occur with brisk upper GI bleeding and rapid intestinal transit.

Upper GI bleeding is composed of acute and chronic bleeding. Chronic bleeding usually presents with melena that has lasted for longer than 1 week. These patients can undergo outpatient evaluation. Acute bleeding that started within 12 hours of presentation can require a more urgent workup. Patients can present with symptoms similar to those of peptic ulcer disease: burning epigastric pain and abdominal tenderness. Other patients present after an episode of severe vomiting. Some patients can be under significant stress in the intensive care unit (ICU) for other causes, and upper GI bleeding develops.

## III. PREOPERATIVE WORKUP

Initially, all bleeding patients are adequately resuscitated and undergo assessment for signs of shock (cool mottled skin, tachycardia, tachypnea, or orthostatic hypotension). Next, a thorough history is taken, paying particular attention to medications (NSAIDs, aspirin, steroids, or anticoagulants), previous surgeries, alcohol use, history of reflux, and any history of ulcer disease. The location, duration, and onset of abdominal pain are ascertained. In the physical examination, symptoms and signs of cirrhosis or portal hypertension (ie, caput medusa, ascites, spider angioma, palmar erythema, or hepatosplenomegaly) especially are evaluated. All patients should have a rectal examination and guaiac slide test.

Patients are resuscitated by means of two large-bore peripheral IV lines. Fluid resuscitation typically is with a balanced salt solution (normal saline or lactated Ringer's solution). This patient is assessed for signs of orthostatic hypotension, which indicates greater than 20% loss of blood volume. Any patient hemodynamically unstable or actively bleeding should be monitored in the ICU. The patient should have a central venous line, possibly a Swan-Ganz arterial line, and a pulse oximetry probe placed. Any patient with any signs of respiratory distress or ongoing hematemesis may be electively intubated before esophagogastroduodenoscopy (EGD). Packed RBCs transfusions may be necessary to keep hematocrit greater than 30% in elderly patients and those with significant comorbidities. The patient should be typed and cross-matched for 4 to 6 units PRBCs. It is imperative that patients have aggressive correction of any coagulopathy if bleeding continues with fresh-frozen plasma and platelet transfusions to keep INR <1.5 and platelet count >50,000/mm$^3$.

A Foley catheter should be placed to monitor urine output and adequacy of resuscitation. Then a NGT is passed. The NGT should be irrigated with at least 500 ml normal saline. Evidence of coffee-ground material or blood from the NGT signifies an upper GI source. However, if bile does not return and the NGT aspirates are clear, one cannot rule out a source distal to the pylorus. Likewise, a bilious, nonbloody aspirate implicates a lower GI source. Occasionally, gastric lavage is necessary to rid the stomach of liquid blood and clots before diagnostic studies (EGD).

**Esophagogastroduodenoscopy.** After hemodynamic stabilization, the patient should undergo an EGD. An EGD can be both diagnostic and therapeutic. The EGD can be used to stop the bleeding by several therapeutic options, including YAG laser, electrocautery (monopolar or multipolar), heater probe, or injection of sclerosing agents (ethanol, epinephrine, or vasopressin).

**Angiography.** Selective visceral angiogram is sometimes used in patients in whom endoscopy cannot be performed or was unsuccessful. The patient must be bleeding at a rate of 0.5 ml/min for successful detection by angiography. Adequate renal function should be assessed before the angiogram. In certain cases, vasopressin, Gelfoam, or coils can be injected as a therapeutic option. A tagged RBC scan can detect slower rates of bleeding, as low as 0.1 ml/min. They are typically not very helpful with upper GI bleeding.

### Preoperative Orders
**Nursing:** NGT irrigation with at least 500 ml normal saline
**Laboratory tests:** CBC, BMP, LFTs, PT, and PTT

NOTE: The hematocrit may not yet have fallen in acute GI bleeding. A patient with a low hematocrit and no signs of hypotension probably has chronic slow bleeding. In significant upper GI bleeding the BUN may be elevated up to around 40 mg/dl.

## IV. CONDUCT OF OPERATION

Because the causes of upper GI bleeding are numerous, only the more common causes will be addressed. Patients need constant assessment of blood loss, urine output, CVP, Hb, HCT, BP, and HR. Poor prognostic indicators include high rates of bleeding, hematemesis, hypotension on admission, and a transfusion requirement of >4 units PRBCs. Patients who require up to 4 units of PRBCs with continued active bleeding within 24 hours will most likely need operative intervention.

**Peptic Ulcer Disease.** Peptic ulcer disease accounts for approximately 50% of upper GI bleeding. NSAID use increases the risk of GI bleeding. Duodenal ulcers are associated with bleeding four times as often as gastric ulcers are. Fortunately, approximately 80% of bleeding stops spontaneously with adequate resuscitation and lavage. EGD should be performed within the first 24 hours, and its therapeutic options are usually successful in stopping the bleeding. If unsuccessful or recurrent hemorrhage occurs, operative intervention is necessary.

Surgical options depend on the hemodynamic status of the patient. The goals of the operations are to at least stop the bleeding and, if the patient's hemodynamics permit, to address the underlying cause of the hemorrhage. Thus, operations can range from simple oversewing of an ulcer to vagotomy (decrease acid production) and drainage procedure (pyloroplasty) or vagotomy and antrectomy (removes gastrin producing cells) with appropriate reconstruction (Bilroth I or II).

**Stress Gastritis.** Stress gastritis occurs in up to 20% of cases and is usually associated with *Helicobacter pylori*. These patients have pain and often have chronic slow blood loss. Patients at risk can be treated with an $H_2$-antagonist, sucralfate, or proton pump inhibitors (PPIs). Resuscitation and supportive management are usually the treatment (bleeding often stops spontaneously). There has also been some success with intraarterial vasopressin injection through the left gastric artery. Surgery is rarely needed, but a vagotomy and pyloroplasty or antrectomy after oversewing the bleeding site is usually effective. Rarely, a subtotal or total gastrectomy is needed.

**Variceal Hemorrhage.** Varicies are another common source of bleeding, often secondary to portal hypertension. Cirrhotic patients should be resuscitated with minimal sodium and overtransfusion avoided. These patients often benefit from a Swan-Ganz catheter. Early endoscopy is used to verify that the varices are the source of the bleeding. Initially, sclerotherapy or banding should be attempted. If it is successful, the patients will need to be treated with chronic sclerotherapy and evaluated for shunt or transplant. If endoscopy is not available or delayed, IV octreotide can be used to stop variceal bleeding. A Sengstaken-Blakemore tube can be used to tamponade the bleeding and can be left in place for 24 hours. If the patient is still bleeding despite the preceding measures, including repeat endoscopic

4

UPPER GASTROINTESTINAL TRACT BLEEDING

maneuvers, a transjugular intrahepatic portoseptemic shunt (TIPS) can be put in place to bridge the patient to a transplant or a possible permanent shunt.

**Mallory-Weiss Tears.** These tears commonly occur in alcoholics and after severe vomiting episodes. These patients will have hematemesis and the acute onset of epigastric pain. Most patients stabilize without the need for operative management. Endoscopic coagulation, injections, or occasionally a Sengstaken-Blakemore tube may be required. If these interventions are unsuccessful, operative management involving an anterior longitudinal gastrotomy and oversewing of the laceration is required.

**Dieulafoy's Lesion.** This lesion is a less common cause of bleeding. It is a 1- to 3-mm artery running through an ulcer-less gastric mucosa. It typically occurs near the esophagogastric junction and can be difficult to visualize endoscopically. The patients have painless bleeding. EGD electrocoagulation and ligation are often successful. Surgical treatment involves a wedge resection of the involved gastric wall.

**Stress Ulcers in the ICU.** These stress ulcers are associated with shock, sepsis, burns (Curling), and CNS tumors (Cushing). These patients have bleeding episodes typically 3 to 5 days after the initial insult. Decreased gastric blood flow causes thinning of the gastric mucosa and eventually gastric bleeding. These patients are treated medically with $H_2$-blockers, PPIs, or sucralfate.

## Postoperative Orders
**Admit to:** ICU
**Diagnosis:** upper GI bleeding
**Condition:** guarded
**Vital signs:** q1h
**Activity:** bed rest
**Allergies:**
**Nursing:** strict I&Os, routine line care, NGT to LCWS, Foley to gravity, check NGT pH q shift and call if less than 4, Pneumoboots
**Diet:** NPO
**IV fluids:** $D_5$/0.45% NS with 20 mEq KCl at 150 ml/h
**Medications:** ranitidine (Zantac) drip; octreotide drip if appropriate; vasopressin drip if appropriate
**Laboratory tests:** CBC, PT, and PTT q shift

## V. DISCHARGE INSTRUCTIONS

Patients can be discharged once they have maintained a stable hematocrit and hemodynamic picture for at least 48 hours. Those patients whose test results are positive for *H. pylori* should undergo appropriate treatment. Also, patients should undergo some form of acid suppression with $H_2$-blockers, PPIs, or sucralfate.

# LOWER GASTROINTESTINAL TRACT BLEEDING

*Todd Ponsky*

Lower gastrointestinal tract (GI) bleeding includes any intraluminal bleeding arising distal to the ligament of Treitz. Although this encompasses most of the GI tract, most cases of lower GI bleeding (70%-80%) originate in the colon. Lower GI bleeding can occur in any age group but is seen most commonly in the elderly. Although lower GI bleeding occasionally is seen as melena, most patients have bright red blood per rectum. Up to 80% of lower GI bleeding are self-limited. However, it is critical to aggressively support these patients with volume resuscitation and localization of bleeding in cases where bleeding continues.

## 5

## I. PATHOPHYSIOLOGY

The most common source of massive blood per rectum is bleeding from an upper GI source, such as a duodenal or gastric ulcer, esophageal varices, or a Mallory-Weiss tear. Although most patients with upper GI bleeding present with melena, massive bleeding may present with red blood per rectum. For this reason, workup of lower GI bleeding always begins by ruling out an upper GI source with nasogastric lavage. Most cases of hematochezia are colonic in origin. Causes of lower GI bleeding include diverticulosis, angiodysplasia, cancer, colonic polyps, hemorrhoids, and colitis. The incidence can be stratified by age group (Table 5-1).

Diverticulosis is the most common cause of acute massive lower GI bleeding when all age groups are considered together. It is also the most likely cause in patients 50 years of age and older. Although diverticuli are more common in the left side of the colon, diverticular bleeding occurs more frequently on the right. GI bleeding is rarely seen in the setting of diverticulitis.

Angiodysplasia is the next most common cause of lower GI bleeding. It is most common in patients older than 65 years of age. Bleeding from angiodysplatic lesions is most common in the right side of the colon, probably because of the thinner colonic wall on that side.

## II. TYPICAL PRESENTATION

Patients presenting with lower GI bleeding require a complete history and physical examination. Tachycardia and orthostatic hypotension are suggestive of significant blood loss. Nausea and vomiting, history of peptic ulcer disease, midepigastric pain, NSAID use, alcohol use, and liver disease may suggest an upper GI source. A history of lower GI bleeding, diverticular disease, or angiodysplasia more likely point to a lower GI source. Patients with intraluminal bleeding secondary to diverticulosis or angiodysplasia

**TABLE 5-1**

MOST COMMON CAUSES OF LOWER GASTROINTESTINAL TRACT BLEEDING

| Age | Cause |
|-----|-------|
| Overall | Diverticulosis |
| >65 y | Angiodysplasia |
| 50-65 y | Diverticulosis |
| <50 y | Hemorrhoids or colonic polyp |

typically have a nontender abdomen. A firm, tender, distended abdomen suggests a more ominous process such as mesenteric ischemia.

A digital rectal and proctopscopic examination should be performed on all patients with lower GI bleeding. This will identify anorectal sources of bleeding such as hemorrhoids. A nasogastric tube should be placed and the stomach lavaged. If this is positive, workup of an upper GI source takes priority.

## III. PREOPERATIVE WORKUP

Evaluation of hemodynamic stability is the first step in the workup of a patient with lower GI bleeding. As always, the airway must be ensured and established if necessary. Patients with massive blood loss may lose consciousness and be unable to protect their airways. These patients require endotracheal intubation and ventilatory support. Once the patient is adequately ventilating, circulation is assessed. Tachycardia, hypotension, and diminished pulses are immediate signs of hypovolemic shock, requiring aggressive volume resuscitation. Two large-bore (16 gauge or larger) peripheral IV lines are placed, and isotonic crystalloid fluid is rapidly infused to restore an adequate blood pressure. A Foley catheter is placed for monitoring of urine output. In patients with known or suspected congestive heart-failure, a central line and pulmonary artery catheter may be necessary for evaluation of hemodynamics. Once patients are hemodynamically stable, the source of bleeding may be identified.

Selective angiography should be performed as soon as possible in patients with brisk lower GI bleeding. Although angiography has the lowest sensitivity of the diagnostic modalities, its high specificity and therapeutic potential make it the test of choice for rapid lower GI bleeding. An angiogram can localize the source of bleeding in 75% of cases but requires a bleeding rate greater than 0.5 ml/min.

Technetium 99m–labeled red blood cell scans are highly sensitive in detecting bleeding rates as low as 0.1 ml/min. However, their use is limited by their low specificity and lack of therapeutic assistance. A bleeding scan has the ability to detect slower bleeding and will ultimately localize more bleeding than an angiogram. A positive bleeding scan only helps to determine the general site of lower GI bleeding but cannot precisely localize it. Thus, a positive bleeding scan should be followed by angiography. A negative bleeding scan indicates that the bleeding has stopped or is too slow for detection. In these cases angiography would be negative as well. These patients should undergo a bowel prep and colonoscopy.

Angiography can be therapeutic with the use of intraarterial vasopressin or embolization. The latter should only be used when operative intervention is planned immediately after angiography, because it leads to bowel infarction in 15% of cases.

Colonoscopy is the test of choice in patients who present with slow to moderate lower GI bleeding. Colonoscopy is difficult in patients with massive lower GI bleeding because of inadequate visualization. However, a rapid bowel prep with 4 L of polyethylene glycol through a nasogastric tube should be started as soon as possible if an urgent colonoscopy is planned. Although endoscopy is a mainstay in treatment of upper GI bleeding, it is much less useful in treating lower GI bleeding. However, in selected cases, bleeding may be cauterized with monopolar, multipolar, or bicap electrocautery, heater probe, or laser.

Small bowel bleeding is difficult to diagnose. When workup of the colon is negative, enteroclysis or enteroscopy may be used to identify small bowel bleeding. Meckel's radionuclide scans may be helpful in younger patients.

## PREOPERATIVE ORDERS

Patients presenting with hypovolemic shock, orthostatic hypotension, need for airway management, or comorbid conditions require intensive care unit admission.

**Admit to:** ICU
**Diagnosis:** lower GI bleeding
**Condition:** guarded
**Vital signs:** q1h (or more frequent if hemodynamically unstable)
**Activity:** bed rest
**Allergies:** NKDA
**Nursing:** sequential compression devices, $O_2$/ventilator prn, Foley catheter
**Diet:** NPO
**IV fluids:** lactated Ringer's at 150 ml/h
**Medications:** IV $H_2$ blocker; home medications (excluding antihypertensives)
**Laboratory tests:** BMP, CBC, T&C for 4 U PRBCs, PT, PTT, CXR, and ECG

### IV. CONDUCT OF OPERATION

There are five indications for surgical intervention in lower GI bleeding:

1. Massive blood transfusion: patients requiring 6 or more units of blood transfusion with a localized lesion
2. Failure of medical therapy: continued bleeding despite attempted angiographic embolization or endoscopic thermal ablation

3. Diffuse disease: widely diseased hemorrhagic bowel or multiple discrete lesions
4. Cancer: patients who have a bleeding lesion suspicious for carcinoma
5. Hemodynamic instability: patients with hemodynamic instability that will not allow for further workup.

Surgical procedures for lower GI bleeding should be selective to the area of colon involved whenever possible. Ideally this should be either a small-bowel resection or a hemicolectomy. Patients with life-threatening bleeding and no identifiable source should undergo a subtotal colectomy. In this 5% of patients, bleeding usually is due to an arteriovenous malformation. Patients who undergo emergency subtotal colectomy have a significantly higher morbidity and mortality compared with patients with identified bleeding sources who undergo segmental resections.

## V. DISCHARGE ORDERS

Patients should return to the emergency department for recurrent bleeding or abdominal symptoms. The patient should be seen in the clinic 1 week after discharge. Patients not requiring surgery should follow up with gastroenterology and surgery.

# INTESTINAL OBSTRUCTION

*Douglas Jones*

One of the most common clinical conditions seen by general surgeons is intestinal obstruction. This occurs when all or part of the luminal contents of the GI tract are blocked.

## I. PATHOPHYSIOLOGY

Two types of intestinal obstructions exist: open and closed. In an open obstruction the GI contents are partially or completely blocked at the distal point of obstruction. However, the GI tract may undergo proximal decompression through vomiting. Closed obstruction refers to a segment of bowel that cannot decompress itself distally or proximally. A closed and open obstruction can be classified as either partial or complete. A complete obstruction occurs if no GI contents or air can pass the point of obstruction. If the GI contents can bypass the point of obstruction, it is a partial obstruction. Strangulation describes an obstruction that compromises blood flow to a segment of bowel. It can result in a nonviable segment of bowel.

Multiple conditions can lead to an intestinal obstruction. Extrinsic lesions such as adhesions, abscesses, and hernias can result in luminal obstruction. In addition, intrinsic lesions such as tumors, diverticulitis, and Crohn's disease and intraluminal processes such as gallstones and intussusception are other causes of obstruction. The most common cause of small bowel obstruction in the United States is postsurgical adhesions. Hernias are the most common cause of bowel obstructions worldwide. The most common cause of large bowel obstruction is a neoplasm.

## II. TYPICAL PRESENTATION

Small bowel obstruction commonly presents with crampy abdominal pain, distention, and obstipation. Vomiting is more pronounced with proximal obstructions, whereas distention is more pronounced with distal obstructions. Colonic obstructions present with constant pain, marked distention, and sometimes vomiting, which usually is feculent.

## III. PREOPERATIVE WORKUP

**History.** The onset and duration of any abdominal pain, nausea and vomiting, diarrhea, and the last time the patient had a bowel movement or passed flatus needs to be determined. Any history of fevers is documented. The nature of the emesis is characterized as clear, bilious, or feculent. Pertinent past medical history includes previous abdominal or pelvic operations, hernias, inflammatory bowel disease, and tumors.

**Physical Examination.** Vital signs are reviewed for signs of fever, tachycardia, or hypotension. In addition, orthostatic vital signs can be helpful in documenting hydration status. The abdomen is examined for distention, tenderness, and the presence of surgical scars. The bowel sounds are characterized either as hyperactive and high-pitched or as hypoactive, which usually signifies a later stage of obstruction. A complete examination includes a search for possible hernias, including incisional, umbilical, inguinal, and femoral, and finally, a digital examination for rectal lesions and gross or occult blood.

**Laboratory Workup.** Laboratory workup includes a basic metabolic panel and a complete blood count. The presence of leukocytosis may be indicative of an ischemic bowel. Occasionally, lactate levels can be helpful, although they are often only elevated in the late stages of the disease.

**Radiographic Studies.** Flat and upright abdominal plain films are obtained. Key points to look for are air-fluid levels, dilated loops of small bowel (>3 cm), bowel wall thickening (>3 mm), air in the colon or rectal lumen (absence suggests complete obstruction), proximal colon dilated more than 8 to 10 cm, and sigmoid colon dilated more than 4 to 5 cm. Occasionally, history and physical examination suggest a bowel obstruction, but plain films are inconclusive. For example, when the lumen of the bowel is completely filled with fluid, no air-fluid levels may be appreciated on plain films. In this case, further workup is necessary.

**Computed Tomography (CT) Scan.** In the case of fluid-filled dilated loops of small bowel, a CT scan can aid in the diagnosis. A CT scan can also localize the transition point between dilated and collapsed loops of bowel. A clear transition point usually indicates the need for surgical decompression. CT scan signs of strangulation include thickening of the bowel wall, pneumatosis intestinalis, portal venous gas, and mesenteric stranding.

**Ultrasonography.** Ultrasonography may be used to identify dilated loops of bowel. Ultrasonography has also been used to detect pneumatosis intestinalis. This is operator dependent and requires a radiologist with a significant amount of experience to make the diagnosis.

**Fluid Resuscitation.** Patients who present with bowel obstructions typically are intravascularly depleted as a result of large amounts of fluid sequestered in the lumen of the GI tract. Nausea, vomiting, and decreased oral intake worsen the extent of dehydration. Fluid resuscitation is imperative. A Foley catheter should be placed for accurate assessment of urine output. Patients with significant cardiac and renal disease may require central venous monitoring for safe resuscitation.

**Nasogastric Tube Placement.** All patients with a bowel obstruction should have a nasogastric tube (NGT) placed. An NGT provides relief of nausea and vomiting and in most cases decreases abdominal pain and distention. This in turn decreases the risk of aspiration.

**Comments.** Bowel obstructions can be managed conservatively or surgically. For partial small bowel obstructions conservative management is usually successful, resolving 60% to 85% of obstructions. In complete bowel obstruction an attempt at conservative management can be made for 24 to 48 hours. However, surgical intervention is indicated if the obstruction has not resolved in 24 to 48 hours or if the patient demonstrates signs and symptoms of or has laboratory findings indicative of strangulation or perforation.

**Preoperative Orders**
    **Admit to:**
    **Diagnosis:** small bowel obstruction
    **Condition:** guarded
    **Vital signs:** q2h × 4 then q4h
    **Activity:**
    **Allergies:**
    **Nursing:** strict I&Os, NGT to low continuous suction, Foley catheter to gravity drainage, routine line care
    **Diet:** NPO
    **IV fluids:** lactated Ringer's 1 to 3 L boluses; the maintenance rate should provide a urine output >30 ml/h
    **Medications:** should be IV; avoid narcotics for serial exams; important home medications can be continued through NGT; antibiotics are not routinely used for simple open obstruction
    **Laboratory tests:** CBC, PT, and PTT; T&C 2 U PRBCs on admission; BMP and CBC q12h to follow electrolytes and WBC count; repeat upright and supine abdominal plain films in 24 hours.

NOTE: Call house officer for temperature >38.3°C, HR >120 bpm, respiratory rate >20 breaths per minute, and SBP <100 mm Hg. Serial abdominal examinations by the house officer are imperative. Changes in temperature, distention, tenderness, or mental status warrant further workup or operative management.

## IV. CONDUCT OF OPERATION

Exploratory laparotomy is performed for bowel obstructions. The incision should provide maximum exposure. Usually a midline abdominal incision will suffice. One should cautiously gain entrance into the abdominal cavity in patients with previous abdominal operations and those with ventral hernias secondary to the possibility of herniated bowel. Once the peritoneal cavity is entered, any peritoneal fluid is evaluated for turbidity, purulence, and color and is sent for Gram's stain and culture with sensitivities. A thorough search of the peritoneum is performed. A systematic way to examine the peritoneal cavity is described later.

The liver is examined by placing the hand over the dome of both lobes. The liver is a site of metastases for different cancers, most notably, colon cancer. The gallbladder is felt for stones or masses. The spleen is checked for any abnormal pathologic findings. The cecum and appendix are located and evaluated for masses and inflammation. The small bowel is run from the ileocecal valve proximally to the ligament of Treitz. Any ischemic changes, masses, or strictures are noted while running the small bowel. Both sides of the mesentery are evaluated at this time. The cecum and the colon are examined distal to the rectum. Any diameter changes, masses, or adherence to adjacent structures should be noted. The sigmoid colon is evaluated for redundancy (a risk factor for sigmoid volvulus). After evaluating the colon, examine the pelvis for inguinal, femoral, and obturator hernias.

Obstructions secondary to adhesions are lysed. If the bowel is obstructed secondary to a mass or is found to be nonviable, a bowel resection is indicated. If it is a segment of small bowel, it may be resected and primarily anastomosed.

For colonic obstructions that require resection, the type of operation depends on whether there is fecal contamination and the location of the obstruction in the colon. For left-sided benign lesions in the setting of no gross contamination, resection with primary anastomosis and a proximal diverting colostomy or ileostomy is the procedure of choice. If the obstruction is secondary to a malignancy, at least 2-cm margins must be obtained. The mesentery must be resected down to its origin during a cancer operation. The left or sigmoid colon is resected if a left or sigmoid colon lesion is causing the obstruction. The proximal colon is brought out as an end colostomy, and the distal colon or rectum is left as a Hartmann's pouch or mucous fistula. The transverse colon is the least common site of colonic obstruction. A segment of the transverse colon is resected, and the colon is primarily anastomosed. The hepatic and splenic flexures can be taken down to relieve tension on the anastomosis. A proximal diverting loop ileostomy is made. For right colon obstructions, a right hemicolectomy with primary anastomosis is recommended. A diverting loop ileostomy is recommended only if there is fecal contamination.

## VARIATIONS OF OPERATION
**Inguinal and Femoral Hernias.** Standard inguinal or femoral herniorrhaphy with groin incision will suffice if the history and physical examination are consistent with a groin hernia as the cause of obstruction. If signs of nonviable bowel are suspected or found intraoperatively, a laparotomy should be performed.

**Sigmoid Volvulus.** Colonic obstruction secondary to a volvulus occurs in the sigmoid colon 65% of the time. The initial treatment for a sigmoid volvulus is rigid proctosigmoidoscopy. This successfully reduces the volvulus in approximately 80% of cases. After reduction of the volvulus, elective sigmoidectomy can be planned. If there are peritoneal signs at initial presentation, proctosigmoidoscopy should not be attempted. A sigmoidectomy with Hartmann's pouch and end colostomy are the procedure of choice.

## POSTOPERATIVE ORDERS

**Admit to:**
**Diagnosis:** small bowel obstruction
**Condition:** stable
**Vital signs:** q2h × 4 then q4h
**Activity:** OOB to chair with assistance
**Allergies:**
**Nursing:** strict I&Os, NGT to LCWS, Foley catheter to gravity drainage, IS × 10 puffs q1h, Pneumoboots and PAS until ambulating, Jackson-Pratt (JP) drain to bulb suction if appropriate
**Diet:** NPO
**IV fluids:** lactated Ringer's 1 to 3 L boluses; the maintenance rate should provide a urine output >30 ml/h
**Medications:** should be IV; perioperative antibiotics
**Laboratory tests:** BMP and CBC qAM

NOTE: Call house officer for temperature >38.3°C, HR >120 bpm, RR >20 breaths per minute, and SBP <100 mm Hg.

## V. POSSIBLE COMPLICATIONS

Perforation and necrosis are possible complications when a patient is managed nonoperatively. Wound infections, anastomotic leak, intraabdominal abscesses, and hemorrhage are possible complications after surgical management.

## VI. DISCHARGE INSTRUCTIONS

Patients should be encouraged to have a diet high in fiber. Patients with an ileostomy should not eat nuts, raw vegetables or fruits, or anything that cannot be cut with a knife. Staples are removed from the incision between postoperative day 8 and 12. Patients with operations that leave the GI tract in discontinuity are eligible for reestablishment of continuity in 2 to 3 months.

# SHOCK

*Jason Brodsky*

The circulatory system is responsible for transporting food and oxygen to the cells and removing waste products of cellular metabolism. When metabolic demand exceeds the ability of blood to deliver oxygen, conversion to the less-efficient anaerobic metabolism occurs. Shock refers to this lack of adequate tissue perfusion. The three types of shock are hypovolemic, cardiogenic, and distributive.

## I. HYPOVOLEMIC SHOCK

Hypovolemia accounts for most cases of shock encountered by the general surgeon. Fluid loss resulting in hypovolemic shock can be either hemorrhagic or nonhemorrhagic. Hemorrhage most often results from trauma. Burns and third space fluid sequestration, as in cases of small bowel obstruction or pancreatitis, are the most common causes of nonhemorrhagic fluid loss. However, it can also result from excessive vomiting, diarrhea, or fluid loss from an enterocutaneous fistula or proximal stoma.

Hypovolemic shock can further be classified as mild, moderate, or severe, on the basis of fluid losses of less than 20%, 20% to 40%, and greater than 40%, respectively.

## II. CARDIOGENIC SHOCK

Cardiogenic shock, or pump failure, results when the heart cannot maintain a cardiac output adequate for tissue perfusion in the face of normovolemia and appropriate vasomotor tone. This form of shock occurs with decreased cardiac contractility. Primary causes are attributed to myocardial abnormalities. It may be seen in the setting of myocardial ischemia, a myocardial infarction, arrhythmias, and severe valvular abnormalities. Secondary causes result from decreased venous return from conditions such as a tension pneumothorax, cardiac tamponade, or acute venal caval obstruction.

## III. DISTRIBUTIVE SHOCK

Distributive shock results when the intravascular space increases. This results in a relative hypovolemic state. The two types of distributive shock are septic shock and neurogenic shock.

Although any microorganism can cause septic shock, it is most commonly associated with gram-negative bacteremia. The lipopolysaccharide endotoxin, a component of the gram-negative cell wall, activates a number of potent vasodilators on its release from injured cell membranes. In its early stages, septic shock is characterized by a hyperdynamic or high cardiac output state. In later stages, when the heart cannot keep up with a rapidly expanding intravascular space, a low output state prevails.

Neurogenic shock occurs when a loss of sympathetic vasomotor tone results in increased intravascular volume. It is most commonly seen as "spinal shock" after traumatic cervical spine transection. It may also be iatrogenically induced after a high spinal anesthetic.

## IV. DIAGNOSIS AND DIFFERENTIATION OF SHOCK

Identification and aggressive treatment of shock are essential to good patient outcome. A patient is in shock when there is any evidence of end-organ hypoperfusion. The most reliable clinical indicator of shock is an altered mental status. Patients will usually have a decreased urine output (except in neurogenic shock). Tachycardia is common as the body tries to increase cardiac output to compensate for the shock state.

In cases of an unclear cause of shock, more invasive monitoring can help to clear the diagnosis. Placement of a central venous catheter allows measurement of central venous pressure (CVP). Normally ranging from 4 to 10 mm Hg, CVP reflects the preload of the right side of the heart. Assuming normal cardiopulmonary anatomy, this number reflects the preload of the left heart, one of the determinants of cardiac performance.

When more accurate information is needed, a pulmonary artery (Swan-Ganz) catheter (PAC) can be placed. Once in place, CVP, pulmonary artery pressure (PAP), wedge (left atrial) pressure, and cardiac output can be determined. When a PAC is used, it is important to use the information to guide a patient's resuscitation, keeping the entire clinical picture in mind. The goal of patient care is to treat the patient and not an individual number.

## V. TREATMENT

Fluid resuscitation remains the mainstay of shock therapy. An adequate circulating blood volume must be restored to ensure end organ tissue perfusion. In initial resuscitation efforts, crystalloid and colloid are equally effective in restoring blood volume. Although colloids have the theoretical advantage of staying in the intravascular space, this benefit is lost after several hours because of shock-associated changes in the endothelium. Because of their significantly lower cost, crystalloids generally should be used for volume resuscitation in shock.

In patients with hypovolemic shock, efforts at restoring blood volume should coincide with an attempt to stop the cause of the hypovolemia. In cases of hemorrhage the site of blood loss should be controlled as possible. In cases of a nonhemorrhagic hypovolemic site, fluid loss is often more chronic and difficult to control requiring ongoing resuscitation. Patients in this group respond quickly to volume repletion and rarely need vasoactive drugs.

In distributive shock, volume resuscitation helps to fill the dilated intravascular space. In these patients, especially those in spinal shock, alpha antagonists may be necessary to restore an adequate blood pressure.

Patients with septic shock should be started on broad-spectrum antibiotics with a regimen including good coverage of gram-negative organisms. A search for sources of infection requiring additional treatment such as abscesses or endocarditis should be undertaken as appropriate. Most cases of neurogenic shock are self-limited, and these patients require supportive care during this time.

Volume resuscitation should be monitored carefully in patients with suspected cardiogenic shock. Although it is vital to ensure adequate preload in these patients to optimize cardiac output, overresuscitation will quickly lead to pulmonary edema and compromise pulmonary status. When in doubt, placement of a CVC or PAC can be helpful in guiding resuscitation. If inadequate perfusion persists after volume resuscitation, beta agonists and other inotropes should be started. Patients refractory to inotropic therapy receive mechanical support. Placement of an intraaortic balloon pump augments coronary blood flow but more importantly decreases afterload, the resistance against which the heart must pump. More invasive devices, such as a ventricular assist device, often commit a patient to heart transplant.

## VI. FOLLOW-UP

Patients with a significant episode of shock require intensive care unit observation. Ongoing resuscitation is often required. Patients with a significant hypotensive episode require a cardiac evaluation. An electrocardiogram and cardiac enzymes are required to rule out myocardial ischemia or infarction. Urine output, blood urea nitrogen, and creatinine should be checked to rule out acute tubular necrosis. Liver enzymes should also be checked to identify "shock liver."

7

SHOCK

# PART III

## Esophagus and Stomach

# ACHALASIA

*Michael Rosen*

Achalasia is a rare disease with an annual incidence of 0.5% to 1.2% per 100,000 people. There is no predilection for race or gender. Pathologic features of achalasia include hypertrophy of the two muscle layers of the esophagus and the nerve fibers, as well as absence of myenteric neural ganglia.

## I. PATHOPHYSIOLOGY

Achalasia (*A*, absence of, and *chalasia*, relaxation) is a motility disorder of the esophagus. It is characterized by a tonically contracted lower esophageal sphincter (LES) and the absence of esophageal body peristalsis. These abnormalities result in a distally obstructed esophagus with no proximal assistance in emptying from the esophageal body. To overcome this obstruction, patients must accumulate a hydrostatic column of fluids and food to bypass the LES. The esophageal body progressively dilates. Eventually, aspiration results as the disease progresses and the esophageal contents overflow into the lungs.

## II. TYPICAL PRESENTATION

Although patients can present at any age, achalasia most commonly is diagnosed in those 20 to 40 years old. The normal sequence of swallowing involves relaxation of the LES to provide an unimpeded path for food to pass into the stomach. Dysphagia, resulting from loss of this relaxation, is the most common presenting symptom. Early in the course of the disease, dysphagia is subtle with complaints of fullness during and after meals. It progresses slowly and becomes more constant. Dysphagia to both solids and liquids distinguishes achalasia from mechanical obstruction resulting from peptic strictures. Heartburn is a common feature that often delays diagnosis, because symptoms are attributed to gastroesophageal reflux while dysphagia goes unrecognized. Despite the increasing feeding difficulties, weight loss is minimal. Pneumonia and bronchitis result from esophageal stasis and pulmonary soilage. The differential diagnosis includes scleroderma, isolated hypertensive LES, diffuse esophageal spasm, and pseudoachalasia. The radiographic and manometric findings of pseudoachalasia are indistinguishable from primary achalasia. This is usually associated with a malignancy of the esophagogastric junction. Patients are older with shorter duration of symptoms and more significant weight loss.

## III. MEDICAL THERAPY

Treatment of achalasia aims to correct the obstructive gradient of the LES. The modalities of treatment can be divided into nonsurgical options, which include pharmacologic agents and pneumatic dilatation, and surgical options both open and by means of minimally invasive techniques.

Pharmacologic agents include nitrates, calcium channel blockers, and botulinum toxin (Botox) injections. Long-acting nitrates are potent smooth muscle relaxants that act on the LES. However, their use is limited by headaches and other side effects that occur with the high doses necessary to achieve relaxation of the LES. Calcium channel blockers are effective in reducing LES pressures. Their short duration of action (60-90 minutes) when taken before a meal keeps the LES open long enough to permit esophageal emptying. Sublingual administration by-passes absorption difficulties resulting from esophageal stasis. *Clostridium botulinum* results in LES relaxation by inhibiting acetylcholine release from the nerve terminal. However, Botox has a limited duration of action (6-8 weeks). In addition, repeated Botox adminstration causes scarring that obliterates the plane between the muscularis and submucosa where the surgical myotomy is performed. Thus, it is best reserved for high-risk operative candidates, including the elderly and sick, as a nonoperative alternative. During pneumatic dilatation, a dilator is passed across the gastroesophageal junction under fluoroscopic or endoscopic guidance. The force from rapid inflation disrupts the muscle fibers of the LES. There is a 65% to 85% success rate with up to two dilatations. The procedure carries a 5% perforation rate.

## PREOPERATIVE ORDERS

**Admit to:**
**Diagnosis:** preoperative Heller myotomy
**Condition:** stable
**Vital signs:** per routine
**Activity:**
**Allergies:**
**Nursing:** strict I&Os; place NGT and use gentle normal saline irrigation until clear; have barium swallow at bedside for OR
**Diet:** clear liquids for 48 to 72 hours preoperatively; NPO after midnight
**IV fluids:**
**Medications:** Ancef, 1 g IV, on call to OR
**Laboratory tests:**

## IV. PREOPERATIVE WORKUP

**Chest X-ray Examination (CXR).** Although plain films may be normal, radiographic findings of achalasia include a mediastinal air–fluid level, increased density from a dilated esophagus full of secretions, absence of a gastric bubble, or evidence of aspiration pneumonia.

**Barium Swallow.** The classic finding of a smoothly tapered distal esophagus leading to a closed LES is known as a "bird's beak." In more advanced disease the esophagus appears more tortuous and dilated.

**Esophageal Manometry.** Esophageal manometry is the most useful test in the workup of achalasia. Findings consistent with achalasia include low pressure, simultaneous repetitive contractions of the esophageal body with no peristaltic waves generated, and failure of the LES to relax during initiation of swallowing. A high resting pressure of the LES is not necessary to diagnose achalasia. In fact, most patients with achalasia have normal resting pressures and fail to relax on swallowing. Esophageal intraluminal pressure is also elevated compared with the gastric pressure secondary to the column of retained food in the lumen.

**Endoscopy.** The primary goal of endoscopy is to rule out malignancy. In achalasia the esophagogastric junction usually appears closed; however, it can accommodate the scope. Esophageal lavage before endoscopy may be necessary to remove retained food particles for adequate visualization.

8

ACHALASIA

## V. SURGICAL ANATOMY

The myotomy for achalasia is performed at the gastroesophageal junction. The lower third of the esophagus consists of two layers of smooth muscle oriented in a circular and longitudinal fashion. There is no serosa on the esophagus. The stomach does have a serosa; it consists of three layers of smooth muscle oriented in a circular, longitudinal, and oblique fashion.

## VI. CONDUCT OF OPERATION

The ideal surgical treatment for achalasia would be one that removes the LES gradient and relieves dysphagia while preventing reflux. Esophageal myotomy can be accomplished by means of an open technique through the chest or abdomen or by a minimally invasive technique using the thoracoscope or laparoscope. Surgical treatment of achalasia is becoming more common as minimally invasive surgical techniques are shown to decrease morbidity and mortality.

### LAPAROSCOPIC HELLER MYOTOMY

After general endotracheal anesthesia is administered, the patient is placed in the supine position with the legs in stirrups. The primary surgeon stands between the legs. The first assistant stands on the patient's left and the second assistant (camera operator) stands on the patient's right. The monitors are placed at the head of the patient. The patient is placed in 30-degree reverse Trendelenburg position.

The abdomen is entered with a Veress needle or the Hasson technique 4 to 5 cm above the umbilicus. Pneumoperitoneum is established, and the camera is introduced. A 10-mm trocar is then placed under direct vision in the right anterior axillary line just below the costal cartilage, where a fan retractor is placed to elevate the left lobe of the liver and gain access to the hiatus. Two ports are placed in the left and right midclavicular lines just cephalad to the umbilicus. The right port is used for dissection while the first assistant places a Babcock clamp in the left trocar to retract the fundus. The final two ports are placed just inferior and on either side of the xiphoid for dissection purposes on the gastroesophageal junction for the myotomy.

The gastrohepatic ligament is divided exposing the hiatus. Dissection begins by dividing the phrenoesophageal ligament anteriorly across the esophagus. The left and right crura are identified, and the dissection is carried as far posteriorly as possible. A 45-degree scope can aid in this part of the procedure. The left hepatic branch of the vagus nerve should be identified and preserved. The mediastinum is entered by bluntly dissecting up the left crura between the esophagus and then in a likewise fashion up the right. This blunt dissection allows mobilization of up to 4 to 6 cm of esophagus into the abdominal space to perform the myotomy. Next, the fundus is mobilized to minimize the tension on the myotomy and aid in the fundoplication by detaching it from its splenic and posterior retroperitoneal attachments.

A Penrose drain is placed around the esophagus, and a clip is applied. This provides the appropriate traction on the esophagus to allow safe dissection. At this point the epiphrenic fat pad is divided to the left of the anterior vagus nerve. The harmonic scalpel is used because of the vascularity of this structure.

The myotomy is performed next. The longitudinal muscle is divided with scissors; then the circular muscle is split after rotating the scissors 90 degrees. The myotomy is begun approximately 4 cm above the gastroesophageal (GE) junction, where the muscle and submucosal planes are most identifiable. With a spreading motion of the scissors, a plane is developed separating the muscularis from the submucosa. The myotomy is carried approximately 6 cm above the GE junction with a 90-degree electrosurgical hook. Care must be taken to avoid the anterior vagus nerve. If encountered, it should be retracted out of the dissection. The myotomy is then carried inferiorly, which is the most important and technically challenging part of the case. The myotomy should be carried approximately 0.5 to 1 cm across the GE junction. This can be recognized by the collarlike oblique muscle on the anterolateral aspect. Great care must be taken at this point, because the plane between the muscle and the submucosa is much less defined, and there are many redundant folds in the stomach making perforation easy. Thus, cautery in this area should be used with caution. If the myotomy is not carried far enough, the patient will have persistent dysphagia, whereas if it is carried too far, the patient will be left with reflux. Some surgeons perform simultaneous endoscopy to enable a better estimate of the gastroesophageal junction. This gives an accurate judgment of how far to carry the myotomy inferiorly. The endoscope also allows better estimation of the depth of the myotomy to prevent inadvertent perforations. After completion of the myotomy, the muscular edges of the myotomy should be undermined to expose 40% to 50% of the esophageal circumference to ensure the edges will not scar together.

The integrity of the esophageal mucosa is tested by filling the distal esophagus and fundus with 250 ml of methylene blue diluted with normal saline. Any areas of perforation can be repaired with interrupted fine absorbable suture.

## VARIATIONS OF OPERATION

Controversy exists as to whether an antireflux procedure is required after a laparoscopic myotomy. The different options will be discussed. The proponents of fundoplication recommend this because of the high incidence of reflux after myotomy. This reflux is most likely a result of the necessary dissection of the crura and the phrenoesophageal ligament distorting the normal architecture of the hiatus and disrupting the natural antireflux mechanism. The anterior fundoplication or the Dor fundoplication is preferred for elderly patients with megaesophagus of greater than 7 cm diameter, because it does not alter the angle of the gastroesophageal junction risking outflow obstruction. First, the angle of His is reapproximated with three interrupted sutures between the fundus of the stomach and the cut edge of the myotomy on the left. Next two to three sutures are placed from the fundus to the diaphragmatic arch to tack the fundus from the arch with each suture moving anteriorly across the esophagus. This is carried down the right side of the myotomy with three more sutures. This rolls the stomach over the myotomy. This should be performed with a 60 F bougie to hold the myotomy open and prevent the fundoplication from narrowing the lumen.

Other surgeons prefer a Toupet or posterior fundoplication. This is recommended for younger patients and those with mild to moderate esophageal dilation less than 7 cm. The advantages of this procedure are that the natural tension lines help to hold open the cut edges of the myotomy, and it is a better long-term antireflux procedure. In elderly patients, however, it is believed to distort the hiatus too much, producing a functional outlet obstruction from the anterior displacement. This is performed by bringing the mobilized fundus behind the esophagus and securing the right free edge of the myotomy with three interrupted 2-0 sutures of either silk or braided nylon. Likewise, the left side is sutured with three sutures. There is no need to suture the stomach to the diaphragm. A bougie is optional, because this fundoplication naturally pulls the lumen open, but it can be helpful to identify the minute uncut tight bands of the myotomy. An NGT is usually placed under direct vision at the end of the case and left in overnight.

## POSTOPERATIVE ORDERS

**Admit to:**
**Diagnosis:** s/p laparoscopic Heller myotomy
**Condition:** stable
**Vital signs:** per routine

**Activities:** ad lib
**Allergies:**
**Nursing:** strict I&Os, NGT to LCWS, IS 10 puffs q1h while awake, Pneumoboots and PAS until fully ambulatory.
**Diet:** NPO until swallow study; advance diet after normal swallow confirmed; liquid diet for first 2 to 3 days, then soft solid diet for the next 3 weeks, then regular diet.

NOTE: If the mucosa has been perforated, keep patient NPO with an NGT for 1 week and study with a barium swallow before feedings are begun.

**IV fluids:** $D_5$/0.45% NS at 85 ml/h
**Medications:** ondansetron (Zofran) and pain medications prn
**Laboratory tests:** routine postop CBC, BMP, and CXR; schedule Gastrografin swallow postoperative day 1 to "evaluate for leak and esophageal emptying"

## VII. POSTOPERATIVE COMPLICATIONS

1. **Delayed esophageal leak** is usually secondary to an inadvertent cautery burn to the esophageal mucosa. Patients commonly have chest pain, fever, and a pleural effusion on CXR. Patients should undergo immediate barium swallow and repair.
2. **Dysphagia** is a result of not carrying the myotomy far enough down on the gastric wall. This can usually be prevented with intraoperative endoscopy to confirm the length of the myotomy. Before reoperation, these patients need esophageal manometry to redefine the pathology and extent of the LES.
3. **Gastroesophageal reflux disease** is a result of the myotomy extending too far down the gastric wall. Patients usually have heartburn. Patients should have a 24-hour pH study. If there is only mild reflux, they can be treated with antacids, but if reflux is severe, they should undergo a partial fundoplication. Chronic reflux can lead to strictures with complaints of dysphagia.
4. **Aspiration pneumonia** is common in these patients because of the large reservoir of food particles in the dilated esophagus.

## VIII. DISCHARGE ORDERS

Patients are discharged postoperative day 1 or 2. Patients may resume regular activity in 1 week. A soft solid diet is given for 3 weeks followed by regular diet. Follow-up is in 1 week for wound check.

# GASTROESOPHAGEAL REFLUX DISEASE AND PARAESOPHAGEAL HERNIA

*Eric E. Roselli*

Gastroesophageal reflux disease (GERD) and paraesophageal hernia (PEH) are two separate yet related problems caused by mechanical dysfunction at the gastroesophageal junction. As such, they can both be treated with the same surgical procedures. By reducing morbidity, recent advances in minimally invasive surgical technique have made these operations more common. Furthermore, there are data to support greater overall patient satisfaction with surgery compared with medical treatment options.

**9**

## I. PATHOPHYSIOLOGY

### GERD

GERD occurs as a result of defective lower esophageal sphincter (LES) function. This is a mechanical problem of a physiologic valve that permits reflux, and thus exposure of esophageal mucosa to the toxic effects of gastric acid and bile. Critical characteristics of LES dysfunction include a low resting pressure defined as less than or equal to 6 mm Hg, a short intraabdominal LES length ($<1$ cm), and a short overall LES length ($<2$ cm). Poor esophageal motility, and thus an ineffective clearance mechanism, also plays a significant role in this dysfunction. This altered esophageal function can be made worse by the damaging effects of reflux and can lead to a vicious cycle of worsening reflux and esophageal mucosal injury. Problems with reflux can also be exacerbated by delayed gastric emptying function.

### PEH

PEH, also known as a type II or III hiatal hernia (not to be confused with a type I simple sliding hiatal hernia), occurs when a portion of the stomach is intrathoracic. Gastric herniation can lead to obstruction with subsequent ulceration, bleeding, gangrene, and perforation in up to 30% of patients. Mortality after perforation approaches 50%. Surgery is indicated whether patients are symptomatic or not.

## II. TYPICAL PRESENTATION

### GERD

Typical GERD symptoms include heartburn, regurgitation, and dysphagia. Patients may describe heartburn symptoms that worsen with bending over or lying down, and this is often accompanied by a bitter taste in the mouth. Many patients also describe severe chest pain, which should be differentiated from angina pectoris, pancreatitis, and cholecystitis. Aspiration during sleep causes waking with hoarseness or chronic cough and asthma. Some patients have mild symptoms and may have one of the complications of GERD including esophagitis, stricture, recurrent aspiration or pneumonia, or Barrett's esophagus. Surgery is indicated for complications, including refractory to medical therapy (histamine [$H_2$] blockers or proton pump inhibitors), symptoms interfering with their lifestyle despite medical therapy, and the need for continuous drug therapy in patients who desire discontinuation of medical therapy. The latter is common in those at a young age, with financial burden, or noncompliance issues because of lifestyle.

### PEH

PEH symptoms typically include cramping abdominal pain and postparandial bloating. Other patients describe early satiety, nausea, shortness of breath, hematemesis, weight loss, and occasionally reflux.

## III. PREOPERATIVE WORKUP

Proper patient and operation selection is paramount to achieving good results. Esophagogastroduodenoscopy (EGD) is important to look for complications, including esophagitis or ulcers, stricture, Barrett's esophagus, and to rule out neoplasia. It also allows measurement of the distance to the GE junction to determine the presence of a short esophagus. All mucosal lesions require biopsy.

A 24-hour pH probe should be performed if no reflux esophagitis is detected on EGD. A positive test demonstrates a distal esophageal pH of less than 4 for more than 4% of the time. Although cumbersome for the patient, this is currently the most reliable test to document acid reflux. This test should be used in patients with reflux symptoms without evidence of esophagitis on endoscopy.

Esophageal manometry guides the choice of operation by determining the extent of fundoplication necessary to complement a patient's adequacy of esophageal peristalsis. Patients with a severe motility disorder or scleroderma should be carefully considered, because they typically have poor responses to surgery.

Barium esophagram is especially important for patients with PEHs. It demonstrates the anatomic relationship of the esophagus, stomach, and diaphragm. This test can demonstrate strictures, which must be addressed preoperatively. Furthermore, a short esophagus is suggested by the presence of an irreducible hiatal hernia in the upright position and should be suspected in patients with a history of stricture requiring dilatation, long segment Barrett's esophagus, a large hiatal hernia (>4 cm at EGD), and PEH.

**PREOPERATIVE ORDERS**

**Nursing:** nasogastric decompression in PEH patients for possible retained gastric contents to avoid aspiration; PAS on call to the OR

**Diet:** NPO after midnight

**Medications:** Ancef, 1 g IV, on call to the OR

## IV. SURGICAL ANATOMY

Four principles important to the reconstruction of a competent gastroesophageal barrier include the following:

1. Restoration of 1.5 to 2 cm of intraabdominal esophagus
2. A functional LES with resting intrinsic pressures of ~15 mm Hg or three times the gastric resting pressure
3. Maintenance of a functional cardioesophageal angle by recreating an intact crural diaphragm and using only the fundus of the stomach to create the valve while avoiding injury to the vagus nerves
4. Matching the degree of resistance provided by the wrap to the peristaltic function or dysfunction of the esophagus.

## V. CONDUCT OF OPERATION

### GERD

**Laparoscopic Nissen fundoplication** is the procedure of choice for uncomplicated GERD and if the patient lacks a history of upper abdominal surgery, a short esophagus, or esophageal dysmotility. Symptomatic relief with medical therapy predicts a good response in this operation.

The patient should be positioned supine with legs abducted or in the lithotomy position, in a steep reverse Trendelenburg position, and with video monitors at the head of the table. The surgeon stands between the legs. The assistant is at the patient's left. The camera holder or liver retractor is at the patient's right.

Five ports are placed as follows:

1. The **camera port** is 10 mm. It is placed just cephalad and to the left of the umbilicus (ie, home plate). It is preferable to use an angled, 30 or 45 degrees, camera.
2. The **surgeon's right hand working port** is 10 mm.
3. **The surgeon's left hand working port** is 5 mm.
   Ports 3 and 4 are placed bilaterally and subcostally at the first and third base positions of a virtual diamond in relation to the camera port (at home plate), with the operative field representing the second base position.

9

GASTROESOPHAGEAL REFLUX DISEASE

4. The **liver retractor** is a 5-mm port. Place the fan retractor through this port in the right lateral subcostal region.
5. The **assistant's working port** is also 5 mm. A grasper should be placed through this port in the left lateral subcostal position for stomach retraction.

Perform a complete dissection of the hiatus region. First, incise the phrenoesophageal membrane and extend the dissection 4 to 6 cm into the mediastinum, taking care to spare the vagus nerves.

Short gastric adhesions and adhesions to the fundus are then divided with a harmonic scalpel. From across and behind the esophagus the fundus is brought around the back of the esophagus from left to right and slid back and forth (the shoeshine maneuver).

The crura are next reapproximated posterior to the esophagus with intracorporeal suturing, usually requiring about three sutures. A 50 to 60 F bougie dilator is then placed down the esophagus, and the wrap is secured with several sutures. It is important to include the anterior wall of the esophagus in at least two of these sutures.

The wrap should be less than 2.5 cm and above the GE junction. The 10-mm port sites should include the fascia in their closure.

## PEH

Laparoscopic PEH repair uses the same approach that GERD does. Main points of the operation include a complete reduction of the hernia contents, which may require extensive mediastinal dissection, excision of the hernia sac, and approximation of the crura without using a mesh repair. In addition, concomitant fundoplication as described to reduce reflux and provide a means of gastropexy should be done.

## TRANSTHORACIC SURGICAL OPTIONS

A transthoracic approach may be indicated in patients with a history of previous antireflux or upper abdominal surgery, short esophagus, or esophageal dysfunction.

**Belsey Mark IV** is a well-proven technique. A left mainstem bronchial blocker or double-lumen tube is placed. The incision is a left posterolateral complete muscle-sparing thoracotomy entering the sixth intercostal space. The lung is retracted superiorly, and the inferior ligament is divided to the level of the inferior pulmonary vein. The mediastinal pleura is divided. The esophagus is isolated with a Penrose drain, and the dissection can be carried to the level of the aortic arch as necessary for esophageal length. Vagal injury is avoided. The phrenoesophageal membrane is then incised circum-ferentially, and the peritoneum is carefully entered. An accessory gastrohepatic artery may require ligation. The distal esophagus and stomach should then be easily delivered into the chest. The antire-flux procedure can then be performed using three rows of three interrupted 2-0 silk sutures 1.5 cm apart to wrap 240 degrees of the fundus around the distal esophagus. The last row is sutured with double-ended needles, which are then passed through the hiatus. The repair is then reduced back into the abdomen without tension, and the previously placed transhiatal sutures are tied to secure the repair to the diaphragm. The posterior hiatus is reapprox-imated with interrupted No.1 silk sutures to allow the easy passage of the distal interphalangeal joint of an index finger. The right pleural cavity is suctioned out if entered, and a left-sided No. 28 chest tube is placed through a separate stab incision and interspace. The thoracotomy is closed in standard fashion.

**Collis gastroplasty** is indicated for treatment of the foreshortened esophagus. Exposure and dissection is performed as for the Belsey procedure. A 50 to 60 F bougie dilator is then inserted by the anesthetist. The lengthening procedure is performed by firing a gastrointestinal anastomosis 50-mm stapler along the bougie onto the proximal stomach beginning at the gastroesophageal junction to create a tubular neoesophagus. The subsequent fundopli-cation—either a Nissen or Belsey Mark IV—is performed around the neoesophagus.

**Laparotomy** is occasionally needed when intraoperative conditions such as difficult anatomy or a bleeding complication warrant conversion to an open procedure. Hand-assisted laparoscopy may be indicated to help reduce a large paraesophageal hernia.

## FUNDOPLICATION OPTIONS

**Toupet** fundoplication is a partial 270-degree wrap used for patients with poor esophageal motility. The leading edge of the fundus is secured to the right anterior esophagus. The left medial fundus is sutured to the left anterolateral esophagus. The fundus is then secured to the crus bilaterally as well.

The **Hill** esophagogastropexy includes a 90-degree plication of the lesser curve around the right side of the esophagus and a posterior esophagogastropexy to the supraaortic median arcuate ligament.

A **Dor** operation consists of a 180- to 200-degree anterior fundopli-cation usually used in conjunction with the Heller myotomy for achalasia.

## POSTOPERATIVE ORDERS

### GERD

**Admit to:** _____ for 23-hour overnight stay

**Diagnosis:** s/p laparoscopic Nissen fundoplication

**Condition:**

9

GASTROESOPHAGEAL REFLUX DISEASE

**Vital signs:** per routine
**Activity:** ad lib
**Allergies:**
**Nursing:** advise the patient to chew food well, avoid bulky foods and raw vegetables in the beginning; it is important to inform and reassure patients of possible gas-bloat, difficulty with burping, and possible need to advance the diet slowly over several days if they experience mild dysphagia due to perioperative swelling
**Diet:** clear liquids the day of surgery and advance as tolerated to a soft diet
**IV fluids:** $D_5$/0.45% NS + 20 mEq KCl at 80 ml/h until tolerating oral intake, then Heplock IV
**Medications:** oral narcotics for analgesia; ondansetron (Zofran) prn
**Laboratory tests:**

**PEH.** As above, except NPO the first night. Then check barium swallow on POD 1 to rule out a leak. The diet may advance as above if the swallow is normal

**Transthoracic Approach.** As for GERD except a portable CXR should be checked in the recovery room. Epidural patient-controlled analgesia should be used until the chest tube is removed on POD 2, and then the patient can be converted to oral analgesics. It is important for the patient to ambulate early; coughing, deep breathing, and the use of the incentive spirometer should be stressed.

## VI. COMPLICATIONS

Mortality is less than 0.5%, and morbidity ranges from 0 to 5%. Complications include early dysphagia in 10% to 30%, which usually resolves spontaneously in 6 weeks. Late dysphagia occurs in 5% to 10% of patients and requires workup with a barium swallow examination. Causes of late dysphagia include a tight wrap, slipped wrap (around the stomach), or herniation of the GE junction. These complications often require reoperation. If none of these is documented, patients often improve with an esophageal dilatation.

Bleeding usually can be dealt with intraoperatively, and splenic injuries are rare. Perforations of the esophagus or stomach are usually identified intraoperatively and can usually be oversewn laparoscopically. Pneumothorax occasionally occurs because of the dissection around the hiatus and can be drained with a red rubber catheter inserted intraoperatively.

Gas-bloat syndrome or diarrhea occurs occasionally and usually improves with diet adjustments and time as patients overcome the habit of swallowing excess air. Although not a complication, the laparoscopic conversion rate ranges from 1% to 12% after an average learning curve of approximately 20 operations.

## VII. DISCHARGE INSTRUCTIONS

Diet is restricted to a GI soft diet with attention to frequent well-chewed meals and avoidance of bulky foods like bread, meats, and raw vegetables. Eventually the diet can be advanced slowly as tolerated without restrictions. Activity should be restricted to no heavy lifting for 2 to 6 weeks, depending on the incision used to avoid hernia. Routine follow-up for trocar site or wound check occurs in 1 to 2 weeks. Follow-up barium esophagram at 8 to 12 weeks is recommended to document anatomy should later problems develop.

# ULCER DISEASE

*Edward Panzeter*

Peptic ulcer disease entails both duodenal and gastric ulcers. Gastric ulcers are further subdivided as follows. Type I gastric ulcers produce no acid and occur along the lesser curvature near the incisura. Type II ulcers are acid hypersecretors and are a combination of both a body gastric ulcer and a duodenal ulcer. Type III ulcers include acid hypersecretors and are prepyloric and usually multiple. Type IV ulcers also produce no acid and are located high on the lesser curvature near the gastroesophageal (GE) junction. Type V ulcers occur anywhere in the stomach and are associated with NSAID/aspirin use.

**10**

## I. PATHOPHYSIOLOGY

Most theories concerning the development of peptic ulcer disease are based on increased acid production or its effects on the gastric/duodenal mucosa. In addition, gastric stasis has been implicated as a risk factor for the development of peptic ulcers secondary to inadequate acid clearance. Environmental factors also play a role in the development of ulcers. NSAIDS disrupt the mucosal barrier of the stomach by inhibiting prostaglandin production. Cigarette smoking has also been linked to ulcer formation. Recently, *Helicobacter pylori* has been implicated as a cause for duodenal ulcer formation. Treatment of *H. pylori* has led to greater cure rates and a decrease in recurrence rates.

## II. TYPICAL PRESENTATION

Patients with ulcers present with a variety of signs and symptoms. Epigastric abdominal pain, aggravated by ingestion of food, is the most common presenting symptom. Other symptoms include nausea, vomiting, anorexia, and weight loss. Physical examination demonstrates epigastric tenderness or frank peritonitis if perforation is present. Hematemesis or guaiac-positive stools are seen in hemorrhagic ulcers. Ulcers are usually diagnosed at the time of upper endoscopy (EGD). Medical treatment of ulcers includes antacids, mucosal defense enhancing medications (sucralfate), lifestyle and diet modifications, $H_2$ antagonists, proton pump inhibitors, and antibiotics specific for *H. pylori*.

## III. PREOPERATIVE WORKUP

All gastric ulcers must be biopsied to exclude malignancy. Benign gastric ulcers are subsequently treated by cessation of ulcerogenic medications and beginning $H_2$ blockers for 8 weeks. If symptoms completely resolve, the patient is monitored clinically, but if symptoms persist, a repeat endoscopy with biopsy and measurement of serum gastrin is performed. If a biopsy is negative, a proton pump inhibitor, e.g., omeprazole, is given for 8 weeks with a follow-up endoscopy at that time. If the ulcer is still present at that time, surgical consultation is obtained.

Duodenal ulcers are initially treated with both $H_2$ blockers for 8 weeks and antibiotics to eradicate *H. pylori*. All patients with duodenal ulcers should be biopsied at the gastric antrum to rule out *H. pylori* infestation. If symptoms resolve, the patient is observed, but a repeat endoscopy is performed for persistent or recurrent symptoms. The patient is again treated against *H. pylori*, advised to stop all ulcerogenic drugs, and a proton pump inhibitor is added for 8 weeks. If symptoms resolve, patients may either be placed on long-term acid suppression with $H_2$ antagonists or be observed. For continued symptoms, a surgical consultation is placed.

Endoscopic therapy is important in patients whose initial presentation is hemorrhage. Endoscopy can be both diagnostic and therapeutic. Therapeutic options for bleeding ulcers include coagulation with heater probe, epinephrine injection, or metal clip application to a vessel. Complications associated with this include perforation (1%-3%), necrosis, or delayed hemorrhage (5%-30%).

Elective ulcer operations are rare today because of the excellent medical regimens available. Current indications for operation are hemorrhage, perforation, obstruction, or intractability. Today, intractability accounts for <5% of ulcer operations and is defined as when a patient's symptoms interfere with normal daily activity despite adequate medical treatment (ie, 12-24 weeks of antisecretory drugs). In addition, elective surgery is performed for ulcer recurrence after initial successful treatment and to exclude malignancy.

## PREOPERATIVE ORDERS

The patient should be adequately resuscitated and IV antibiotics started before patient is taken to the OR. An NGT should be placed in the emergency room and lavage performed to identify the source of upper GI bleeding if it is present.

**Admit to:**
**Diagnosis:** PUD
**Condition:** stable
**Vital signs:** per routine
**Activity:** OOB to chair with assistance, or ad lib
**Allergies:**
**Nursing:** I&Os, NGT to LCWS, Foley to gravity to monitor urine output, IS × 10 puffs q1h while awake
**Diet:** NPO
**IV fluids:** to keep urine output at 30 ml/h
**Medications:** ranitidine (Zantac) 50 mg IV q8h; antibiotics on call to OR
**Laboratory tests:** CBC, BMP, LFTs, PT, PTT, amylase, lipase, ECG, KUB with upright CXR, T&C 4 U of PRBCs

## IV. SURGICAL ANATOMY

The stomach is located in the left upper quadrant of the abdomen extending from the gastroesophageal junction at the esophageal hiatus to the pylorus. The stomach is lateral to the left lobe of the liver, medial to the spleen, and bounded posteriorly by the pancreas and retroperitoneum. The stomach has a rich vascular arcade consisting of the left and right gastric arteries supplying the lesser curvature and the left and right gastroepiploic arteries supplying the greater curvature. The stomach has a dual venous drainage system, the portal system and the systemic system via the esophageal veins. Neural input to the stomach is through the vagus nerves, anterior (left) and posterior (right), and the celiac axis for sympathetic stimulation.

The duodenum extends from the pylorus to the ligament of Treitz and is retroperitoneal in location. The duodenum has four portions: the first or duodenal bulb, which overlies the gastroduodenal artery; the second or descending portion, which courses along the pancreas and is where the ampulla of Vater is located; the third or transverse portion, which lies between the aorta and the superior mesenteric artery; and the fourth or ascending portion. The blood supply is varied and is derived from both the celiac and superior mesenteric artery axes by way of the gastroduodenal artery and the superior or inferior pancreaticoduodenal arteries. Venous drainage is through the portal system.

## V. CONDUCT OF OPERATION

The goals of an ulcer operation are to correct the emergent problem, prevent ulcer recurrence, exclude malignancy, and limit operative morbidity. Because most ulcer operations today are emergent, controversy exists concerning the need to include a definitive ulcer operation at the time of emergent surgery. Definitive repair should be avoided when shock, significant comorbid medical conditions, or perforation >24 hours is present. The emergent operation of choice in a perforated ulcer is a Graham patch or placement of an omental pedicle within the perforated area, not closing the ulcer and reinforcing the closure with omentum. In addition, ligating the offending vessel best treats bleeding ulcers.

### VARIATIONS OF OPERATION

Traditional ulcer operations include vagotomy (either truncal or selective) with drainage (either pyloroplasty or gastrojejunostomy), highly selective vagotomy without drainage, vagotomy with antrectomy, or subtotal gastrectomy. Drainage procedures are necessary with truncal or selective vagotomy, because the antral nerves of Latarjet are denervated; therefore, the emptying of solids is reduced. These ulcer operations are performed at the time of emergent ulcer surgery if the patient is stable. Truncal vagotomy consists of division of the left vagus nerve proximal to hepatic branches

**10**

**ULCER DISEASE**

**TABLE 10-1**

ADVERSE EFFECTS OF SURGERY FOR ULCER REPAIR

| | Highly Selective Vagotomy | Vagotomy and Antrectomy | Vagotomy and Drainage |
|---|---|---|---|
| Morbidity | 5%-10% | 15%-20% | 5%-10% |
| Mortality | 0%-1% | 0%-2% | 0%-3% |
| Ulcer recurrence | 1%-25% | 0%-2% | 1%-12% |
| Dumping | 0%-6% | 1%-25% | 1%-12% |
| Diarrhea | 0%-5% | 1%-22% | 2%-20% |

and the right vagus nerve proximal to its celiac branches. Selective vagotomy consists of division of the nerves of Latarjet just distal to the hepatic or celiac vagal branches. Highly selective vagotomy involves division of the vagal nerves to the parietal cells and does not require a drainage procedure. Antrectomy involves resection of the parietal cell mass and reconstruction with either a Bilroth I (gastroduodenostomy) or Bilroth II (gastrojejunostomy), depending on the pliability of the duodenum. Finally, subtotal gastrectomy is resection of 70% to 75% of the distal stomach with a Bilroth II reconstruction. Table 10–1 describes the results of the three ulcer operations

## POSTOPERATIVE ORDERS

**Admit to:**
**Diagnosis:** s/p gastric ulcer surgery
**Condition:** stable
**Vital signs:** per routine
**Activity:** OOB to chair with assistance
**Allergies:**
**Nursing:** I&Os, NGT to LCWS, Foley to gravity, Pneumoboots, PAS
**Diet:** NPO
**IV fluids:** D$_5$/0.45% NS with 20 mEq KCl at 125 ml/h
**Medications:** ranitidine (Zantac) 50 mg IV q8h, pain medication, perioperative antibiotics
**Laboratory tests:** CBC, PT, PTT, BMP

## VI. COMPLICATIONS

Complications are divided into short- and long-term complications of ulcer surgery. Short-term complications include rebleeding of the ulcer, gastroparesis, duodenal stump blowout, and leaks. Rebleeding of ulcers is greatest with simple oversewing of the ulcer or vagotomy and pyloroplasty, whereas vagotomy and antrectomy reduce this risk. Gastroparesis is common after upper intestinal surgery and is usually treated conservatively, although reglan or erythromycin may be of some benefit. The upper GI tract is often examined first to identify any functional obstruction. Duodenal stump blowout can occur and presents with severe abdominal sepsis requiring reoperation. Occasionally, a tube duodenostomy is necessary to control a difficult duodenum. Leaks or fistulas after closure of an ulcer or pyloroplasty are uncommon, occurring <5% of the time. Reoperation is usually unsuccessful, and conservative management with total parenteral nutrition, bowel rest, drainage, and antibiotics is the usual course of action.

Long-term complications of ulcer surgery include recurrent ulcers, dumping syndrome, diarrhea, malabsorption, and bile reflux gastritis (Table 10-1). Recurrent ulceration after surgery is common, with the results given earlier. Most recurrent ulcers are managed medically, but marginal ulcers or ulcers at the gastrojejunostomy anastomosis often require reoperation. Tachycardia, diaphoresis, hypotension, and abdominal pain occurring shortly after meals characterize dumping syndrome. Symptoms usually improve with time, but sometimes additional surgery, such as conversion to a Roux-en-Y, is necessary for correction of this problem. Recently, octreotide has been used to control dumping syndrome. Diarrhea usually occurs 30 minutes after a meal and is watery. This also improves with time, and reoperation is often unsuccessful. Most patients after antrectomy have vitamin $B_{12}$ deficiency and need exogenous $B_{12}$ injections. Bile reflux gastritis consists of bilious vomiting, abdominal pain, and bile gastritis on biopsy. Treatment consists of conversion of a Bilroth anastomosis to a Roux-en-Y.

**10**

**ULCER DISEASE**

## VII. DISCHARGE ORDERS

Patients are ready for discharge after ulcer surgery when they are hemodynamically stable and tolerating a diet. Depending on the type of operation performed and on whether a definitive procedure was obtained, patients may require *H. pylori* treatment or long-term acid suppression treatment.

# GASTRIC CANCER

*Conrad Simfendorfer*

Although the incidence of gastric cancer has declined dramatically in the United States in the last 50 years, it still remains among the top 10 leading causes of cancer-related deaths in the United States. It is estimated that 24,000 new cases of gastric cancer were diagnosed in 1994, with a death rate of approximately 7.5 per 100,000. Despite diagnostic advances such as dual-contrast radiography and endoscopy, the disease is often not recognized until it is at an advanced stage, and with the exception of early gastric cancer, which is usually (>90%) cured with surgery alone, survival at 5 years remains 20% to 30%.

**11**

## I. PATHOPHYSIOLOGY

The incidence of gastric cancer varies widely from country to country, as well as regionally, suggesting a strong environmental factor in the development of gastric cancer.

The disease seems to be correlated with a high intake of preserved food, which contains high levels of nitrates, nitrites, and salt, which can act as gastric irritants.

There is growing evidence that *Helicobacter pylori* and chronic gastritis play a role in the development of gastric cancer. Chronic *H. pylori* infection, if untreated, may lead to chronic atrophic gastritis with metaplasia, with an associated high risk of gastric cancer.

Adenomatous gastric polyps, although rare, carry a potential for the development of gastric malignancy. The risk of cancer developing in adenomatous polyps is thought to be between 10% and 20%, and is greatest for polyps that are 2 cm or greater in diameter. Patients with multiple polyposis or recurrent adenomas should be considered for subtotal or total gastrectomy. Those with malignancy and multiple polyps should undergo total gastrectomy.

Previous gastric operations may increase a person's risk for gastric cancer threefold. Several studies with long-term follow-up indicate that the relative risk does not increase for up to 15 years after gastric resection.

Gastric adenocarcinomas occur in two histologic subtypes—intestinal and diffuse. Intestinal-type tumors have a glandular appearance resembling colonic carcinoma, with diffuse inflammatory cell infiltration and frequent intestinal metaplasia. It is more common in populations at high risk and occurs more frequently in men and older patients. In contrast to intestinal-type neoplasms, diffuse-type tumors are composed of tiny clusters of small uniform cells, have less inflammatory infiltration, more lymphatic invasion, frequent intraperitoneal metastases, and carry a poorer prognosis. This form tends to occur more frequently in women, younger patients, and in populations with a relatively low incidence of gastric cancer.

Patients with gastric adenocarcinoma should undergo surgical resection, either subtotal gastrectomy or total gastrectomy, to maximize the chances for cure in patients with localized disease and to provide palliation to patients with advanced malignancy. Distal subtotal gastrectomy for early lesions has a 5-year survival rate of 90% or greater. For more advanced lesions, the extent of gastric resection, the necessity for lymphadenectomy or splenectomy, and the role of adjuvant chemo-radiotherapy remains controversial.

## II. TYPICAL PRESENTATION

Unfortunately, the symptoms of gastric cancer are not specific and can closely resemble those of benign gastroduodenal diseases, mainly gastric ulcer. Recent studies have shown that weight loss and epigastric abdominal pain are the most common symptoms. Other symptoms include nausea, anorexia, dysphagia, and melena. Approximately 10% of patients present either with acute upper gastrointestinal hemorrhage or with disseminated disease, including supraclavicular or pelvic adenopathy, ascites, jaundice, or hepatomegaly.

Physical examination in early gastric cancers is most often normal. One third may have guaiac-positive stool. Abnormal physical findings, such as cachexia, abdominal mass, hepatomegaly, and lymphadenopathy, usually indicate advanced disease.

## III. PREOPERATIVE WORKUP

**Endoscopy.** Flexible fiberoptic endoscopy is the most accurate diagnostic method currently available for the diagnosis of gastric cancer, with a diagnostic accuracy of 87% and 94% when biopsies are obtained. Early lesions may appear as small, plaquelike lesions, polypoid, or as shallow ulcers. More advanced lesions are typically ulcerated with irregular elevated margins and shaggy necrotic centers. Diffuse-type cancers have extensive tumor plaques or large polypoid masses. Linitis plastica is recognized by a nondistensible stomach.

**Barium Study.** Double-contrast (air and barium) studies have up to a 90% diagnostic accuracy, that is a sensitive and cost-effective test for the detection of gastric cancer. Findings usually include ulceration, gastric mass, loss of mucosal detail, and distortion of the gastric sihouette.

**Computed Tomography Scan.** Increasingly, CT has been used as both a primary diagnostic method and to assess extragastric spread. Although controversial in its use for staging, CT can readily demonstrate metastatic involvement of the liver, spleen, pancreas, and adrenal glands. But it is less reliable with regard to tumor invasion of adjacent organs or the presence of lymphatic metastasis.

**Ultrasonography.** Endoscopic ultrasonography is proving to be highly sensitive in evaluating gastric submucosal lesions and differentiating them from benign disease processes, such as leiomyomas, which are smooth, round hypoechoic masses that are contiguous with muscularis propia.

## PREOPERATIVE ORDERS

Patients should remain NPO the night before surgery. A routine bowel preparation should be administered, unless obstruction is suspected. Otherwise, these patients should undergo a workup similar to that for other major abdominal operations.

## IV. SURGICAL ANATOMY

The stomach is a large irregular piriform sac between the esophagus and the small intestine, lying just beneath the diaphragm, resting in the supine position, on the stomach bed, formed by the pancreas, spleen, left kidney and suprarenal gland, transverse colon, and its mesocolon. The stomach is entirely covered by peritoneum and is located in the left hypochondriac and epigastric regions of the abdomen. It has a lesser and greater curvature and is divided into the cardia, fundus, body, and pylorus. It receives its blood supply from the right and left gastric, right and left gastroepiploic, short gastric, and gastroduodenal arteries.

## V. CONDUCT OF OPERATION

The patient is placed in the supine position, and general anesthesia with endotracheal intubation is induced. The abdomen is prepped and draped sterilely. A nasogastric tube is placed. An upper abdominal midline incision is made, extending from the xiphoid process to the umbilicus or a point below the umbilicus.

## SUBTOTAL GASTRECTOMY

After the peritoneal cavity is entered, the abdominal contents are examined carefully, for extension of tumor and evidence of adenopathy. The greater omentum is retracted anteriorly and superiorly to expose the transverse colon. Electrocautery is used to detach the greater omentum from the colon, allowing access to the lesser sac. The stomach is then lifted, and the peritoneum over the superior aspect of the pancreas is incised, exposing the celiac axis. The left gastric artery is identified at its origin from the celiac axis, and the artery is doubly ligated and divided. Lymph nodes in the area may be mobilized for inclusion in the specimen.

The gastrohepatic ligament is divided, and the stomach is retracted inferiorly and to the right to expose the right gastric artery. This is then dissected, ligated, and divided. Then the right gastroepiploic vessels are identified at the inferior aspect of the antrum, dissected, divided between clamps, and ligated. The stomach is then lifted anteriorly to expose the duodenum, and several small vessels between the duodenum and pancreas are carefully dissected.

Attention is then returned to the greater curvature, and tumor location is assessed to select a site for transection that will give a 6-cm margin proximal to gross tumor. The short gastric vessels are usually divided up to a point just distal to the most inferior short gastric vessel. The stomach wall is cleared on the greater and lesser curvature at the point of transection. A stapler is placed across the stomach, a large Payr clamp is placed distal to the stapler, and a scalpel is used to transect the stomach adjacent to the stapler. A row of interrupted seromuscular sutures is placed to oversew the stapled edge. A stapler is then placed across the duodenum just distal to the pylorus, a small Payr clamp is placed proximal to the stapler, and a scalpel is used to transect the duodenum adjacent to the stapler. The staple line is then oversewn in an interrupted fashion.

Attention is then made toward the formation of a gastrojejunostomy. A short loop of jejunum is brought anterior to the colon. An opening is made in the greater curvature of the stomach, 1 cm proximal to the staple closure, to allow entry of one tip of a side-to-side stapler. An opening is made on the antimesenteric border of the jejunum, the side-to-side stapler is introduced into the stomach and jejunum, and care is taken to avoid interposing tissue between both organs. The stapler defect is closed with interrupted through-and-through sutures, then the gastrojejunostomy is oversewn with interrupted seromuscular sutures. The operative site is inspected for bleeding, all instruments and sponges are removed from the abdomen, and the incision is closed in the usual fashion.

## TOTAL GASTRECTOMY

After an upper midline incision and thorough inspection of the abdomen, the stomach is completely devascularized and mobilized, with the dissection extended to include at least a proximal centimeter of duodenum. The duodenum is divided with a gastrointestinal anastomosis (GIA) stapler. The stomach and esophagus are left attached until placement of the posterior row of anastomosis.

Attention is then directed to the reconstruction of an esophagoenteric continuity, most often through a Roux-en-Y esophagojejunostomy. A minimum of 18 inches of roux loop is required to prevent bile reflux esophagitis. A transection is made as proximal as possible with preservation of the vascular arcades to both sides of the jejunum, using the GIA stapler. The anastomosis can be made in either an antecolic or retrocolic manner, selecting a route that causes the least tension.

The esophagojejunal anastomosis is performed using a hand-sewn, double-layer, interrupted, 3-0 silk suture. The nasogastric tube is placed through the anastomosis into the jejunal limb before placing the anterior row of sutures.

Then the jejunojejunostomy is performed either with a GIA-TA-55 stapler or by a hand-sewn double-layer technique. The mesenteric defect is closed. Finally, the abdomen is closed after inspection for bleeding and removal of instruments and sponges.

A variation of the esophagojejunal anastomosis exists through the creation of a jejunal pouch. The distal jejunum is brought up in the antecolic position, and traction sutures are placed to form a 15-cm jejunal loop. A GIA stapler is passed through enterotomies and fired, creating a jejunal pouch for gastric replacement. An end-to-end anastomosis (EEA) instrument is passed through the open enterotomies and the center rod extended at the apex of the jejunal loop. The anvil is secured into place, the esophagus is gently passed over the anvil, and the esophageal purse string is tied around the rod. The cartridge and anvil are approximated, and the EEA instrument is fired. The enterotomy is then closed with a staple device. The Roux-en-Y is then completed with a 5- or 10-cm GIA stapler. Extended resection, mainly resection of the stomach, perigastric nodes, and lymph nodes along the named arteries of the stomach, should be performed when there is gastric serosal involvement or when local regional lymph nodes are involved. Controversy exists regarding further nodal resection, mainly celiac and periaortic, as well as routine splenectomy.

## VARIATIONS OF OPERATION

Although laparoscopic gastrectomy and partial gastrectomy are feasible alternatives to traditional open surgery and have been succesfully performed for benign conditions of the stomach, malignancy remains a contraindication, except when performed in the confines of a prospective study.

## POSTOPERATIVE ORDERS

**Admit to:** general surgery
**Diagnosis:** s/p gastrectomy
**Condition:** stable
**Vital signs:** q4h with pulse oximetry q shift
**Activity:** bed rest, OOB in AM
**Allergies:**
**Nursing:** strict I&Os, NGT to LIWS with sign posted over bed "Do not manipulate NG tube," Foley to gravity, PAS, IS × 10 puffs q1h
**Diet:** strict NPO
**IV fluids:** D$_5$/lactated Ringer's at 125 ml/h

**Medications:** Pepcid 20 mg IV q12h
Morphine 2-8 mg IV q3h prn
Compazine 10 mg IV q6h prn
**Laboratory tests:** CBC, BMP

## VI. POTENTIAL COMPLICATIONS

In addition to the usual complications that may follow large abdominal surgery, mainly infection and hemorrhage, gastrectomies may be complicated by a number of postgastrectomy syndromes. These fortunately only affect 1% to 3% of cases severely.

Dumping syndrome is believed to be caused by the unmetered entry of ingested food into the proximal small bowel. Early dumping symptoms include nausea, epigastric discomfort, borborygmi, palpitations, and, occasionally, dizziness and syncope. Late dumping symptoms occur 1 to 3 hours after a meal and may include the preceding symptoms, as well as reactive hypoglycemia. Most patients will have improvement of their symptoms over time. Only about 1% of patients may need octreotide before meals to improve their symptoms.

Alkaline reflux gastritis is a diagnosis reserved for patients with postprandial epigastric pain, evidence of reflux of bile into the stomach, and histologic evidence of gastritis. The only proven treatment is diversion of intestinal contents from contact with the gastric mucosa through a Roux-en-Y gastrojejunostomy with an intestinal limb of 50 to 60 cm. This is effective in eliminating bilious vomiting, but patients usually report recurrent or persistent epigastric pain.

## VII. DISCHARGE ORDERS

Patients are discharged to home once they can tolerate a regular diet and can ambulate without assistance. They should refrain from strenuous activity for 4 to 6 weeks. Patients are encouraged to resume a regular diet but initially to consume small, frequent meals. Patients are instructed not to drive while taking narcotics. Occasionally, $B_{12}$ supplementation is necessary. Patients are generally seen in follow-up in 1 to 2 weeks.

# PART IV

## Small and Large Intestine

# APPENDECTOMY

*Jason Brodsky*

Appendectomy is one of the most common operations performed by general surgeons. Historically, patients underwent an operation solely on the basis of the history and physical examination. Currently, computed tomography (CT) and ultrasonography are used for diagnostic purposes. Despite these radiologic advances, the diagnosis of appendicitis remains a cornerstone of general surgery, incorporating a thorough history and basic physical examination skills.

**12**

## I. PATHOPHYSIOLOGY

1. **Acute appendicitis** due to obstruction of the appendiceal lumen is the most common indication for appendectomy. In the young, obstruction often results from lymphoid hyperplasia, resulting from either systemic or local infection. The latter is often caused by *Shigella* or *Salmonella* infection. In adults, fecaliths commonly cause appendiceal obstruction. Other causes include tumors and parasitic infestations. Regardless of cause, obstruction leads to bacterial overgrowth, inflammation, and appendiceal wall thickening. The resultant increase in appendiceal wall tension secondary to edema leads to ischemia, necrosis, and eventual perforation.
2. **Normal appendix during operation for acute appendicitis.** An appendectomy should be performed during exploration for presumed acute appendicitis. The exception to this is suspected Crohn's disease with involvement of or near the base of the appendix. A negative appendectomy rate of 15% is acceptable to avoid appendiceal perforation. Perforations of the appendix are associated with a significantly higher morbidity and mortality than that seen with negative explorations.
3. **Interval appendectomy** follows the nonoperative therapy of acute appendicitis. Occasionally, a perforated appendix will spontaneously form a walled-off abscess in the right lower quadrant. Nonoperative therapy with percutaneous drainage and intravenous broad-spectrum antibiotics resolves most of these abscesses. The appendix is then removed electively 6 to 8 weeks after drain removal.
4. **Incidental appendectomy** remains controversial. The decision to perform this procedure is made by the attending surgeon on an individual basis. In a clean case or when prosthetic materials are used, an appendectomy should not be performed. In determining whether to perform an incidental appendectomy, it is important to consider the patient's age, because the incidence of appendicitis decreases with increasing age.

## II. TYPICAL PRESENTATION

Appendicitis presents in a number of ways depending on the location of the appendix. Appendicitis classically presents with periumbilical pain localizing to the right lower quadrant. Anorexia is a hallmark symptom, and most patients experience nausea at some point during their course. Physical examination typically reveals fever in conjunction with a tender abdomen. Pain is most severe overlying McBurney's point (a point one third of the distance between the anterior superior iliac spine and umbilicus). Peritoneal signs are common. Examiners might induce pain in the right lower quadrant when palpating the left lower quadrant (Rovsing's sign), when rotating the hip internally (obturator sign), or when extending the hip (psoas sign). Focal tenderness may be present on rectal examination. The overall course of appendicitis is 24 to 36 hours from the onset of symptoms to perforation.

## III. PREOPERATIVE WORKUP

Diagnosis of appendicitis is classically made on the basis of the history and physical examination. Most decisions to operate for appendicitis require no additional studies. However, a CBC is usually obtained. It typically shows an elevated WBC count with a left shift. Hematocrit may also be elevated because of dehydration. Urinalysis is often obtained as part of the workup to rule out pyelonephritis or kidney stones as a cause for the patient's symptoms. White blood cells may be seen in the urine if the appendix is retrocecal and irritates the adjacent ureter.

In cases in which the diagnosis is unclear, management options include hospital admission or radiologic evaluation. Patients admitted for observation should remain NPO and undergo serial examinations every 1 to 2 hours. Radiologic evaluation may entail ultrasonography or a CT scan.

Ultrasonographic examination, typically used in children, may demonstrate a thickened (>10 mm) appendiceal wall and a distended, noncompressible appendiceal lumen. However, ultrasonography is operator dependent, and appendiceal visualization may be limited by obesity or bowel distention. CT findings suggestive of appendicitis include inflammatory changes in the right lower quadrant, a distended appendix with a thickened wall, and free air localized to the right lower quadrant.

Once the diagnosis of appendicitis is made, patients should receive a second-generation cephalosporin with anaerobic coverage (cefoxitin or cefotetan). Pain medication is given as needed, and other standard preoperative preparations for abdominal surgery are made.

### PREOPERATIVE ORDERS
**Admit to:**
**Diagnosis:** acute appendcitis
**Condition:** stable
**Vital signs:** per routine

**Activity:** bed rest

**Allergies:**

**Nursing:** I&Os, Foley to gravity and NGT to LCWS if necessary, Pneumoboots and PAS, IS q1h while awake

**Diet:** NPO

**IV fluids:** $D_5$/0.45% NS with 20 mEq KCl at 125 ml/h

**Medications:** cefotetan 1 g IV q8h; no pain medications if undergoing serial examinations

**Laboratory tests:** CBC, LFTs, PT, PTT, BMP, UA, ECG, CXR

## IV. SURGICAL ANATOMY

The appendix is a blind pouch of intestine located on the posteromedial border of the cecum. Length averages 9 cm, with a range of 2 to 20 cm. The base of the appendix is found at the confluence of the three taeniae coli of the ascending colon. The mesentery of the appendix is called the mesoappendix and contains the appendiceal artery, a branch of the ileocolic artery. At the distal portion of the appendix, the artery lies on the appendix itself. Lymphatic drainage is through the ileocolic nodes.

## V. CONDUCT OF OPERATION

The patient is placed in the supine position, and general anesthesia with endotracheal intubation is induced. The abdomen is prepped and draped sterilely. A 4- to 5-cm incision is made at the level of McBurney's point, with the medial corner at the lateral edge of the right rectus abdominus muscle. Cautery is used to incise Scarpa's fascia to expose the fascia of the external oblique muscle. This is incised sharply along the course of its fibers (superolateral to inferomedial). A muscle-splitting technique is then used with two Kelly clamps. Each clamp is sequentially placed and spread at right angles to the other until the fascia of the internal oblique is identified. This too is incised, and the internal oblique and transversus abdominis are split in a similar manner. The transversalis fascia and peritoneum are then grasped between tonsil clamps and incised sharply, avoiding injury to any underlying structures. Once the peritoneal cavity is entered, the incision is dilated with appendiceal retractors.

A finger placed in the incision sweeps the appendix and delivers it into the wound. If the appendix is not seen, the cecum is grasped gently with a Babcock clamp and delivered through the incision. The taenia coli are then followed proximally to identify the base of the appendix. Once the appendix is delivered, the mesoappendix is sequentially divided between hemostats and ligated with 3-0 silk ties. Once the base of the appendix has been adequately exposed, it is clamped and doubly ligated at its base with a 0 chromic tie. Two ties are used with knots placed on opposite sides of the appendiceal base. The appendix is amputated and passed off the table as a specimen. The mucosa of the appendiceal stump is cauterized to prevent mucocele formation. The abdomen is irrigated with warm normal saline, with special attention to the right lower quadrant, the right colic gutter, and the pelvis.

The peritoneum, transversalis, internal oblique, and external oblique are each closed with a running 2-0 Vicryl suture. The wound is irrigated again. In cases of perforated appendicitis, the wound is left open to prevent wound infection. In nonperforated appendicitis, Scarpa's fascia is closed with interrupted 3-0 Vicryl sutures, and the skin is reapproximated with a running subcuticular 4-0 Vicryl suture. Benzoin, Steri-Strips, and sterile dressings are applied.

## VARIATIONS OF OPERATION

**Laparoscopic Appendectomy.** Laparoscopic appendectomies are commonly performed in females or when the diagnosis is uncertain. The laparoscopic approach enhances visualization of other intraabdominal organs to identify other possible sources of pathology. Preparation and positioning of the patient is similar to an open appendectomy. The patient should void before induction of anesthesia or a Foley catheter is placed. A Hasson technique is used at the umbilicus, and a 5-mm trocar is placed in the superior midline. One additional 12-mm port is required. Locating this port in the left lower quadrant laterally along the bikini line allows good cosmesis without sacrificing exposure in most cases. If the appendix is located in a particularly cephalad position, a right upper quadrant or upper midline position enhances exposure for retraction and dissection. The mesoappendix with the appendiceal artery is dissected from the base of the appendix. An endovascular stapler is used to divide the mesoappendix. A GIA stapler is then used to divide the appendix. Alternatively, sutures or endoloops can be used.

**Pediatric Patients.** In this population the operation is essentially the same, only the size of the incision should be smaller, appropriate to the child's size. Pediatric surgeons are more likely to close these wounds primarily or place drains at the surgical site.

## POSTOPERATIVE ORDERS

In cases of nonperforated appendicitis, no further antibiotics are necessary. The patient may have sips of clear liquids until bowel function is confirmed at which point the diet is advanced as tolerated. If the patient tolerates oral intake, oral pain medication is used. Early mobilization and ambulation are essential. An incentive spirometer is helpful in preventing atelectasis.

Perforation of the appendix is associated with increased morbidity. Patients should remain on postoperative intravenous antibiotics. For most patients continuing the cephalosporin is adequate. With severe spillage of enteric contents, triple antibiotic coverage (ampicillin, gentamicin, and metronidazole) is used. These patients remain NPO following their operation, and their diet is advanced with resolution of their ileus and return of bowel function.

**Admit to:**
**Diagnosis:** s/p appendectomy
**Condition:** stable
**Vital signs:** per routine
**Activity:** ad lib
**Allergies:**
**Nursing:** ambulate q shift, Pneumoboots, PAS until fully ambulating, IS, I&Os
**Diet:** sips of clear liquids when tolerating oral intake or NPO
**IV fluids:** $D_5$/0.45% NS with 20 mEq KCl at 125 ml/h Heplock
**Medications:** PCA; antibiotics if appropriate
**Laboratory tests:** CBC, BMP in AM

## VI. POTENTIAL COMPLICATIONS

Although wound infections occur in only 5% to 10% of cases of nonperforated appendicitis, this rate can reach 50% in those whose appendices have perforated. The most common serious complication after appendectomy is an intraabdominal abscess, which occurs in 3% to 10% of patients. It is especially prevalent in cases of perforated appendicitis. An abscess should be suspected when patients show persistent leukocytosis, fever, or ileus. A CT scan is the most sensitive test, although it may not be helpful less than 7 days postoperatively. Appendiceal stump blowout is uncommon but could lead to abscess formation. Enteroenteric and enterocutaneous fistulas are also possible but occur in less than 1% of patients.

## VII. DISCHARGE ORDERS

Patients are discharged to home once they can tolerate a regular diet and ambulate without assistance. By the time of discharge, they should be afebrile and their white blood cell count should return to normal. In these cases, patients are given no dietary restrictions at the time of discharge. Activity should not be strenuous, and patients should not lift heavy objects until seen in follow-up. Patients are instructed not to drive while taking narcotic medication. Oral pain medication, preferably an NSAID is prescribed. Although narcotics may be given for severe pain, patients are advised of the medication's adverse effect on bowel function and encouraged to limit their use of these drugs. Patients are seen in follow-up 1 to 2 weeks after their operation.

12

APPENDECTOMY

# DIVERTICULAR DISEASE

*Hani Baradi*

Diverticular disease is prevalent in Western countries, affecting 10% by age 40 and 65% by age 80 years. Diverticula are more common in the colon than any portion of the gastrointestinal (GI) tract. Sigmoid colon involvement accounts for 95% of diverticular disease. The descending, transverse, and ascending colon are involved in decreasing order of frequency.

## I. PATHOPHYSIOLOGY

13

Diverticula are related to a fiber-deficient diet causing high colonic intraluminal pressure that leads to mucosal herniation through weak points in the colon wall. Classically, diverticula are located at the site blood vessels penetrate into the colon wall. This is the inherent weak point, allowing herniation of mucosa and submucosa through the circular muscle. The propensity to involve the sigmoid is explained by Laplace's law, which states that pressure within a tube is inversely proportionate to radius.

Diverticula are classified as true if all layers of the colonic wall are involved, including the muscle layers, or false if only the mucosa and submucosa herniate through the muscular layer. Typically, colonic diverticula are acquired and false. However, congenital colonic diverticula, which are single, true, and usually on the right side, also exist.

## II. TYPICAL PRESENTATION

1. Diverticulosis is the presence of multiple false diverticula. It is asymptomatic in 80% of patients and detected incidentally on barium enema or colonoscopy. However, diverticulosis can result in severe lower GI hemorrhage, necessitating surgical intervention.
2. Diverticulitis occurs when one or more diverticula become inflamed, resulting in surrounding pericolitis. Patients present with left lower quadrant abdominal pain, fever, nausea, and vomiting. Physical findings include abdominal distention, left lower quadrant tenderness, and occasionally a palpable mass. Occult blood is present in stool. Leukocytosis is mild to moderate. Urinary symptoms may herald a colovesical fistula with pneumaturia and feces in urine. Free perforation can lead to peritonitis. Patients with a single episode of diverticulitis can be managed conservatively. However, after the second episode, surgical resection is indicated because of the likelihood of a subsequent complication.

## III. PREOPERATIVE WORKUP

Plain abdominal films show ileus and free air if perforation has occurred. Diagnosis of acute diverticulitis is confirmed by CT scan, which will demonstrate the diverticula and pericolic abscess. Barium enema and colonoscopy are kept in abeyance until recovery from an acute attack for fear of perforation. Cystoscopy may reveal edema of the bladder wall in colovesical fistula.The patient with diverticulitis may need hospitalization, NPO, NGT, IV fluids, and systemic antibiotics against anaerobes and gram-negative organisms.

## PREOPERATIVE ORDERS

The usual preoperative assessment is done, including cardiac, pulmonary, hepatic, and renal status.

**Diet:** Clear liquids 48 hours before surgery and NPO after midnight

**Nursing:** Mechanical bowel preparation with polyethylene glycol is done the day before surgery; incentive spirometry teaching; consent for a possible colostomy should be obtained and the stoma site marked preoperatively

**Medications:** neomycin and erythromycin, 1 g each, at 1, 2, and 11 PM the day before surgery (IV metronidazole plus a second-generation cephalosporin or aminoglycoside are given at induction of anesthesia and repeated at appropriate intervals during surgery to maintain adequate tissue level)

## IV. SURGICAL ANATOMY

Below the iliac crest the colon acquires a mesentery and becomes the sigmoid colon. The sigmoid colon continues inferiorly down to S3, where it loses the mesentery and becomes the rectum. The sigmoid is separated from the bladder in males and the uterus in females by the small bowel.

Blood supply is by two to four sigmoidal arteries from the left colic artery, a branch of the inferior mesenteric artery. Venous drainage is through the inferior mesenteric vein to the portal vein. Lymphatic drainage is to the inferior mesenteric nodes.

## V. CONDUCT OF OPERATION

A Foley catheter and an NGT are placed after induction of anesthesia, and the patient is placed in Lloyd-Davies stirrups to allow use of the end-to-end anastomosis (EEA) stapler through the anus. The abdomen is prepped and draped in a sterile fashion. A midline incision is used to enter the abdomen, and a Thompson retractor is applied. The left colon is mobilized by dividing the white fascial line of Toldt. The omentum is divided from medial to lateral, and the splenocolic ligament is cut between clamps. The left ureter is identified. The proximal level of resection is chosen on the basis of the involvement, and a gastrointestinal anastomosis (GIA) stapler is used to transect the colon. The distal end of the resection is the rectosigmoid junction.

The mesentery is divided, and vessels are ligated at the origin of the inferior mesenteric artery. The specimen is removed, and a colorectal anastomosis is constructed using an EEA stapler through the anus or a hand-sewn technique. The peritoneal cavity is washed with saline, and the abdomen is closed with nonabsorbable fascial sutures.

## VARIATIONS OF OPERATION

1. **Interval one-stage resection:** done after resolution of an acute attack. The bowel is prepped preoperatively, and the involved segment is removed down to the rectosigmoid junction with primary anastomosis.
2. **Hartmann's procedure:** if there is obstruction, inflammatory adhesions, gross infection, or the bowel is loaded with stool, the involved area is resected, the rectum is closed at the peritoneal reflection, and the left colon is brought out as a left iliac fossa colostomy. This can be reversed at a later date. In selected obstruction cases the bowel can be cleaned by on-table lavage, placing a catheter at the appendix stump and washing the colon with saline to allow primary anastomosis. Colovesical fistulas are cured with the resection of diseased bowel and fistula closure.
3. **Three-stage procedure:** now rarely performed. It involves a transverse colostomy and drainage of the paracolic abscess followed by left colon resection with colostomy diversion, and finally, a colostomy takedown.

## POSTOPERATIVE ORDERS

**Admit to:**
**Diagnosis:** s/p bowel resection
**Condition:** stable
**Vital signs:** per routine
**Activity:** ad lib, encourage ambulation
**Allergies:**
**Nursing:** NGT to LCWS, Foley to gravity, Pneumoboots until fully ambulating, IS q1h while awake; stoma nurse consult if appropriate
**Diet:** NPO until passing flatus, then clear liquids
**IV fluids:** $D_5$/0.45% NS with 20 mEq KCl at 125 ml/h
**Medications:** antibiotics for at least 24 hours or longer if there are signs of infection; adequate pain medication
**Laboratory tests:**

## VI. POSSIBLE COMPLICATIONS

1. Wound complications: infection, hematoma, or dehiscence
2. Anastomotic leak with intraabdominal abscess or colocutaneous fistula
3. Prolonged ileus or early bowel obstruction

## VII. DISCHARGE ORDERS

Patients are instructed to avoid heavy lifting for 8 weeks. Driving is allowed after they stop narcotic analgesia. They may shower but should avoid soaking the wound in a bath for a week. Wound sutures or staples are removed in 7 to 10 days. A follow-up appointment is given in 2 weeks.

# COLON CANCER

*Hani Baradi*

Colon cancer ranks second after cancer of the lung in incidence and death rates. The incidence increases with age from 0.39/1000 persons per year at age 50 to 4.5/1000 persons per year at age 80. Adenocarcinoma accounts for 95% of colon tumors. Multiple synchronous tumors are found in 5% of patients, and the cumulative risk of metachronous tumors is 30% after 5 years. The distribution of colon cancer involvement is rectum 30%, right colon 25%, sigmoid 20%, left colon 15%, and transverse colon 10%.

**14**

## I. PATHOPHYSIOLOGY

Carcinogenesis of the colon is a multistep process. Heredity factors—oncogenes—make cells susceptible to cancer. Mutations or loss of tumor suppressor genes activates these oncogenes. In addition, promoters such as bile acids stimulate the growth of benign neoplasms.

### GENETIC PREDISPOSITION TO COLON CANCER

1. Familial adenomatous polyposis: loss of a segment on the long arm of chromosome 5 and deletion of genes from chromosomes 17 and 18
2. Autosomal dominant hereditary nonpolyposis colorectal cancer (HNPCC)
   a. Cancer family syndrome (CFS; Lynch 2): early onset at age 20 to 30, right colon dominance, and associated extracolonic adenocarcinomas such as endometrial cancer
   b. Hereditary site-specific colon cancer (HSSCC; Lynch 1): with same features except lacks extracolonic cancers

Some conditions that can predispose patients to colon cancer are ulcerative colitis, Crohn's colitis, radiation, polyps, and ureterocolostomy. Likewise, a high-fat, low-fiber diet is associated with increased risk of colon cancer. The proposed mechanism for this association is secondary to dietary fat enhancing cholesterol and bile acid synthesis by the liver. Anaerobic colonic bacteria convert these bile acids into secondary bile acids, which are known promoters of carcinogenesis. Fiber is converted by colonic bacteria into ligans that protect against colon cancer.

Colon cancer may spread in the following ways:

1. **Direct extension:** carcinomas grow circumferentially and may cause complete obstruction before diagnosis. This occurs predominately in the smaller caliber left colon. It takes approximately 1 year to encircle three fourths of the colon circumference. Longitudinal submucosal spread is by way of the lymphatics and rarely extends

beyond 2 cm. The lesion may involve neighboring structures or cause colon perforation.

2. **Hematogenous metastasis:** by way of the portal vein to the liver or tumor embolization through lumbar and vertebral veins to the lungs.
3. **Lymph node metastasis:** most common form of tumor spread.
4. **Transperitoneal seeding:** causing peritoneal carcinomatosis or Blumer's shelf in the pelvic cul-de-sac.

## II. TYPICAL PRESENTATION

Obstruction or peritonitis accounts for 25% of colon cancer presentations.

**Right colon cancer:** tumors can attain a large size before detection secondary to the large caliber and thin wall of the right colon. Also, the fluid fecal content makes obstruction unlikely. Typical presentations include anemia, right iliac fossa mass, leading point for an intussusception, or incidental discovery during an operation for other indications.

**Left colon cancer** usually presents with alteration in bowel habits, pain, blood within the stool, or a palpable mass.

**Sigmoid cancer** causes pain, tenesmus, and bladder symptoms.

**Transverse colon cancer** can be mistaken for gastric carcinoma. It presents with anemia and weakness.

**Metastatic disease:** liver metastasis presents with hepatomegaly, ascites, and carcinomatosis peritonei. The supraclavicular area should be examined for metastatic nodes.

## III. PREOPERATIVE WORKUP

**Laboratory Findings.** Carcinoembryonic antigen (CEA) is not a screening tool but correlates with postoperative recurrence. Failure of CEA to return to normal is a poor prognostic sign.

**Imaging Studies.** CXR and CT scan of the abdomen and pelvis are done to assess metastasis to the liver and lymph nodes. Barium enema may reveal an apple core appearance of the colon.

**Colonoscopy.** A colonoscopy is done to biopsy the lesion and look for synchronous tumors.

### PREOPERATIVE ORDERS
**Admit to:**
**Diagnosis:** preoperative colon resection
**Condition:** stable
**Vital signs:** per routine

**Activity:** ad lib

**Allergies:**

**Nursing:** I&Os, IS teaching; PAS to protect from DVT; bowel preparation using polyethylene glycol is essential, except in patients with a complete colon obstruction, in which case it is done as an on-table lavage; possibility of a stoma is discussed and its site marked by the ET specialist

**Diet:** restriction to fluids 48 hours before the operation and fasting after midnight the day before surgery

**Medications:** systemic antibiotics—metronidazole plus a second-generation cephalosporin or gentamicin—are given at the start of surgery to cover anaerobes and gram-negative bacteria

**Laboratory tests:** UA, CBC, LFTs, CEA, CXR, CT, barium enema

**14**

**COLON CANCER**

## IV. SURGICAL ANATOMY

The colon is 4 to 6.5 feet long. The ascending and descending colon segments are fixed to the retroperitoneum, whereas the transverse and sigmoid colon are suspended by a mesentery. The greatest lumen diameter is at the cecum decreasing progressively to the sigmoid. The superior mesenteric artery supplies the right colon by the ileocolic and right colic branches and the transverse colon up to its midpoint by the middle colic artery. The inferior mesenteric artery supplies the left colon by the left colic and sigmoid arteries. Colic arteries bifurcate and form arcades, so that the marginal artery forms an anastomosis between the superior and inferior mesenteric arteries. A complete anastomosis is only present in 15% to 20% of cases. Lymphatic drainage follows major arteries. The superior mesenteric vein drains the right colon, and the inferior mesenteric vein drains the left colon. Both empty into the portal vein.

## V. CONDUCT OF OPERATION

After induction of anesthesia and insertion of the endotracheal tube, nasogastric and Foley catheters are placed, and the abdomen is prepped and draped in a sterile fashion. A midline abdominal incision is used to enter the peritoneum. The peritoneum, liver, and lymph nodes are palpated for metastases. The operation is designed to remove the tumor with adequate margin and its draining lymph nodes by dividing the major blood vessels supplying the involved segment (no-touch technique—Turnbull).

Tumors of the cecum and the ascending colon are resected by a right hemicolectomy. This entails ligation of the ileocolic, right colic, and the right branches from the middle colic artery. For hepatic flexure cancer, an extended right hemicolectomy is performed by ligating the middle colic artery at its origin. Care must be taken during mobilization of the right colon to avoid injury to the right ureter, gonadal vessels, inferior vena cava, superior mesenteric vein, and duodenum. For transverse colon cancer, a transverse colectomy is performed by dividing the middle colic artery at its origin. Splenic flexure tumors are treated with segmental resection by dividing the left colic artery and preserving the middle colic artery. Splenic injury should be avoided during mobilization of the splenic flexure. Descending colon cancers require a left hemicolectomy, which includes the midtransverse colon to distal sigmoid colon. For sigmoid cancer, a segmental resection can be done ligating the sigmoidal artery near its origin. The choice of anastomotic technique (hand-sewn versus stapled) depends on the surgeon's preference.

## VARIATIONS OF OPERATION

Emergency operation for obstruction or perforation due to unprepped colon and size discrepancy between colonic segments may require a temporary stoma. Another alternative is on-table lavage.

## POSTOPERATIVE ORDERS

**Admit to:**
**Diagnosis:** s/p colectomy
**Condition:** stable
**Vital signs:** per routine
**Activity:** ad lib
**Allergies:**
**Nursing:** strict I&Os, NGT to LCWS, IS q1h while awake, ambulate q shift, Pneumoboots until fully ambulatory; patients with a stoma should receive ET
**Diet:** NPO until passing flatus
**IV fluids:** $D_5$/0.45% NS with 20 mEq KCl at 125 ml/h
**Medications:** antibiotics for 24 hours after surgery, PCA
**Laboratory tests:**

## VI. POSSIBLE COMPLICATIONS

Postoperative bowel obstruction that does not resolve within 14 days may require reexploration. A contrast study can differentiate mechanical obstruction from ileus.

The incidence of anastomotic leak is 3% to 5% and presents with fever, increasing abdominal pain, distention, and leukocytosis. Typically, this occurs on the fifth to seventh postoperative day. CT scan or Gastrografin enema is used to confirm the diagnosis. Small leaks can be treated with NPO, hyperalimenation, and IV antibiotics, whereas large disruptions need reoperation and a colostomy. Other complications include urinary tract infection, wound sepsis, deep venous thrombosis, and pulmonary complications.

## VII. DISCHARGE INSTRUCTIONS

The patient will need yearly colonoscopy during the first 2 years, because 80% of recurrences occur during this time. If colonoscopy is negative in the second year, it should be repeated every other year. History and physical examination, CEA, fecal occult blood, LFTs, CT of the abdomen, and CXR are done yearly.

# INFLAMMATORY BOWEL DISEASE

*Hani Baradi*

## CROHN'S DISEASE

Crohn's disease is a chronic, transmural inflammation that can involve the entire gastrointestinal (GI) tract. The cause is unknown; however, infectious or immunogenetic causes are suspected. The most common sites of involvement are the terminal ileum and proximal colon. The disease is characterized by a waxing and waning course. There is no predilection for either gender, and age of onset is biphasic with an early (15-30 years) and late (55-60 years) peak incidence. Crohn's disease is prevalent in Western countries, especially among Ashkenazi Jews. Familial aggregation occurs in 10% to 30% of cases. Cigarette smoking has been associated with increased disease risk.

**15**

### I. PATHOPHYSIOLOGY

Macroscopically, the involved bowel segments are rigid and thick walled because of the fibrosis and edema narrowing the bowel lumen. The mesenteric fat "creeps" along the bowel wall, eventually reaching the antimesenteric edge. The serosa appears granular. The mesentery is short, thick, and edematous with adjacent enlarged lymph nodes. Inflammation can extend to adjacent structures, resulting in fistulas, sinuses, and abscesses. The mucosa of the bowel contains cobblestoning, aphthoid, and longitudinal ulcers with narrowing of the lumen and proximal dilatation of the uninvolved bowel.

Microscopically, there are noncaseating granulomas away from ulcerations, in lymph nodes and other organs with lymphoid aggregation, in the submucosa and subserosa. Fissures and ulcers extend into muscularis propria with transmural inflammation.

### II. TYPICAL PRESENTATION

Symptoms include intermittent abdominal pain, diarrhea, hematochezia, anorexia, nausea, vomiting, and malnutrition. Extraintestinal manifestations may be present in the skin (pyoderma gangrenosum and erythema nodosum), eyes (conjunctivitis, iritis, and uveitis), joints (arthritis and ankylosing spondylitis), and liver (sclerosing cholangitis and hepatitis). Perianal disease is found in 50% of ileocolitis cases and may be the initial presentation in one third of the cases. Fistulas, fissures, and abscesses are typical manifestations of perianal disease.

**Complications**

1. Small bowel obstruction from adjacent fibrosis
2. Fistulas: enteroenteric, enterocutaneous, enterovesical, or enterovaginal
3. Intraabdominal abscesses
4. Toxic megacolon
5. Perforation and peritonitis
6. Gastrointestinal bleeding
7. Increased risk of bowel carcinoma

Surgery is not curative for Crohn's disease and is focused on complications including intestinal obstruction, bleeding, perforation, failure of medical therapy, intestinal fistulas, fulminant colitis, malignant changes, and perianal disease.

## III. PREOPERATIVE WORKUP

**Laboratory tests** show anemia, leukocytosis, hypoproteinemia, and elevated ESR and acute-phase proteins.

**Colonoscopy and EGD** reveal the disease extent and provide biopsies.

**Radiologic examination** includes barium studies, fistulograms, CT scan for masses and abscesses, and ERCP for hepatobiliary involvement.

**Attention to nutritional status** is important because patients may be malnourished and may require perioperative TPN.

### PREOPERATIVE ORDERS

**Nursing:** enemas night before surgery until clear; possibility of stoma is discussed with the patient

NOTE: In cases of obstruction do not attempt bowel cleansing.

**Diet:** clear liquids 48 hours before surgery; NPO after midnight day before surgery

**Medications:** parenteral prophylactic antibiotics are given perioperatively; stress-dose steroids if patient was treated with prednisone within preceding 6 months

## IV. CONDUCT OF OPERATION

A Foley catheter and a nasogastric tube are placed after induction of anesthesia, and the abdomen is prepped and draped in a sterile technique. Abdominal exploration must be complete and requires division of all adhesions with examination of the entire bowel. Visible changes of the disease are identified with narrowing of the lumen, thickened wall, serositis, and mesenteric fat creeping. Proposed sites of resection are determined on the basis of gross disease and should be chosen conservatively. Microscopic disease at resection margins does not compromise anastomosis healing. Length of uninvolved bowel should be measured.

**Ileocecal resection** is the procedure of choice for ileocecal disease with primary ileotransverse anastomosis.

**Segmental resection:** short segments of small or large bowel involvement can be treated with resection and primary anastomosis.

**Colectomy with ileorectal anastomosis** should be performed only in cases of diffuse colitis with rectal sparing.

**Temporary loop ileostomy** can be used as diversion in severe perianal disease.

**Proctocolectomy and ileostomy** is used for colonic and anal disease failing to respond to medical treatment.

**Ileostomy with blowhole colostomy (Turnbull procedure)** for temporary decompression and drainage of toxic megacolon, achieved with loop ileostomy and blowhole transverse colostomy.

**Strictureplasty** used to avoid excessive bowel resection. Strictured areas are incised along its length and closed transversely.

**Perianal disease** treated by drainage of abscesses and seton placement around fistulas.

## POSTOPERATIVE ORDERS

**Admit to:**
**Diagnosis:** s/p bowel resection
**Condition:** stable
**Vital signs:** per routine
**Activity:** ad lib
**Allergies:**
**Nursing:** strict I&Os, NGT to LCWS until flatus is passed, Pneumoboots until fully ambulatory, Foley to gravity, IS q1h; stoma nurse consult if appropriate
**Diet:** NPO
**IV fluids:** $D_5$/0.45% NS at 125 ml/h
**Medications:** steroid taper; slow antibiotics for 24 hours postoperatively; PCA
**Laboratory tests:**

## V. POSSIBLE COMPLICATIONS

Anastomotic leaks with intraabdominal abscesses and enterocutaneous fistulas may require percutaneous drainage and long-term total parenteral nutrition.

**15**

**INFLAMMATORY BOWEL DISEASE**

## VI. DISCHARGE INSTRUCTIONS

Patients require life-long surveillance because the disease is incurable. Clinical recurrence affects 20% at 2 years and 40% to 50% at 4 years after surgery; 30% undergo reoperation in 5 years.

# ULCERATIVE COLITIS

Ulcerative colitis is a diffuse inflammation of the colonic and rectal mucosa. It is characterized by remission and exacerbation of rectal bleeding and diarrhea. The incidence is highest in developed countries with a predilection for Jews. Both sexes are affected equally. Most cases are diagnosed between age 15 and 40. Familial patterns are present in 10% to 25% of cases. The cause is unknown; however, infectious, immunologic, dietary, environmental, vascular, allergic, and psychogenic factors are currently under investigation.

## I. PATHOPHYSIOLOGY

The disease is confined to the mucosa and submucosa. Involvement is continuous, with the rectum always affected. The remainder of the colon is involved in a varying extent. Occasionally, with pancolitis, the ileum is inflamed as a result of backwash ileitis in 10% of cases. The mucosa is infiltrated, with polymorphonuclear leukocytes forming crypt abscesses that coalesce and form ulcers. Undermining of adjacent mucosa by ulcers gives a pseudopolypoid appearance. In severe forms, inflammation extends to muscularis and serosa causing toxic megacolon. With time, dysplasia or carcinoma in situ develops.

## II. TYPICAL PRESENTATION

1. **Mild:** 60% of cases, involving the distal colon (80%) or pancolitis (20%) with less than four bloody loose bowel movements a day.
2. **Moderate:** 25%, with more than four bowel movements a day but no systemic signs.
3. **Fulminant:** 15%, sudden onset of bloody diarrhea more than four times daily with one or more signs of systemic illness: fever more than 37.5°C, tachycardia more than 90 bpm, hypoalbuminemia less than 3 g/L, and weight loss more than 3 kg.

Extraintestinal manifestations involve the eye (iritis, uveitis, conjunctivitis, episcleritis, keratitis, retinitis, and retrobulbar neuritis), joints (arthritis and ankylosing spondylitis), skin and mucus membranes (stomatitis, gingivitis, erythema nodosum and pyoderma gangrenosum), and liver (pericholangitis, fatty infiltration, hepatitis, cirrhosis and sclerosing cholangitis).

Complications: toxic colitis, perforation, severe bleeding, strictures, and colon cancer.

Surgery is indicated in 20% of cases for the following:

1. Fulminating disease
2. Acute perforation: 50% mortality
3. Chronic disease with anemia, diarrhea, tenesmus, and urgency
4. Steroid-dependent disease
5. Severe dysplasia on colonoscopy
6. Severe hemorrhage or stenosis
7. Extraintestinal manifestations

## III. PREOPERATIVE WORKUP

**Laboratory Findings.** Findings will include anemia, leukocytosis, elevated ESR, hypoalbuminemia, and electrolyte depletion.

**Imaging Studies.** Plain films of the abdomen detect megacolon with a diameter of more than 6 cm or free air in the case of a perforation. Barium enema may show ulceration, pseudopolyps, and loss of haustrations (lead-pipe appearance).

**Colonoscopy.** A colonoscopy is done to evaluate the disease extent and obtain biopsy specimens to rule out cancer. It should be avoided in toxic disease because of perforation risk.

### PREOPERATIVE ORDERS

**Diet:** nutritionally depleted patients should receive a 10- to 14-day course of TPN

**Medications:** stress-dose steroids for those patients receiving long-term steroid therapy; perioperative antibiotics

**Nursing:** complete bowel preparation with 1 gallon of polyethylene glycol 1 day before surgery, except in cases of obstruction; possibility of stoma discussed and site marked by stomal nurse

## IV. CONDUCT OF OPERATION

### TOTAL ABDOMINAL COLECTOMY AND ILEOSTOMY

This procedure is used in emergency situations or if the diagnosis of ulcerative colitis versus Crohn's disease cannot be established. The rectum is either brought out at the lower end of the wound as a mucous fistula or closed beneath the skin to avoid rectal breakdown and intraabdominal abscess. Advantages include quick recovery, histologic evaluation of the colon, and subsequent restorative surgery after stopping steroids, and optimization of nutritional status. It is contraindicated in anal sphincter dysfunction, severe rectal disease, dysplasia, or cancer.

## PROCTOCOLECTOMY AND PERMANENT ILEOSTOMY

This procedure is associated with the fewest complications. However, there is a 20% long-term risk of adhesions and 5% to 10% risk of delayed perineal wound healing. It is curative, with no anastomosis to heal, requires a single operation, and eliminates the fear of incontinence. The disadvantage is a permanent ileostomy.

## PROCTOCOLECTOMY WITH ILEAL-POUCH ANAL ANASTOMOSIS (IPAA)

An ileal pouch is created using a gastrointestinal anastomosis stapler in J, S, or W shape and anastomosed to the anus with an end-to-end anastomosis stapler. Mucosectomy of the upper anal canal with anastomosis at the dentate line removes all at-risk mucosa and subsequent risk of cancer, but it may result in imperfect continence with nocturnal seepage. The alternative is a double-stapled anastomosis to the upper anal canal with better continence, but it carries a theoretical cancer risk and need for annual anoscopy and biopsies. A temporary diverting loop ileostomy is used to reduce the incidence of pelvic sepsis and ileal pouch and ileoanal anastomotic dehiscence. The ileostomy is taken down in 3 months after a Gastrografin study that demonstrates a healed anastomosis and good anal manometry.

## ILEOSTOMY WITH A CONTINENT INTRAABDOMINAL KOCK POUCH

This is a reservoir of ileum with a spout made by inverting the efferent ileum on itself to give a continent valve below the skin. Passing a catheter through the valve empties the pouch. This procedure is rarely used because of a high complication rate.

## POSTOPERATIVE ORDERS

**Admit to:**
**Diagnosis:** s/p bowel resection
**Condition:** stable
**Vital signs:** per routine
**Activity:** ad lib
**Allergies:**
**Nursing:** I&Os, NGT to LCWS, stoma nurse consult
**Diet:** NPO until passing flatus
**IV fluids:** $D_5$/0.45% NS with 20 mEq KCl at 125 ml/h
**Medications:** antibiotics for 24 hours; slow steroid taper
**Laboratory tests:**

## V. POSSIBLE COMPLICATIONS

Possible complications are anastomotic leak, intraabdominal infection, pouchitis, ileostomy complications (retraction, prolapse, parastomal hernia, and skin irritation), and sexual dysfunction after proctectomy.

# PART V

## Anorectal

# FISTULA IN ANO

*Floriano Marchetti*

By definition, a fistula is an abnormal communication between two epithelial-lined surfaces. In a fistula in ano the communication is between the anal canal and the perianal skin. Fistula in ano occurs in 30% to 60% of patients with an anorectal abscess. Although abscess is the acute manifestation of anorectal sepsis, fistula is considered the chronic sequelae of the same process.

## I. PATHOPHYSIOLOGY

**16**

Anal fistulas do not heal spontaneously, and if left untreated, they will lead to recurrent abscess formation and possibly sepsis. Fistulas are reportedly found in up to 76% of patients with a recurrent abscess. Men are involved more frequently than women (2:1 to 7:1), with the highest incidence between the third and fifth decade. Fistulas can be simple, with a single short tract, or complex, with long tract and multiple openings.

Fistulas can also be secondary to multiple systemic conditions. Some of the causes include Crohn's disease, chronic ulcerative colitis, tuberculosis, foreign body, neoplasms, lymphogranuloma venereum, trauma, and radiation.

Despite the several classification systems proposed over the years, the most accepted one is the Parks classification. This centers on the fistula's relationship to the anal sphincters and is divided into intersphincteric 70%; transsphincteric 23%; suprasphincteric 5%; and extrasphincteric 2%.

### INTERSPHINCTERIC FISTULA

Intersphincteric fistula is the most common type, and it is the intermediate form that might progress into the other types. It develops in the intersphincteric plane and in its simplest form progresses downward until it opens in the perianal skin (*simple low tract*). The fistula might also progress upward, remaining in the intersphincteric plane and more proximally between the longitudinal muscle of the distal rectum and the internal anal sphincter (IAS) (*high blind tract*). The fistula can further extend and erode into the rectum (*high tract with rectal opening*). In some cases the fistula develops predominantly upward without opening in the perineum (*high tract without perineal opening*). The infection in this latter form of fistula might also spread in the supralevator plane (*extrarectal extension*) and may be seen as a supralevator abscess.

### TRANSSPHINCTERIC FISTULA

A transsphincteric fistula develops from an abscess in the intersphincteric plane, which subsequently perforates the external anal sphincter (EAS) to reach the ischioanal fossa and then the perineal skin, usually more lateral than a intersphincteric fistula. The EAS can be penetrated at different levels, and the treatments vary according to the level of involvement of the EAS. A transsphincteric fistula can also develop a secondary tract extending upward in the ischioanal fossa and even penetrate the supralevator plane (*high blind tract*). A probe passed into the external perineal opening can reach the apex of this secondary tract, thus missing the primary opening in the anal canal. Another danger in probing this fistula is the associated risk of inadvertently entering the lower rectum, thus turning a relatively minor fistula into a much more complicated iatrogenic extrasphincteric fistula.

## SUPRASPHINCTERIC FISTULA

Suprasphincteric fistulas originate in the intersphincteric plane but instead of progressing toward the perineum, they spread upward over the EAS and the puborectalis muscle; then they track downward through the puborectalis to cross the ischioanal fossa and open in the perineal skin. Rarely, this fistula is seen with a more significant extension in the supralevator space (*high blind track*), which could also spread in a horseshoe fashion.

## EXTRASPHINCTERIC FISTULA

In this type of fistula the secondary tract of a transsphincteric fistula spreads upward through the ischioanal fossa and across the levator ani to perforate to low rectal wall. This fistula may also result from trauma, inflammatory bowel disease, or pelvic inflammation. In most cases the extrasphincteric fistula is the result of reckless probing of a transsphincteric fistula with secondary perforation of the rectum.

## II. TYPICAL PRESENTATION

Patients with fistula in ano present with complaints of purulent discharge (65%) from a perianal opening, pain (34%), swelling (24%), and diarrhea (5%). These patients commonly have a history of an anal abscess that has burst open spontaneously or has required repeated surgical drainage.

A perianal fistula can be noted as a skin opening on the perianal area, usually with some granulation tissue or indurated scar and erythema. However, the external opening can be missed unless palpation of the area yields the expression of some purulent or serosanguinous fluid. Multiple skin openings are seen with complex fistulas. The internal opening can be difficult to locate.

On digital examination the fistulous tract can be identified with palpation of an indurated cord, and the internal opening might be felt as a small indurated area or a pit in the anal canal. By use of a probe through the external orifice, the internal opening can be located. Occasionally, the opening in the crypt is not patent at the time of the probing. The risk of opening a false passage into the anal or rectal mucosa is significant and should be avoided. Probing is best accomplished in the operating room. A "low" opening is found when the angle at which the probe is held is approximately 30 degrees from the skin, whereas the angle is wider, around 80 degrees or more, when a high fistula is encountered. Probing is successful in 80% of cases; when it fails, the injection of methylene blue mixed with diluted peroxide is usually helpful.

## III. PREOPERATIVE WORKUP

**16**

**FISTULA IN ANO**

**Endoscopy.** All patients with a fistula should undergo anoscopy and rigid proctoscopy. The internal opening can be visualized on anoscopy, whereas proctoscopy will allow examination of the rectal mucosa to look for associated conditions such as Crohn's disease or rectal cancer. A rigid proctoscope can also reveal the presence of a higher, rectal internal opening.

**Radiology.** Radiologic evaluation of a patient with an abscess or fistula in ano is of little value in the acute setting. In patients with recurrent fistulas, several radiologic techniques are useful. Fistulography has not proven to be sufficiently accurate in 84% of patients. Other studies have found some value in selected patients for the definitive management. Endoscopic ultrasound (EUS) is useful in the evaluation and treatment of complex fistulas. The injection of hydrogen peroxide seems to enhance the accuracy of EUS. Magnetic resonance imaging's (MRI) role in the assessment of anorectal suppurative disease is growing. Studies show high concordance rates between MRI and surgical findings. Other studies have also shown MRI accuracy is significantly superior to that of EUS in the classification and evaluation of fistula in ano.

**Preoperative Orders**
    **Check coagulation studies:** PT, PTT, CBC
    **Fleets enema** before surgery

## IV. SURGICAL ANATOMY

The **Goodsall's rule:** "When an external opening is posterior to a coronal plane dividing the anus in anterior and posterior halves, the fistula tract can be traced back to an internal opening in the posterior midline. When the opening is anterior to this plane, the fistula proceeds in a radial fashion in the anal canal." The Goodsall's rule has been challenged by findings of many anterior fistulas (70%) originating from the midline within the anterior half of the anal canal.

## V. CONDUCT OF OPERATION

There are several general principles in the surgical treatment of fistulas. The primary internal opening of the fistula must be identified. The fistulous tract must be eradicated along with the crypt responsible for the infection. The relationship between the fistula tract and the EAS and the puborectalis muscle must be assessed. Only once this relationship is known can an accurate classification of the fistula be made and the treatment planned accordingly. The minimal amount of muscle should be divided to unroof the fistula. The EAS can be divided with impunity in its lower half, provided that normal sphincter function is present preoperatively. Identify the presence of side tracts. Good drainage of the secondary tracts is fundamental, especially when a high fistula is present. Finally, assess the presence of secondary disease.

Before embarking in treating a fistula in ano, one should ensure that the sphincter function is adequate. The key to preserving continence is the conservation of the anorectal ring. The division of this part of the sphincter complex will likely render the patient incontinent.

In general with the exception of a superficial fistula, fistulotomy (division of the lower part of the IAS) should be performed in the operating room, with either regional or general anesthesia. The patient is placed in prone position unless the fistula is anterior and involving the genitalia, in which case the lithotomy position is preferable. The perineal area is then prepped and infiltrated with local anesthetic (lidocaine 0.5%, marcaine 0.25%, epinephrine 1:200,000).

A blunt tip probe is inserted into the skin opening to delineate the course of the tract and identify the internal opening. This is a delicate maneuver, during which it is quite easy to open a false passage in the anorectal mucosa. With an anoscope or a Ferguson retractor, the anal canal should be inspected and probed to localize the internal opening. If, despite all this, the internal opening is not found, injecting the external opening with a 50/50 solution of hydrogen peroxide and methylene blue can aid in localization. Next, the level at which the primary tract traverses the EAS is assessed (high or low fistula). With the probe in place, a finger passed into the anal canal and its relationship with the EAS and more important with the puborectalis muscle (PRM) is identified. In more than 90% of patients the fistula tract is well below the level of the PRM: in these cases the fistulotomy can be extended upward to the most cephalad level of the fistula tract without endangering continence. However, a more conservative approach limiting the extent of the muscle division to the lower portions of the IAS and EAS and using a seton to encircle the proximal portion of the EAS and the involved PRM will further preserve continence.

In the treatment of a low fistula the tissue over the probe (which includes the lower portions of IAS and EAS) is divided with the bovie and the granulation tissue is curetted. The skin edges are then excised, and the incision is left open to heal by secondary intention; others recommend the marsupialization of the edges for faster healing. No packing of the wound is necessary.

For the treatment of horseshoe fistula the classical approach consists of laying open all the complex tracts around the anus followed by scrupulous removal of all infected, granulation tissue. With the probe in the primary tract in the posterior midline, again the lower part of both sphincters is divided. The edges may be marsupialized or left open after trimming the skin edges. A more conservative approach includes a posterior midline incision between the anus and the coccyx, with division of the IAS to allow for the removal of the crypt involved. The anococcygeal ligament is then opened along the axis of its fibers to expose the tract in the deep postanal space; a partial fistulectomy of a T-shaped tract is then carried out for 1 to 1.5 cm. The secondary openings of the fistula are then widened and the skin edges excised to allow for adequate thorough curettage and drainage of the secondary tracts. Better functional results in terms of continence are achieved with this more conservative approach.

## VARIATIONS OF OPERATION

**Advancement Rectal Flap.** This operation is generally used in the treatment of very high transsphincteric fistulas or suprasphincteric fistulas or in patients who have previously had traditional treatments fail. Other indications include rectovaginal fistula and Crohn's fistulas.

In brief, it consists of excision of the internal opening, followed by raising a full-thickness rectal flap. The main tract is then curetted, and the defect in the sphincter is repaired with absorbable sutures. After this, the flap is placed over the previous tract area and sutured in place with absorbable sutures. The use of perioperative antibiotics is indicated, and a diverting stoma is recommended by many authors.

**Seton.** The use of a seton is advisable with high transsphincteric fistulas or suprasphincteric fistulas when a large division of EAS or PRM is required to adequately treat the fistula. After the lower portion of the IAS and EAS is divided, the seton is passed by use of a dull-head probe around the upper part of the sphincter with or without the PRM.

There are three definite advantages in using the seton. The seton stimulates fibrosis next to the sphincter, which will help keep the edges of the muscle in close approximation when, later on, the sphincter is divided, thus limiting the gaping and improving continence preservation. It also allows determination of how much muscle is actually involved above the level of the primary tract. Finally, the seton functions as an excellent drain.

Nonabsorbable suture or a rubber band is used with reported similar results. Once the seton is placed, it can be used for drainage, which will allow a delayed single or staged division of the muscle encompassed in the

16

FISTULA IN ANO

seton 6 to 8 weeks later. The seton causes enough fibrosis to hold the sphincter together after its division. Other authors advocate using the seton as a cutting tool by tying the seton very tightly around the sphincter. The seton is progressively tightened, thus gradually dividing the muscle by pressure necrosis. This will also cause fibrosis, which will hold the muscle edges together. A third function of the seton is to keep it in place for longer periods to achieve perfect drainage without dividing the EAS.

## POSTOPERATIVE ORDERS

Patients undergoing fistulotomies rarely require admission. Thus, postoperative orders consist of stool softeners, adequate pain medicine, and lidocaine gel. Patients should be encouraged to take sitz baths at least three times a day.

## VI. COMPLICATIONS

The most common complication after fistulotomy is incontinence. The incidence of incontinence is inversely proportional to that of recurrence. In particular, the division of the sphincter, whether primary or staged, is associated with higher incidence of incontinence (up to 62%) but very low (0%) recurrence rates, whereas the use of the seton without sphincter division is associated with minimal incontinence problems but with recurrence rates of 12% to 34%.

## VII. DISCHARGE ORDERS

Patients should follow-up in 2 to 3 weeks for wound checks. Again, sitz baths and stool softeners should be advised.

# PERIRECTAL ABSCESS

*Floriano Marchetti*

Perirectal abscesses are a result of a loculated infectious process in one of the perirectal spaces. These abscesses can result in systemic illness, including sepsis.

## I. PATHOPHYSIOLOGY

The process leading to the formation of an abscess in the acute form, and of a fistula in ano in the chronic form, originates from an infection of the anal glands. This is the result of an obstruction of the gland's duct, which leads to stasis and subsequent infection. The evidence that the primary internal opening of the fistula is always found at the dentate line supports this theory.

Once the infection is established, the inflammatory process will extend according to the path of least resistance. From the intersphincteric plane, however, the infection may extend caudally, cranially, or find its way through the barrier of the external anal sphincter and penetrate the ischioanal space. A horseshoe fistula/abscess develops when the process circumferentially involves the ischioanal space. This occurs with posterior midline fistulas penetrating the deep postanal space and then extending toward the ischioanal fossa bilaterally.

Anorectal abscesses are more common in men (2:1 to 3:1). The presentation of an anorectal abscess may vary according to the space involved. Thus, anorectal abscesses are classified on the basis of location into five types: perianal, ischioanal, intersphincteric, supralevator, and deep postanal space. In addition, the horseshoe abscess can be considered separately from an ischioanal and deep postanal space abscess.

Perianal abscesses seem, in most series, to be the most frequent type, with a 48% incidence vs. ischiorectal (22%), intersphincteric (12%), and supralevator (9%). Perianal abscesses usually originate in the intersphincteric plane and then extend caudally to form in the subcutaneous tissue in the vicinity of the anal verge. Clinically, they present with erythema, induration, or fluctuation in the perianal area.

Supralevator abscesses are rare (2.5% of abscesses in most series) and the most difficult to diagnose. This often leads to delay in diagnosis from a few days to 2 to 3 weeks. Clinically, they manifest with severe perianal or gluteal pain. The correct treatment of this entity depends largely on the cause; thus before any treatment is begun, the correct origin should be determined. Supralevator sepsis can originate as a cephalad extension of an intrasphincteric abscess, cephalad extension of a ischioanal abscess, or transsphincteric fistula downward extension of a pelvic sepsis (appendicitis, diverticulitis, Crohn's disease, gynecologic disease, or malignancy).

Deep postanal space abscesses are usually secondary to transsphincteric fistulas originating on the posterior midline. The pain, which is mostly posterior, may radiate to the sacrum and coccyx or buttocks; in some cases it may present in a sciatic distribution. Physical examination might fail to reveal signs other than posterior tenderness, and thus the diagnosis can be frequently missed. The patient will return with a more superficial abscess or after spontaneous drainage. This abscess can also communicate with the ischioanal fossa on each side (horseshoe abscess).

## II. TYPICAL PRESENTATION

Acute anal or perineal pain is usually the presenting symptom in patients with anorectal abscess. In the presence of persistent anal pain, the possibility of an undiagnosed intersphincteric abscess should be entertained until proven otherwise. The pain is typically unrelenting, continuous, and throbbing. Sitting, defecation, movements, coughing, and sneezing exacerbate the pain. Swelling in the perianal region is also common on presentation. Patients note bright red blood per anus and commonly report a recent episode of diarrhea. Systemic symptoms such as fever, chills, and malaise usually follow the pain.

In the presence of an acute anorectal abscess, the inspection of the perineum might be inconspicuous, in particular with an intersphincteric abscess. More frequently, signs of inflammation are apparent with swelling and erythema. On palpation, pain and tenderness might hinder an accurate assessment. However, a tender mass is usually appreciated in the perianal region or the ischioanal fossa. Rectal examination may be impossible without anesthesia, especially when the abscess lies in the intersphincteric plane. In these circumstances it can be difficult to differentiate the pain of an abscess from that of a fissure in ano. However, pain due to an anal fissure is not continuous and occurs with defecation. In addition, inguinal adenopathy is usually absent with a fissure, whereas it is often present with an abscess. When the pain is severe and no source can be identified or a satisfactory and thorough examination is precluded because of patient discomfort, the patient should undergo an examination under anesthesia (EUA).

## III. PREOPERATIVE WORKUP

Most of the preoperative workup for rectal abscess consists of localization by physical examination. Occasionally, a perirectal abscess can be difficult to localize, and then radiologic studies can aid in the diagnosis. Particularly, computed tomography scan and magnetic resonance imaging can be useful in determining the location of the abscess cavity, as well as providing the possibility for directed drainage if appropriate.

### PREOPERATIVE ORDERS

  **Diet:** NPO if going to the OR for drainage
  **Medications:** routine antibiotics
  **Coagulation studies:** PT, PTT, CBC

## IV. SURGICAL ANATOMY

### MUSCLES

The internal anal sphincter (IAS), the more superficial of the two muscle layers of the anal canal, is the caudal continuation of the circular layer of the rectum. It is a smooth muscle, capable of providing an involuntary, persistent, tonic contraction.

Surrounding this layer there is a more complex layer of striated muscles including the levator ani, puborectalis, and external anal sphincter (EAS) muscles. The intersphincteric plane is the space between the EAS and IAS sphincters and is partially occupied by the conjoined longitudinal muscle (CLM). This is the caudal extension of the longitudinal muscle layer of the rectum joined by fibers of the levator ani and puborectalis muscles. Fibers from the CLM cross inferior to the EAS and insert in the perianal skin and are referred to as corrugator cutis ani.

### ANAL GLANDS

Anal glands are related to the pathogenesis of anal fistulas. The glands are distributed around the anal canal. In adults, they are mostly lodged in the submucosal layer (80%) but can extend into both the IAS (8%), CLM (8%), and EAS (2%). The glands are lined by stratified columnar epithelium with goblet cells (mucus-secreting) and open directly into the anal crypts at the level of the dentate line.

### ANORECTAL SPACES

There are three anorectal spaces. The ischioanal space contains areolar fat, important nerves, and vessels and is essentially contained below the levator ani muscle. It surrounds the anal canal with its anterior boundaries represented by the superficial and deep transverse perineal muscles. It is medially demarcated by the lateral and inferior surfaces of the EAS and levator ani muscles, respectively. The lateral boarder is the obturator internus muscle and its fascial insertion into the ischium. The floor of this space is delineated by the transverse septum. The supralevator space is contained between the peritoneum above and the levator ani muscle inferiorly. It extends on each side to surround the rectum. Finally, the deep postanal space is the area delineated by the levator ani superiorly and the anococcygeal ligament inferiorly. In essence, it is the continuation above the anococcygeal ligament of the right and left ischioanal spaces. Any infection in one of the ischioanal spaces spreads through this space to reach the contralateral ischioanal space to form the so-called horseshoe abscess-fistula.

## V. CONDUCT OF OPERATION

### PERIANAL ABSCESS

In the treatment of perianal abscess, antibiotics alone have proven to be ineffective. Perianal abscess necessitates surgical drainage, and this can be

**17**

PERIRECTAL ABSCESS

achieved in the office or the emergency room. The patient is placed in either the jackknife or lateral decubitus positon. The area is sterilely prepped and then a solution of 0.5% lidocaine, 0.25% marcaine, and adrenaline (1:200,000) is injected locally to anesthetize an area of at least 2 × 2 cm of skin. Despite the common practice of a linear, single incision, a cruciate incision is recommended over the area of fluctuance, as close as possible to the anal verge. The skin edges are to be excised to prevent them from closing the incision, thus blocking the drainage. Packing is not necessary unless bleeding is present and no electrocautery is available. The packing can be removed in several hours or the following day.

## ISCHIOANAL ABSCESSES

Ischioanal abscesses can still be treated on an outpatient basis with local anesthesia. Some authors do recommend treating these abscesses in the operating room. In general, more extensive abscesses benefit from general anesthesia. Again, a cruciate incision is recommended; an index finger should sweep the cavity to ensure breaking of any loculations and adequate drainage of the cavity. No packing is necessary, and the skin edges are excised as seen with perianal space abscesses. Counter incisions might be necessary when a very large cavity is encountered.

## INTERSPHINCTERIC ABSCESSES

Intersphincteric abscesses may be difficult to diagnose, given the scarcity of external signs of inflammation. An EUA is in order often to obtain a diagnosis given the difficulty of achieving good exposure. Simple drainage of the abscess will result in a high rate of recurrence. The abscess has to be laid open, and this entails the division of the IAS up to the dentate line or higher if the cavity has a more cephalad extension.

## SUPRALEVATOR ABSCESS

A supralevator abscess, which originates from an intersphincteric fistula or abscess, should be drained intrarectally by dividing the IAS. Draining this abscess through the ischioanal fossa would turn it into a suprasphincteric fistula. If the supralevator abscess derives from an ischioanal abscess or transsphincteric fistula, it should be drained externally through the ischiorectal fossa. An extrasphincteric fistula is likely to follow if drained transrectally. When the abscess is secondary to pelvic sepsis, percutaneous radiologic drainage is recommended followed by appropriate definitive treatment of the underlying pathology.

## DEEP POSTANAL SPACE ABSCESS

Regional or general anesthesia is necessary for a deep postanal space abscess. The treatment consists of placing a probe through the internal opening in the posterior midline, which is regularly present. Then the tissues over the probe are incised, thus including the distal IAS and the superficial and subcutaneous EAS, sparing its coccygeal attachment. Others recommend dividing only the IAS and sparing the EAS. This could be achieved by just spreading the superficial EAS to enter the space by a midline incision between coccyx and anus, followed by a second incision on the posterior midline of the anal canal dividing only the IAS.

## HORSESHOE ABSCESSES

Horseshoe abscesses (HA) can develop in any of the anorectal spaces. Regional or general anesthesia is indicated for these patients also. Intersphincteric HA are treated by dividing the IAS at the site of the abscess, thus exposing the crypt responsible for the infection. Supralevator HA are rare; considerations are similar to those for the supralevator abscess. If the abscess derives from an ischioanal abscess, a bilateral external drainage should be performed. The treatment of HA in the ischioanal fossa is similar to that for the deep anal space abscesses with the addition of paraanal counter incisions to drain the anterior extension of the abscess as proposed by Hanley.

## VARIATIONS OF OPERATION

An alternative approach in selected patients (no serious systemic disease, and no severe sepsis) is the use of catheter drainage. Preparation is the same as for the cruciate incision; a stab incision is made to provide immediate drainage of pus and symptomatic relief. Then a 10 to 16 F de Pezzer (ie, mushroom) catheter preferably, or alternatively a Malecot or a Foley catheter, is inserted over a stiff probe into the cavity. The shape of the abscess when using a mushroom-type catheter will hold the drain in place, thus avoiding sutures. The catheter is then shortened to leave 2 to 3 cm protruding outside of the cavity so that the catheter does not fall into the cavity. Clinical judgment should dictate the appropriate time for removal of the catheter; this will depend on the size of the cavity, the type and the amount of drainage, and the evidence of granulation tissue around the tube.

## POSTOPERATIVE ORDERS

Since most of these procedures are performed in the office or emergency department setting, these patients are rarely admitted. In this setting there is no role for antibiotics, because drainage of the abscess cavity is adequate therapy. However, certain exceptions include rheumatic or acquired valvular heart disease; immunosuppressed patients; the presence of extensive soft tissue infection such as with involvement of perineum, groin, thigh, or abdominal wall; and in diabetic patients. The idea of administering antibiotics and holding the drainage of an abscess in the absence of fluctuation is flawed, because it causes an unnecessary delay in the treatment, which might lead to further extension of the sepsis.

**Admit to:**
**Diagnosis:** s/p perirectal abscess drainage
**Condition:** stable
**Vital signs:** per routine
**Activity:** ad lib
**Allergies:**
**Nursing:** I&Os, drains to gravity, pack wound tid if appropriate, sitz
    bath tid
**Diet:** as tolerated; diabetic diet if appropriate
**IV fluids:** Heplock
**Medications:** antibiotics if appropriate
**Laboratory tests:** CBC

## VI. COMPLICATIONS

The primary complication of perirectal abscesses is inadequate drainage and recurrence. This can be minimized by adequate incisions and drainage at the primary treatment. However, if the patient does have a recurrence, then another drainage procedure is necessary. Another, complication of recurrent perirectal abscess formation is a fistula in ano, which will be discussed separately. Incontinence can occur if the external anal sphincter is completely transected.

## VII. DISCHARGE ORDERS

The patient should be advised to take warm sitz baths three times per day and after each bowel movement. If pain is significant, the patient can be given a lidocaine topical gel. The wound should be packed three times a day if necessary. Follow-up is in 2 to 3 weeks to check the wound and evaluate for the presence of fistulas.

# HEMORRHOIDS

*Keith Zuccala*

Normally all persons have hemorrhoidal tissue. It is classified as hemorrhoids only when patients have clinical symptoms.

## I. PATHOPHYSIOLOGY

The exact cause of hemorrhoids is unknown, but there are several theories regarding their cause. The most common assumption is that hemorrhoids are related to an enlargement of the vascular cushion secondary to engorgement of the vascular bed. This is thought to be caused by prolonged straining, lifting, increased abdominal pressure, and weak pelvic floor support. As the cushions become engorged, they can thrombose and are especially susceptible to localized trauma during defecation of hard stools.

**18**

## II. TYPICAL PRESENTATION

The presentation varies based on whether the abnormal hemorrhoidal tissue is "internal" or "external." **Internal hemorrhoids** (those above the dentate line) are rarely painful and usually present with bleeding or prolapse. Patients may also complain of rectal fullness and mucous or bloody drainage.

Internal hemorrhoid classification
| | |
|---|---|
| First degree | Bleeding |
| Second degree | Bleeding and prolapse with spontaneous reduction |
| Third degree | Bleeding with prolapse requiring manual reduction |
| Fourth degree | Bleeding with incarceration (nonreducible) |

Internal hemorrhoids rarely cause pain unless they become incarcerated (fourth degree) and are thrombosed.

**External hemorrhoids** may develop a skin tag with repeated engorgement and stretching of the overlying skin. Rarely do external hemorrhoids bleed unless they erode through the skin. External hemorrhoids frequently are painful, because even small engorgement or thrombosis stretches the overlying anoderm, which has a rich sensory innervation.

One of the most important concepts to remember regarding the presentation of hemorrhoids is that their presentation is hardly pathognomonic or specific. Many other anorectal problems (and gastrointestinal problems in general) can present with hematochezia, pain with defecation, and abnormal discharge. A thorough workup should be initiated before one confidently diagnoses abnormal hemorrhoidal tissue as the true cause of a patient's symptoms.

## III. PREOPERATIVE WORKUP

In general, most hemorrhoids can be treated nonoperatively. This requires behavior modification and changes in dietary habits, which reveals why hemorrhoids are so prevalent and also why they can be difficult to treat. Simple behavior modifications such as better hygiene and avoidance of straining during defecation can significantly reduce the symptoms of inflamed hemorrhoids. It is also important to keep stool soft, formed, and regular. Dietary modifications include increased dietary fiber (or bran or psyllium) and staying well hydrated. Dietary modifications should be the primary therapy in the treatment of hemorrhoids, even those that may require surgical care. Usually, first- and second-degree hemorrhoids respond to dietary modification, softening of stool, and avoidance of prolonged straining on the commode. Increased water consumption is also vital as previously mentioned. If conservative measures fail after a 1- to 2-month trial, "operative" intervention is required.

### PREOPERATIVE ORDERS

**Nursing:** Fleets enema 4 hours before operation
**Diet:** clear liquid diet for 48 hours before operation; NPO after midnight

## IV. SURGICAL ANATOMY

Hemorrhoids are "normal" tissue found at the end of the anal canal, which becomes pathologic after chronic trauma. This tissue, often referred to as a vascular cushion, is actually composed of vascular, smooth muscle, elastic, and connective tissues. Hemorrhoidal tissue is most prominent at the right anterolateral and posterolateral positions and the left lateral position. If this orientation is always remembered, even large, prolapsed hemorrhoids, whose base may be difficult to precisely identify, can be treated successfully.

Generally, there are two types of hemorrhoids, internal and external. Differentiation between the two is based on where the hemorrhoid is located in relationship to the dentate line; those above are considered internal and those below are external.

## V. CONDUCT OF OPERATION

"Operative" intervention may require surgery in the classic sense but usually involves other mechanical modalities. The most common mechanical intervention is rubber band ligation. This can be performed only on internal hemorrhoids because of the lack of pain fibers in the overlying mucosa. This procedure may be performed in the office setting as an outpatient procedure using an anoscope. The internal hemorrhoid is suctioned into a cylinder at the end of the anoscope, and then a rubber band is placed at the base of the hemorrhoid. The hemorrhoid becomes ischemic, necroses, and eventually sloughs off, leaving a scar that should not reprolapse or bleed. Usually the tissue sloughs in about 1 week and may be accompanied by some minimal bleeding. Rarely is intervention required for hemostasis. One quadrant can be banded every 2 weeks or so. Very seldom should multiple sites be treated at one time. Other interventions such as photocoagulation, chemical sclerosis, cryosurgery, and direct-current coagulation have been described, but none have proven to be superior or as safe as rubber band ligation.

Surgical excision may be performed on larger (third- and fourth-degree) hemorrhoids, external hemorrhoids, or thrombosed, painful hemorrhoids. The patient is given general anesthesia and then placed in a prone, jackknife position on the operating room table. Using either sharp dissection (scalpel, etc) or electrocautery with a needle tip, the hemorrhoid is elliptically excised at its base. The dissection should stay very superficial avoiding the underlying sphincter. The defect is then closed with a running absorbable (chromic 4-0) suture. Adequate visualization and retraction is essential and a digital rectal examination should always be done before the start of the procedure. It is also advisable to inject the base of the hemorrhoid with local anesthetic with epinephrine to help elevate the mucosa and also to provide some measure of hemostasis and postoperative analgesia.

### VARIATIONS OF OPERATION

Patients seen in the emergency setting with an acutely, thrombosed, painful, external hemorrhoid can obtain relief with excision of the tissue. This is performed using local anesthetic with epinephrine; however, the wound is usually left open. Incision and evacuation alone of the clot is not recommended, because there is a risk of recurrence and rebleeding. If the thrombosis occurred more than 48 hours before being seen by the surgeon, conservative measures (laxatives, sitz baths, stool softeners) will provide better results.

### POSTOPERATIVE ORDERS

Patients go home the same day if the surgery or banding is uncomplicated. Often a topical anesthetic cream or ointment is applied at the end of surgery. The tube should be sent home with the patient, and they can apply the topical anesthetic after each sitz bath.

### VI. COMPLICATIONS

Rubber band ligation is an essentially safe procedure, but there are occasionally perilous complications. Urinary retention is a common postprocedure complication. It is very rare after a single banding, but if multiple hemorrhoids are banded, the incidence may be as high as 10% to 20%.

18

HEMORRHOIDS

Surgical excision may carry a rate of 33% or higher. Usually, this occurs when the internal sphincter is injured and goes into spasm. Avoiding injury to the sphincter and avoiding excess intravenous fluid administration can reduce the incidence of urinary retention.

Sphincter injury can occur if too vigorous a dissection/excision is performed, which can lead to incontinence and life-long misery. Also, multiple excisions of the dentate line/anoderm can result in circumferential scarring with anal stenosis. For this reason, only a few hemorrhoids should be excised at a time, and an island of mucosa should remain between each excision.

Certainly, the common complications of any invasive procedure are relevant, including bleeding, anesthetic complications, and infection. Perineal sepsis and even death have been reported after rubber band ligation in which too thick a piece of tissue was ligated. Patients with undo pain, fevers, chills, or urinary retention should be advised to return to the emergency department immediately. Rarely does bleeding occur, but if it is arterial, a return trip to the operating room will be mandated; therefore it is always advisable to ensure total hemostasis has been achieved at the end of the first procedure.

These patients also are at risk for fecal impaction if too large an excision is performed and inadequate analgesia is provided.

## VII. DISCHARGE INSTRUCTIONS

Patients should take a sitz bath three times a day and after each bowel movement. They should be discharged with a prescription for a stool softener and dietary instruction (more bran or fiber in diet, 8 glasses of water a day, avoid straining). Heavy narcotics should be avoided, because these can lead to constipation. straining and worsening of the hemorrhoids. Nonsteroidal antiinflammatory drugs should also be avoided, because they may contribute to postoperative (or postbanding) bleeding. Follow-up is in 1 week or sooner if the condition worsens. Patients should be made to void before discharge, because urinary retention can be a problem.

# RECTAL CANCER

*Floriano Marchetti*

Rectal cancer occurs in 75% of patients without risk factors and 25% of patients with associated risk factors. These risk factors include family history without a genetic syndrome (15%-20%), inherited genetic syndromes (hereditary nonpolyposis colon cancer [HNPCC] and familial adenomatous polyposis [FAP], 4%-7% and 1% respectively), personal history 1%, and other risks including inflammatory bowel disease (IBD) 1%.

## I. PATHOPHYSIOLOGY

Most colorectal cancers follow the adenoma to carcinoma sequence. The earlier a cancer is detected, the better the prognostic outlook. Thus, the goal is to detect any malignant or premalignant lesion (polyp) at an early stage. This involves routine screening. The screening program depends on the patient's risk for colorectal cancer (CRC).

Average-risk patients should begin a screening program at age 50. This includes an annual fecal occult blood test (FOBT) performed with two samples of each of three consecutive stools. A positive test should mandate a colonoscopy or a flexible sigmoidoscopy with an air-contrast barium enema (ACBE). In addition, a flexible sigmoidoscopy is performed every 5 years. All polyps are biopsied. If an adenoma or carcinoma is found, then a repeat colonoscopy is performed to examine the remainder of the colon. Finally, a complete colonoscopy is necessary every 10 years.

Patients at increased risk are followed-up on the basis of the reason for their higher risk of colorectal cancer. Patients with a first-degree relative with CRC should undergo the aforementioned protocol for average-risk patients; however, this screening should begin at 40 years of age. More commonly, these patients are offered an initial colonoscopy.

Patients with a history of adenomatous polyps should undergo a repeat colonoscopy at 3 years. After a negative colonoscopy, it should be repeated every 5 years. Patients having undergone a curative resection for CRC should have a colonoscopy within 1 year from surgery. With a normal result the colonoscopy is repeated in 5 years.

Patients with a family history of FAP should initially undergo genetic testing and counseling. If they are a carrier of the FAP gene, flexible sigmoidoscopy every year should begin at puberty. The development of polyposis should prompt surgical intervention. Patients with a family history of HNPCC should have a colonoscopy every 1 to 2 years starting at 20 to 30 years of age and then every year after 40. Patients with IBD should undergo a colonoscopy with random biopsies after 8 years from diagnosis of pancolitis or after 15 years when left-sided colitis is present.

## II. TYPICAL PRESENTATION

Patients with colorectal cancer can present with a myriad of vague abdominal complaints. This can entail crampy abdominal pain, discomfort, or severe pain and tenderness in the face of an obstructing lesion. Patients can present with weight loss and complain of dark stools or bright red blood per rectum.

In addition to a usual history and physical examination, previous anorectal procedures and any continence problems should be ascertained. The digital examination is essential to evaluate the lesion. If it is within reach of the finger, it should be assessed for extension, distance from the anal verge, and especially for mobility in relation to the deeper planes. A complete history should include evaluation of metastatic disease and lymphadenopathy.

## III. PREOPERATIVE WORKUP

The preoperative workup for rectal carcinoma consists of two phases. Initially, the local tumor is assessed; then evidence of systemic disease is evaluated to accurately stage the tumor. The staging system for rectal cancer based on the TNM classification system is shown in Table 19-1.

### ASSESSMENT OF LOCAL TUMOR

Rigid proctoscopy provides direct visualization of the lesion and will allow the accurate measurement of the distance of the lesion from the anal verge. Biopsies of the lesion should be taken as well.

The assessment of the depth of the invasion in the rectal wall and the presence of lymph node metastasis is of fundamental importance in the staging and thus in the therapeutic decisions. The most accurate method to determine the level of invasion is controversial. Both computed tomography (CT) and magnetic resonance imaging (MRI) have a role in advanced-stage disease and when there is invasion into the surrounding structures. The accuracy of CT is reportedly 70% for depth of invasion, whereas the accuracy for detecting metastatic lymph nodes is only 40% to 50%. MRI is offering promising data, especially with the use of endoanal coils. Accuracy for depth of invasion is 70% to 90% and for lymph node metastasis is approximately 57% to 90%.

Endorectal ultrasonography (EUS) uses a rotating probe (7.5-10 MHz transducer) to define the layers of the rectal wall and determine the depth of invasion. Accuracy for depth of invasion is 81% to 94% and for lymph node involvement is 58% to 83%.

### EVALUATION OF SYSTEMIC DISEASE

Chest radiographs are taken to rule out gross lung metastatic disease and establish a baseline picture of the lungs for postoperative follow-up.

TABLE 19-1

## TNM STAGING OF RECTAL AND COLORECTAL CANCER

### STAGING OF RECTAL CANCER

**Primary Tumor**

Tx  Primary tumor cannot be assessed

T0  No evidence of primary tumor

Tis Carcinoma in situ

T1  Submucosal invasion

T2  Invades muscularis propria

T3  Invades subserosa or nonperitonealized

T4  Directly invades other organs or structures and/or perforates viscus

**Lymph Nodes**

Nx  Nodes cannot be assessed

N0  No nodal metastases

N1  1 to 3 pericolic or perirectal nodes positive

N2  4 or more pericolic or perirectal nodes positive

N3  Metastasis in a node along a named vascular trunk pericolic or
    perirectal tissues or apical node metastasis

**Distant Metastases**

Mx  Metastasis cannot be assessed

M0  No distant metastasis

M1  Distant metastasis

### STAGING OF COLORECTAL CANCER

| 0   | Tis   | N0         | M0 |
|-----|-------|------------|----|
| I   | T1    | N0         | M0 |
|     | T2    | N0         | M0 |
| II  | T3    | N0         | M0 |
|     | T4    | N0         | M0 |
| III | Any T | N1, N2, N3 | M0 |
| IV  | Any T | Any N      | M1 |

CT scan and ultrasonography (US) of the abdomen and pelvis are sensitive for liver metastasis: 60% with US and 70% to 95% with a contrast-enhanced CT. In addition, the CT scan can provide assessment of the local extension of the cancer within the pelvis. A colonoscopy is performed to evaluate the rest of the colon to rule out any synchronous lesions.

## PREOPERATIVE ORDERS

**Admit to:**

**Diagnosis:** colorectal cancer

**Condition:** stable

**Vital signs:** per routine

**Activity:** ad lib

**Allergies:**

**Nursing:** I&O, preoperative teaching from endostomal nurse

**Diet:** NPO after midnight
**IV fluids:** $D_5/0.45\%$ NS with 20 mEq KCl at 125 ml/h after midnight
**Medications:** Golytely bowel prep; neomycin and erythromycin PO;
    antibiotics on call to OR
**Laboratory tests:** CBC, LFT's, BMP, PT, PTT, UA, ECG, CXR, CEA level

## IV. SURGICAL ANATOMY

The rectum begins approximately 15 cm from the anal verge. It is defined by the level of the confluence of the taenia on the colon. The rectum has three separate blood supplies. They consist of a superior hemorrhoidal branch of the left colic artery, the middle colic artery a branch of the internal iliac artery, and the inferior rectal artery a branch of the internal pudendal artery.

## V. CONDUCT OF OPERATION

Rectal cancer is amenable to local therapy, low anterior resection (LAR) or coloanal anastomosis (CAA), and abdominoperineal resection (APR). The distance of the lesion from the anal verge is the most important factor in determining the appropriate operation. Cancer of the upper third of the rectum is routinely treated with LAR; lesions in the middle third of the rectum still carry some controversy concerning the best treatment. Cancers in the lower third were classically treated with APR. Recently, a very low anterior resection or a CAA has been offered to selected patients with cancer in the middle and lower third of the rectum. Studies have proven that a lower margin of 2 cm provides adequate clearance. Thus, in selected patients, LAR is now the standard treatment for tumors of the middle and lower third of the rectum, and only 10% to 20% of these patients undergo APR currently. Other factors influencing the choice of surgery are body build, gender, obesity, local spread, perforation, abscess, size and fixation of the lesion, histologic grade, presence of obstruction, adequacy of bowel preparation, and general medical condition.

Low anterior resection entails a full mobilization of the rectum with transection of both lateral stalks. The expression "very low or extended LAR" is reserved for those instances when the anastomosis is at or just above the level of the levator ani. The patient is placed supine on the operating table in a slight Trendelenburg position, and the legs are placed in either Lloyd-Davies or Allen stirrups. A vertical incision is used below the umbilicus and carried down to the level of the pubis, and a self-retaining retractor is placed. The sigmoid is divided from the peritoneal reflection along the white line of Toldt up to the proximal descending colon and down to the cul-de-sac, using the electrocautery or the scissors. The sigmoid mesentery is then dissected medially with a sponge stick until the left gonadal vessels are identified. The left ureter is identified as it passes just medial to the gonadal vein at the level of the iliac crest. The peritoneum is then incised on the right side of the sigmoid at the base of the mesentery, and this is continued down to the cul-de-sac. The incision is then extended upward to the level of the inferior mesenteric artery (IMA) origin from the aorta. The index finger is then wrapped around the IMA, and its remaining peritoneal attachments are divided carefully with either the bovie or scissors. When the origin of the IMA is free, the vessel is clamped. The left ureter should be clearly identified to avoid inadvertently clamping it at this time. The IMA is then divided at the origin from the aorta, and its proximal stump is ligated with a double No. 1 absorbable tie. Ligating the IMA at the origin is not required for a better cure, but rather to allow for better mobilization of the descending colon. Next, the left colic artery is clamped, divided, and ligated to provide good collateral blood supply through the Riolan arcade followed by ligation of the inferior mesenteric vein. The bowel is divided proximally at the junction of the descending colon and sigmoid between Bainbridge and Kocher clamps. The sigmoid-rectum is then stretched, and retrorectal areolar tissue is identified and then entered with both blunt and sharp dissection. The sympathetic chain (hypogastric nerves) is to remain posterior to the plane of dissection. The dissection is brought laterally in a concave sweep around the rectum. This will develop the lateral stalks. The rectosacral fascia (Waldeyer's fascia) is then encountered and divided with bovie or scissors. The dissection is then extended downward until the tip of the coccyx is reached. The dissection is then brought laterally to divide the lateral ligaments of the rectum; very rarely it is necessary to ligate vessels at this level. The dissection continues anteriorly, and the rectovesical/rectovaginal reflection is incised. Then the dissection continues behind the seminal vesicles and distal to the prostate in men. In women the dissection proceeds downward between the rectum and the vagina until the lower edge of the pubis is palpated. The mobilization of the rectum must include radial clearance of the tumor, which may be more important than the distal margin clearance. A high local recurrence rate has been found when radial clearance is not achieved. Metastatic deposits have been found in the mesorectum up to 4 cm from the tumor. The dissection of the rectum has to include the whole mesorectum in a parallel fashion to the rectum, avoiding coning down distally.

Once the mobilization of the rectum is completed, a stapler (PI#33) is placed as low as possible and fired. The rectum above the stapler line is divided with the knife and removed. Alternatively, the rectum is clamped with a right-angle clamp and divided.

A purse-string suture is placed on the distal descending colon and subsequently tightened around the anvil of a circular stapler introduced in the colon. The circular stapler is then introduced from the anus and cautiously advanced until the staple line is well extended. The stapler is then opened until the tip perforates the rectum wall just posterior to the staple line. The descending colon is pulled down, and the anvil is secured to the tip of the stapler and locked. The stapler is then closed, and the two ends are approximated ensuring that the vagina in females and the seminal vesicles in males are not caught in between the two ends. After the stapler is fired and removed from the anus, the two donuts are checked for completeness and sent to pathology. The anastomosis is checked by injecting air in the rectum while the pelvis is filled with saline.

## VARIATIONS OF OPERATION

Local therapy consists of three options: transanal excision, transanal endoscopic microsurgery (TEM), and endocavitary radiation (ECR). Transanal excision can be done with patients prone or in stirrups, determined by the location of the tumor (anterior or posterior quadrants, respectively). Essential steps of the procedure include adequate exposure with appropriate retraction, full-thickness excision of the lesion, and assurance of a 1-cm circumferential margin. The defect can be closed with absorbable sutures or be left open. Mortality rates approach zero.

Transanal endoscopic microsurgery can be performed up to 20 cm in the rectosigmoid using special proctoscopes. The rectum is insufflated with $CO_2$. Through multiple ports, special instruments are introduced to excise the lesion and to primarily close the defect.

Endocavitary radiation may be used for both cure and palliation. A low-voltage system is used to limit the depth of penetration, thus allowing larger doses of radiation compared with external beam radiation. A total of 9000 to 15,000 cGy is administered in three to five doses. No general anesthesia is required, and the procedure is performed on an outpatient basis.

## POSTOPERATIVE ORDERS

**Admit to:**
**Diagnosis:** s/p low anterior resection
**Condition:** stable
**Vital signs:** per routine
**Activity:** OOB to chair with assistance
**Allergies:**
**Nursing:** I&Os, NGT to LCWS, Foley to gravity, IS × 10 puffs q1h while awake, PAS and Pneumoboots until ambulating, ostomy to bag drainage if necessary, routine line care
**Diet:** NPO then clear liquids when passing flatus
**IV fluids:** $D_5$/0.45% NS with 20 mEq KCl at 125 ml/h
**Medications:** PCA, perioperative antibiotics for 24 hours
**Laboratory tests:** CBC, BMP in AM

## VI. COMPLICATIONS

Mortality after LAR is low (1%-3%), whereas complications are more common and include transient urinary dysfunction (3%-15%), sexual dysfunction in men (5%-70%), ureter injury, and presacral hemorrhage.

Anastomotic leak occurs in 5% to 10% of cases with a colorectal anastomosis, but subclinical leaks occur in up to 50%. Anastomotic stricture occurs in 5% to 20%.

## VII. DISCHARGE INSTRUCTIONS

Patients can be advised of the 5-year survival rates after LAR of 72% for stage I, 54% for stage II, 39% for stage III, and 7% for stage IV. Local recurrence tends to occur in the first 2 years after surgery and varies from 5% to 30% in the different series. Severe pelvic pain, bowel obstruction, and severe bilateral lower extremity edema are the main symptoms. Thus, patients should undergo intensive follow-up in the first 2 years with visits every 3 months for the first year and then every 6 months until 5 years. These follow-up appointments should include a routine physical examination and history, and a carcinoembryonic antigen level. A colonoscopy should be done at 1 year to evaluate for local recurrence at the anastomosis.

On the basis of the recommendations of the National Institute of Health Consensus panel, stage II and III rectal cancers should receive postoperative chemoradiation. Postoperative radiation has been shown to reduce the risk of local recurrence both with advanced lesions and microscopic residual disease (40% to 11% with a dose of 60 Gy compared with lower doses).

19

RECTAL CANCER

# PART VI

## Hepatobiliary and Pancreas

# CHOLECYSTECTOMY

*Michael Rosen*

The gallbladder exists to store and concentrate bile. Removal of the gall-bladder results in an increase in enterohepatic cycling of bile salts and is one of the most common surgical procedures performed by the general surgeon.

## I. PATHOPHYSIOLOGY

The gallbladder stores bile produced by the liver, concentrates the bile, and then excretes it after stimulation by local hormones. The absorption of water, sodium chloride, and sodium bicarbonate leads to a 10-fold concentration of bile salts, bile pigment, and cholesterol in the gallbladder lumen compared with the intrahepatic bile. The gallbladder mucosa, by secreting mucus, is also important in protecting the gallbladder from injuries secondary to the lytic action of bile. The gallbladder fills with bile as a result of the increased pressure in the biliary tree because of contraction of the sphincter of Oddi. The gallbladder stores and concentrates bile until stimulation occurs in response to meals or cephalic stimulation. Release of bile from the gallbladder depends not only on coordinated contraction of the gallbladder but also on relaxation of the sphincter of Oddi. Rhythmic contractions occur in response to cholecystokinin/pancreozymin (CCK), which is released from the duodenum in response to fatty foods. Normal contraction of the gallbladder occurs four to six times a day, and absence of the gallbladder leads to increased enterohepatic cycling.

The average adult liver secretes approximately 250 to 1000 ml of bile daily. Bile is composed of electrolytes, bile salts, proteins, cholesterol, fats, and bile pigments. The color of bile depends on a breakdown product of red blood cells, bilirubin, which is secreted into the bile independent of the bile salt pool. Most of the dry weight of bile is composed of the organic compounds of bile salts, cholesterol, and phospholipids. Bile salts are synthesized in the liver from cholesterol before conjugation. Bile salts aid in the digestion and absorption of fats, and most are reabsorbed in the terminal ileum. This makes up the enterohepatic circulation, and less than 5% of this circulating bile salt pool is delivered to the colon.

Bile also contains cholesterol and lecithin in concentrations lower than that in plasma. Cholesterol is insoluble in bile, and the solubility of cholesterol depends on bile acids and lecithin. Changes in the rate of solubility depend on the concentration of bile acids and phospholipids. Insolubility of cholesterol is also thought to be from supersaturation, an important factor in the formation of cholesterol stones. Most patients with gallstones in Western cultures have stones composed predominantly of cholesterol. When the concentration of bile salts and lecithin decreases relative to the concentration of cholesterol in bile, cholesterol supersaturation occurs, with the development of cholesterol crystals. Factors that are important in the formation of cholesterol stones include obesity, hormones, bacteria, reflux of intestinal and pancreatic juices, bile stasis, and metabolic abnormalities.

Pigmented stones are another variety of gallstones. Pigment stones form as a result of an increase or alteration in the solubility of unconjugated bilirubin. Multiple disease processes predispose patients to the formation of pigment stones. Two types of pigment stones exist based on the percentage of certain insoluble inorganic components. Black pigment stones, which are more highly associated with hemolysis, cirrhosis, and increased age, have a higher percentage of inorganic components. Brown pigment stones are associated with stasis, infection, and infestation with parasites. Brown stones are also located throughout the intrahepatic and extrahepatic biliary tree, whereas black stones are usually located exclusively in the gallbladder. Other factors associated with the formation of brown pigment stones include long-term parenteral nutrition and extensive ileal resection.

## II. TYPICAL PRESENTATION

Cholecystitis, or inflammation of the gallbladder wall, is secondary to gallstones in 95% of patients. After this initial obstruction of the cystic duct, several clinical scenarios may take place. The stone can pass through the cystic duct into the common bile duct, relieving the initial symptoms of biliary colic but predisposing patients to cholangitis and gallstone pancreatitis. The impacted cystic duct stone may also fall back into the gallbladder lumen, relieving the symptoms of biliary colic. This latter situation occurs commonly in patients with symptomatic gallstones, because 60% to 75% of patients will report episodes of similar symptoms without progressing to acute cholecystitis. The gallstone can also remain impacted in the cystic duct. As a result of the cystic duct obstruction, the gallbladder bile is absorbed, and the gallbladder eventually becomes filled with secreted mucinous material. This clinical situation is called hydrops, and aspiration of the gallbladder at the time of surgery reveals either clear or white bile. The clinical findings of cholecystolithiasis are based on the degree of inflammation that occurs in the gallbladder wall. Mild to severe inflammatory changes of the gallbladder wall may occur, as well as progression to gangrene and perforation of the gallbladder. Obviously, these different clinical states will have varying degrees of symptoms.

Approximately 20% of all patients who undergo cholecystectomy for symptomatic cholecystitis will have acute cholecystitis. Vigorous contractions of the gallbladder, after stimulation by CCK, secreted in response to ingestion of a fatty meal, will lead to pain in the right upper quadrant and epigastrium. In many patients, pain will radiate to the back or subscapular region. Approximately 75% of patients with acute cholecystitis will give a history of previous symptoms. If cystic duct obstruction continues with resultant inflammation and edema of the gallbladder wall, patients will develop other symptoms, such as fever, vomiting, anorexia, and localized pain to the right upper quadrant. On physical examination, the patient with acute cholecystitis may have localized right upper quadrant tenderness or, if more progressed, a tense, tender, and palpable gallbladder. A positive Murphy's sign may be helpful in confirming the diagnosis of acute cholecystitis. Cessation of deep inspiration will occur after deep palpation in the right upper quadrant because of the diaphragmatic motion forcing the tender gallbladder into the examiner's hand. Laboratory examinations are less diagnostic for acute cholecystitis. The white blood cell count, serum transaminase levels, pancreatic enzymes, and bilirubin levels may be moderately elevated.

Chronic cholecystitis represents the process of recurrent inflammation of the gallbladder secondary to repeated obstruction of the cystic duct from gallstones. Chronic inflammation also leads to scarring of the gallbladder and progression to a nonfunctioning gallbladder. The diagnosis of chronic cholecystitis is based on both clinical and radiologic evaluations. The symptomatology of chronic cholecystitis includes recurrent episodes of biliary colic, occasionally initiated by the ingestion of fatty foods, as well as increased bloating, flatulence, and dyspepsia. Patients with chronic cholecystitis may confuse these symptoms with other disease processes, such as irritable bowel disease, reflux esophagitis, or constipation.

## III. PREOPERATIVE WORKUP

The differential diagnosis of acute cholecystitis includes hepatitis, pancreatitis, appendicitis, myocardial ischemia, pneumonia, peptic ulcer disease, diverticulitis, and renal stones. Laboratory examinations should help exclude hepatitis, pancreatitis, and renal stones. A chest x-ray examination will help differentiate pneumonia or pneumonitis from acute cholecystitis, and an electrocardiogram and serum cardiac enzymes will identify a myocardial infarction or ischemia. A long retrocecal appendix may mimic acute cholecystitis, although history and clinical course should help differentiate these two disease processes. Acute cholecystitis should not progress to the extent of appendicitis over time, and this may help differentiate these two disease processes.

The diagnosis of acute cholecystitis not only depends on history and clinical examination but also on radiographic studies. The "gold standards" for diagnosis of this disease are ultrasonography and scintigraphy. Oral cholecystography, computed tomography (CT), endoscopic retrograde cholangiopancreatography (ERCP), intravenous cholangiography, and plain radiographs are of limited value in the initial diagnosis of acute cholecystitis. Plain radiographs of the abdomen are rarely diagnostic for patients with acute cholecystitis, because fewer than 15% of gallstones are radiopaque. In patients with progression of their gallbladder disease to emphysematous cholecystitis, air will be visualized on plain radiographs in the gallbladder lumen or gallbladder wall secondary to gas-forming organisms.

Ultrasound examination of the abdomen in the patient with acute cholecystitis will usually reveal gallstones and gallbladder wall thickening and

**20**

**CHOLECYSTECTOMY**

tenderness. Ultrasonography has been shown to be almost 90% sensitive in the diagnosis of acute cholecystitis, with a specificity and accuracy of 98% and 96%, respectively. Other findings on ultrasound examination include pericholecystic abscesses or fluid collections. Calcification of the gallbladder wall secondary to multiple episodes of inflammation can also be seen, but this is more likely to be associated with chronic cholecystitis.

Radionucleotide scanning or scintigraphy will help confirm the diagnosis in the patient with suspected acute cholecystitis. Radionucleotide imaging, like ultrasonography, is safe, noninvasive, and reasonably rapid. The various agents are taken up by the liver and excreted into the bile and are eventually concentrated in the gallbladder. After delivery of the agent, excretion into the bile ducts occurs, and visualization of the gallbladder usually takes place within 15 to 45 minutes, as long as the cystic duct is patent and the gallbladder has normal function. Nonabsorption by the gallbladder will lead to nonvisualization and a positive radionucleotide scan impression. Radionucleotide scanning has an accuracy of approximately 95%, with a sensitivity and specificity of 92% and 97%, respectively.

Cholecystectomy is the preferred therapy for patients with acute cholecystitis. Not only does it remove the inflamed organ, it also eliminates the possibility of further stone formation in most patients. Emergency cholecystectomy is rarely required and is reserved for those patients who either have a complication of acute cholecystitis or are severely septic. Most patients can undergo surgery within 24 to 48 hours of their presentation to the hospital once the diagnosis is established and the patient is stabilized for surgery.

## PREOPERATIVE ORDERS

**Admit to:**
**Diagnosis:** acute cholecystitis
**Condition:** stable
**Vital signs:** per routine
**Activity:** ad lib
**Allergies:**
**Nursing:** I&Os
**Diet:** NPO
**IV fluids:** $D_5$/0.45% NS with 20 mEq KCl at 125 ml/h
**Medications:** heparin, 5000 U SC on call to OR
cefotetan, 1 g IV, q12h
**Laboratory tests:** CBC, LFTs, amylase, lipase, BMP, CKs with isoenzymes, PT, PTT, UA, CXR, ECG, RUQ ultrasound

## IV. SURGICAL ANATOMY

The gallbladder lies on the undersurface of the liver, bound to its fossa by vessels, connective tissue, small biliary communications, and lymphatics. The gallbladder may have a mesentery so that it lies separate from the liver parenchyma, or it may be deep within the liver as an intrahepatic gallbladder.

There are four regions of the gallbladder: the fundus, the body, the infundibulum, and the neck. The gallbladder terminates in the cystic duct, which then enters the extrahepatic biliary tree. The cystic duct can join the common hepatic duct to form the common bile duct in a variety of fashions. Classically, the cystic duct enters from a lateral point. The cystic artery typically arises from the right hepatic artery and courses superoposterior to the cystic duct. The triangle of Calot is defined by the common hepatic duct, cystic duct, and the edge of the liver. Within the triangle, the cystic artery is usually identified.

## V. CONDUCT OF OPERATION

Cholecystectomy can be performed in either an open or laparoscopic fashion. Laparoscopic cholecystectomy has become the "gold standard" and has been proven to be a safe and efficacious procedure in the management of gallstone disease. Most surgeons will attempt laparoscopic cholecystectomy in patients with acute cholecystitis.

The patient is placed in the supine position with both arms tucked in at the sides. A Foley catheter and orogastric tube are placed to decompress the bladder and stomach before trocar insertion. The surgeon stands on the patient's left side, the first assistant is on the right, and the camera operator stands to the left of the surgeon.

The abdomen is entered using the open technique. A 2-cm linear infraumbilical incision is made. The subcutaneous fat is dissected until the median raphe is identified as it enters into the linea alba. This is grasped with a Kocher clamp and brought into the wound. Next, a second Kocher clamp is applied inferiorly. The linea alba is cut with a Mayo scissors approximately 1.5 cm. Two stay sutures are placed at the superior and inferior aspects of the fascia. The peritoneum is entered with a Hasson trocar. The stay sutures are secured on the trocar. The abdomen is insufflated to 15 cm $H_2O$. The camera is placed, and the other trocars are placed under direct visualization after the abdominal wall has been transilluminated and vascular structures are avoided. A 10-mm trocar is placed in the epigastrium just to the right of the falciform ligament. Two 5-mm ports are placed in the right upper quadrant in the midclavicular and anterior axillary lines and used for retraction.

The gallbladder is initially grasped at the fundus with the most lateral trocar and retracted to the right upper quadrant to expose the porta hepatis. Next the midclavicular trocar is used to grasp the infundibulum to provide retraction. The epigastrium port is the main operative port, and at this time it is used to bluntly remove the peritoneum and adhesions surrounding the gallbladder and cystic duct. Care should be taken to stay high on the gallbladder and avoid using cautery to prevent common bile duct injuries. The infundibulum should be retracted laterally to open the hepatoduodenal ligament.

Once the peritoneal attachments of the hepatoduodenal ligament are removed, one proceeds to identify the cystic duct gallbladder junction. This is done with gentle blunt spreading motions. The duct should be dissected as proximal to the gallbladder neck as possible to provide adequate length for clipping and dividing this structure without disturbing the common bile duct. Once the cystic duct is clearly identified, the cystic artery is dissected out superoposteriorly. This should be freed up to allow placement of two clips proximally and one distally. After the artery and duct are clearly identified and are seen going on to the gallbladder wall, a proximal clip is placed on the cystic duct as close to the gallbladder as possible. Next, a cholangiogram can be performed to further delineate confusing anatomy or evaluate for common bile duct stones.

The cystic duct and cystic artery are then clipped and divided. Next the gallbladder is dissected off the liver bed. This is performed using hook cautery, with the infundibulum being retracted to provide traction for safe division. After the gallbladder is removed and the liver bed is examined for bleeding or bile, the gallbladder is taken out of the abdomen using the Endocatch bag. The abdomen is then irrigated, taking care to avoid suction in the porta for fear of dislodging the clips. All trocars are removed under direct vision, and the fascia is closed in the umbilical port.

## VARIATIONS OF OPERATION

Conversion to open cholecystectomy is not considered a complication and is required in fewer than 10% of cases. Conversion is required when there is extensive inflammation or bleeding, a variability in the biliary anatomy, or a suspected iatrogenic injury. Previous abdominal surgery, obesity, pregnancy, and severe inflammation are not considered contraindications to laparoscopic cholecystectomy. Patients who are not stable for general anesthesia, those with a bleeding diathesis, and those with suspected gallbladder malignancy should not undergo laparoscopic cholecystectomy.

The use of intraoperative cholangiography has been a heavily debated topic among biliary surgeons, even before the advent of laparoscopy. Cholangiography is used to identify occult common bile duct stones and to delineate biliary anatomy. Proponents of selective cholangiography cite many articles in the literature detailing cases of biliary tract injury despite the use of cholangiography. These authors propose that detailed dissection of the cystic duct will decrease the chances of bile duct injury, and without preoperative markers of common bile duct stones, such as persistent jaundice or stones evident on ultrasonography, cholangiography merely adds risk and time to the operative procedure. Those surgeons who routinely use cholangiography, regardless of the preoperative laboratory or radiographic findings, cite the advantages of delineating the complete biliary anatomy and the possibility of identifying occult common bile duct stones, which exist in 4% to 10% of patients. Also, these authors agree that the percentage of bile duct injuries might not decrease with routine cholangiography, but the severity of these injuries will be much decreased.

Patients with acute cholecystitis who are not stable for surgical intervention can be treated with cholecystostomy. This procedure can be performed percutaneously or by means of an open surgical technique under local anesthesia. This is a temporizing procedure, although in many cases of acute acalculous cholecystitis, the procedure can be curative. Complications of cholecystostomy include bile leak or peritonitis, injury to surrounding organs, bleeding, and continued intraabdominal sepsis. Patients who do not respond to percutaneous or open drainage of the gallbladder will require surgical intervention. Most patients who will eventually have a good outcome show clinical improvement within 48 hours of the procedure. Cholecystostomy is considered a temporizing procedure, although it may obviate the need for cholecystectomy in patients with acalculous cholecystitis.

**20**

**CHOLECYSTECTOMY**

## POSTOPERATIVE ORDERS

**Admit to:**
**Diagnosis:** s/p laparoscopic cholecystectomy
**Condition:** stable
**Vital signs:** per routine
**Activity:** ad lib
**Allergies:**
**Nursing:** I&Os, Pneumoboots, PAS until fully ambulatory, IS q1h while awake
**Diet:** as tolerated
**IV fluids:** $D_5$/0.45% NS with 20 mEq KCl at 100 ml/h; Heplock when tolerating oral intake
**Medications:** antibiotics if appropriate
**Laboratory tests:** none

## VI. COMPLICATIONS

Common bile duct injury is a serious complication of laparoscopic cholecystectomy. It is an avoidable complication usually related to improper surgical techniques. With liberal use of cholangiography, the cystic duct gallbladder neck junction should always be identified; the clips should never be placed without clearly identifying the structure (even in the face of bleeding) and converting to an open procedure if the surgeon is unsure of anatomy or uncomfortable with proceeding with the laparoscopic approach so this dreaded complication can be avoided. Common bile duct injuries are best treated immediately with biliary bypass procedures.

Another more common complication of laparoscopic cholecystectomy is bile leaks. These are commonly a result of a leak from the liver bed or loss of control of the cystic duct stump. Treatment includes drainage either percutaneously by means of CT or ultrasonographic guidance or by stent placement with ERCP. With adequate drainage, these leaks usually spontaneously resolve.

## VII. DISCHARGE INSTRUCTIONS

Most uncomplicated laparoscopic cholecystectomies are performed as out-patient procedures. Patients should be discharged with adequate pain medication. They should be instructed that shoulder pain is normal for up to 48 hours; any signs of fever or drainage from the wounds should prompt a call to the office. Patients should not drive until they are not taking narcotics. Patients should have a follow-up appointment in 1 to 2 weeks for a wound check.

# ACUTE PANCREATITIS

*Michael Tarnoff*

Acute pancreatitis represents a broad spectrum of clinical and pathologic disease. Although there is no strict definition, pancreatitis always entails some degree of acute parenchymal inflammation in association with variable involvement of adjacent organs and tissues. Patients diagnosed with any form of pancreatitis should be approached with caution and mandate close surveillance. Most acute pancreatitis is clinically benign and self-limited. Despite this, there is no surgical disease so capable of abrupt deterioration and catastrophic consequences as pancreatitis. As a result, an in-depth understanding of the potential severity of this clinical entity is vital to the practice of general surgery.

## I. PATHOPHYSIOLOGY

The nomenclature used to describe the spectrum of disease classified as pancreatitis is confusing but can be summarized as follows. Acute self-limited pancreatitis refers to parenchymal inflammation with no pancreatic necrosis or permanent ductal or parenchymal changes. Pancreatic necrosis may complicate any case of acute pancreatitis. In the absence of systemic signs of infection, this is referred to as sterile pancreatic necrosis. Secondary infection of necrotic pancreatic tissue is known as infected pancreatic necrosis. The coalescence of several areas of infected pancreatic necrosis is referred to as pancreatic abscess. Hemorrhagic pancreatitis refers to the situation in which pancreatic necrosis or severe inflammation causes erosion of the regional blood supply with subsequent hemorrhage into the retroperitoneum. When repeated episodes of acute pancreatitis lead to permanent ductal or parenchymal damage, the disease is known as chronic pancreatitis.

Ninety percent of acute pancreatitis occurs secondary to alcohol or gallstone disease. The former predominates in urban regions, whereas the latter prevails in all other populations. The exact mechanism by which alcohol use leads to pancreatic inflammation remains obscure. Alcohol is a known stimulant of secretin and sphincter of Oddi contraction. The most widely accepted theory for the development of alcohol-mediated pancreatitis relates to the pancreatic exocrine hypersecretion resulting from the release of secretin after alcohol intake. This event, coupled with partial ampullary obstruction, may lead to most cases of alcoholic pancreatitis. Other theories include alcohol-mediated protein plugging of the pancreatic duct or a direct toxic effect of circulating triglycerides released after alcohol intake.

The clinical association of midepigastric abdominal pain, elevated serum levels of the pancreatic enzymes amylase and lipase, and cholelithiasis is termed gallstone pancreatitis. The mechanism by which gallstones lead to pancreatitis is also poorly understood. Studies that use endoscopic retrograde pancreatography (ERCP) have revealed that nearly 90% of patients with gallstone pancreatitis have a common channel. This common channel is formed by the union of the pancreatic and common bile duct. It is widely believed that gallstone obstruction of this channel leads to mechanical outflow obstruction of the pancreatic duct. Fixed mechanical obstruction is not a prerequisite, however. The mere migration of gallstones past the pancreas causes reflux of bile into the pancreatic duct. Bile reflux is believed to be the trigger for pancreatic inflammation in these cases.

Hypertriglyceridemia is a well-known yet poorly understood factor in the development of some cases of acute pancreatitis. Ischemia stemming from systemic hypotension, embolic events, or coronary artery bypass can lead to pancreatic inflammation. Pancreatic duct obstruction from malignancy, cysts, or pancreatic divisum are associated with pancreatitis. Numerous medications have been implicated as causative agents in the development of rare cases of acute pancreatitis.

## II. TYPICAL PRESENTATION

Most patients with acute pancreatitis present with a chief complaint of midepigastric abdominal pain that radiates to the back. It is mandatory to attempt to define the cause of acute pancreatitis, because treatment is cause dependent. The history of the present illness should include questions directed toward establishing any of the previously described causative factors. Alcohol-induced pancreatitis usually follows episodes of binge drinking, whereas gallstone pancreatitis typically occurs after a large meal. The systemic nature of acute pancreatitis leads to numerous associated findings, all of which should be sought in the history of the present illness. Pleural effusions can develop as a result of secondary diaphragmatic irritation leading to complaints of shortness of breath or hiccups. Extensive retroperitoneal inflammation may induce adynamic ileus resulting in nausea, vomiting, or anorexia. These symptoms can also occur when severe pancreatic inflammation leads to pseudocyst formation and obstruction of the duodenum. Rarely, when pancreatic necrosis has led to secondary infection or hemorrhage, patients may present with signs of sepsis or hypovolemic shock.

Physical findings in acute pancreatitis are generally nonspecific. Vital signs are typically stable but can be variable in rare cases involving infection or hypovolemia. Hypovolemia can result from third space fluid sequestration or hemorrhage. Jaundice is an unusual finding but may be present when concomitant common bile duct obstruction occurs from gallstones, malignancy, or pseudocyst. Asymmetric breath sounds may result from pleural effusion. Abdominal findings are variable and may include distention or upper abdominal fullness or mass. Discoloration of the abdominal flanks and umbilicus is known as Grey-Turner's and Cullen's sign, respectively. These physical findings occur with severe hemorrhagic pancreatitis and represent retroperitoneal blood, which dissects into the respective tissue plane.

## III. NONOPERATIVE MANAGEMENT

Most patients with acute pancreatitis can be managed nonoperatively. Oral intake should be withheld until the clinical signs of inflammation resolve. This usually manifests as resolution of abdominal pain and tenderness and normalization of serum levels of amylase and lipase. When oral intake is begun before symptom resolution, there is a higher incidence of infectious complications and recurrent parenchymal inflammation.

Nasogastric suction is useful in patients with concomitant adynamic ileus but has never been shown to shorten the course of the disease. There is no well-defined role for histamine receptor antagonists or somatostatin in the treatment of these patients.

Careful monitoring of fluid and electrolyte balance is essential in patients with acute pancreatitis. Hypovolemia from third space fluid sequestration is common and should be corrected with balanced salt solution. Central venous pressure monitoring may be helpful in patients with comorbid conditions such as chronic renal failure or cardiopulmonary disease or in patients who fail to respond to initial fluid resuscitation. Close monitoring of serum sodium, potassium, calcium, and magnesium is essential to safe management.

The role of antibiotics in patients with acute pancreatitis is controversial. There is no proven benefit to the use of prophylactic antibiotics in patients with acute self-limited pancreatitis. Patients found to have sterile pancreatic necrosis do, however, benefit from the use of prophylactic broad-spectrum antibiotics. Imipenem-cilastatin has been shown to reduce the risk of subsequent infectious complications of sterile necrosis and should be used in this setting.

Pain management is best accomplished with narcotic analgesics other than morphine. Morphine is a known stimulant of sphincter of Oddi contraction and may exacerbate pancreaticobiliary obstruction. It is vital to maintain vigilance over the status of the patient's abdomen in this setting. Analgesics of any kind should be used sparingly and only after the extent of intraabdominal pathology has been fully appreciated. Patients with persistent abdominal symptoms should be reevaluated at regular intervals without systemic analgesics, which can mask clinical findings.

## IV. PREOPERATIVE WORKUP

### BLOOD CHEMISTRY

Measurement of the serum amylase and lipase is the time-honored objective means of diagnosing acute pancreatitis. These enzymes are the product of the exocrine secretion of the pancreas. Extravasation of exocrine secretions occurs even with mild pancreatic inflammation. Resorption of the extravasated secretions leads to increased serum values. Hyperamylasemia typically occurs within 24 hours of the onset of inflammation and resolves by 7 days. Prolonged elevation of the serum amylase or lipase suggests pancreatic pseudocyst.

There are several pitfalls in relying on serum amylase to diagnose pancreatic inflammation. First, hyperamylasemia is not specific for pancreatitis and can be seen in perforated peptic ulcer disease: acute appendicitis; salpingitis; salivary gland disorders including mumps, parotitis, and sialoadenitis; renal failure; and pneumonia. Second, the half-life of amylase creates a diagnostic window through which hyperamylasemia is only present between 24 hours and 7 days from the onset of inflammation. This leaves the potential for false-negative results (10%). Last, hyperamylasemia does not occur in patients with hypertriglyceride-induced pancreatitis. Additional serum measurements of the amylase s-isoenzyme and urinary amylase enhance the specificity of hyperamylasemia in the diagnosis of pancreatitis.

Serum lipase is a more specific marker for pancreatic inflammation than serum amylase. In addition, the half-life of lipase is longer and permits more accurate detection of elevated levels than does serum amylase measurement. Despite this, hyperlipasemia can also be seen in cases of perforated peptic ulcer disease, acute cholecystitis, and intestinal ischemia. Each of these clinical entities should be excluded. Ultimately, the combination of hyperamylasemia and hyperlipasemia coupled with appropriate clinical parameters can be relied on for an accurate diagnosis of pancreatitis.

A complete blood count should be analyzed in all patients with acute pancreatitis. Common findings may include an elevated white blood cell count secondary to associated inflammation or infection. Hemoconcentration is also possible as a result of third space fluid loss. Rarely, patients may be anemic as a result of hemorrhagic pancreatitis.

The basic metabolic panel is also useful. Hyperglycemia can occur and results from a relative state of hypoinsulinemia and hyperglucagonemia. Patients with severe fluid deficit can have azotemia. Hypocalcemia is not infrequent and results from associated hypoalbuminemia, deposition of calcium in the inflamed retroperitoneum (also known as fat saponification), and a relative skeletal resistance to parathyroid hormone.

## RADIOGRAPHY

Plain chest radiographs should be obtained in all patients with pancreatitis. It is important to exclude pulmonary sequela of pancreatitis, including pleural effusion or atelectasis. In addition, upright chest films can be useful in detecting free intraabdominal air in a patient with hyperamylasemia and abdominal pain.

Abdominal radiography, including plain upright and supine views, is nonspecific but can provide useful information in these patients. The most common finding on plain abdominal radiographs is a nonspecific bowel gas pattern. Adynamic ileus can occur and appears as dilated small and large small bowel loops with air-fluid levels throughout. The finding of a solitary dilated jejunal loop is known as the sentinel loop sign and signifies localized ileus secondary to adjacent inflammation. The colon cutoff sign refers to a focally dilated loop of transverse colon with no air distally. This also results from localized irritation from adjacent retroperitoneal inflammation. Other findings include retroperitoneal air secondary to necrotizing infection, obliteration of the psoas muscle border as a result of inflammation, or abscess or right upper quadrant calcification resulting from gallstones.

The role of abdominal computed tomography (CT) in the evaluation of patients with pancreatitis is well established. Patients with acute, self-limited pancreatitis do not need radiographic study beyond a right upper quadrant ultrasonogram to evaluate the biliary tree. Any patient with a prolonged course or any patient suspected of having pancreatic necrosis should undergo dynamic abdominal and pelvic CT scan with oral and intravenous contrast. This study permits assessment of pancreatic parenchymal viability and effectively evaluates the severity of retroperitoneal inflammation and the presence of a pancreatic pseudocyst.

## RANSON'S CRITERION

Ranson's criterion is a well-established scoring system that predicts mortality in patients with pancreatitis not related to gallstones. Recently, modified criteria have been derived, which provide similar predictions for patient with gallstone-mediated pancreatitis. Ranson's prognostic signs are summarized in Table 21-1.

In patients presenting with two or fewer of the prognostic indicators listed, there is no associated mortality, and these patients require only supportive care. Patients who present with 3-4 signs have a 15% mortality, with 50% of these individuals requiring intensive care monitoring. Intensive care is mandatory for patients who present with five to six signs, because mortality in this group approximates 50%. Those patients who have seven or more prognostic indicators invariably have a higher mortality and a prolonged hospital course.

### TABLE 21-1
**RANSON'S CRITERIA**

| At Admission | During Initial 48 h |
| --- | --- |
| Age >55 y | Hematocrit fall >10% |
| White blood cells >16,000/mm$^3$ | Blood urea nitrogen elevation >5 mg/dl |
| Blood glucose >200 mg/dl | Serum Ca fall to <8 mg/dl |
| Serum lactate dehydrogenase >350 IU/L | Arterial $P_{O_2}$ <60 mm Hg |
| Aspartate aminotransferase >250 U/dl | Base deficit >4 mEq/L |
| | Estimated fluid sequestration >6 L |

21

ACUTE PANCREATITIS

**PREOPERATIVE ORDERS**
**Admit to:** ICU
**Diagnosis:** pancreatitis
**Condition:** guarded
**Vital signs:** q1h
**Activity:** bed rest
**Allergies:**
**Nursing:** strict I&Os, NGT to LCWS, Foley to gravity, IS q1h while awake, Pneumoboots.
**Diet:** NPO
**IV fluids:** $D_5$/NS at 125 ml/h
**Medications:** antibiotics if indicated
**Laboratory tests:** CBC, amylase, lipase, BMP, Ca, $PO_4$, Mg, triglycerides, alcohol level, PT, PTT, LFTs, ABGs, CXR, KUB (flat and upright), RUQ ultrasound "rule out gallstones"

## V. SURGICAL ANATOMY

The pancreas is completely retroperitoneal and lies posterior to the stomach and lesser omentum. The gland consists of four portions. The pancreatic head lies adjacent to the duodenal loop. The uncinate process arises from the head as a posterior inferior extension, passes posterior to the superior mesenteric vein (SMV), and ends at the right lateral portion of the superior mesenteric artery (SMA). The pancreatic neck lies adjacent to the head and represents the portion of the pancreas directly anterior to the SMV. The body of the pancreas lies to the right of the neck, and the pancreatic tail consists of that portion of the gland in contact with the splenic hilum. The tail of the gland lies in a position superior to the head as the pancreas courses obliquely from right to left.

The blood supply of the pancreas has several origins. The pancreatic head shares a common blood supply with the duodenum. The anterior and posterior pancreaticoduodenal arcades branch from the superior and inferior pancreaticoduodenal vessels, respectively, and provides the major blood supply to this region. These latter vessels branch from the celiac and SMA, respectively. The body and tail of the pancreas receive blood from the dorsal and transverse pancreatic arteries, which branch from the splenic and gastroepiploic arteries. The posterosuperior and posteroinferior portion of the body are supplied by the superior and inferior pancreatic arteries.

The venous drainage parallels the arterial supply and uniformly drains into the portal venous system. The lymphatic drainage of the pancreatic head is to the subpyloric, portal, mesocolic, mesenteric, and aortocaval regions. The body and tail primarily drain into the retroperitoneum or the splenic hilum.

## VI. OPERATIVE INDICATIONS

There are three general indications to operate on pancreatitis: treatment of infection, uncertainty of diagnosis, and treatment of concurrent biliary tract disease. With the exception of patients undergoing surgery for treatment of biliary tract disease, patients who require operative intervention to treat pancreatitis have typically become debilitated and require extensive and prolonged care.

In 5% of patients with pancreatitis, infectious complications develop, ranging from infected necrosis to pancreatic abscess. Any patient with systemic inflammatory signs, a pancreatic fluid collection, or pancreatic necrosis should undergo CT-guided aspiration with immediate Gram stain to exclude the lesser sac as the source of the infection. When the Gram stain is positive for bacteria, additional intervention is necessary.

Patients with infected necrosis or pancreatic abscess usually require operative debridement and drainage. Percutaneous drainage is a viable option in select patients whose infected collections appear uniform and homogeneous on CT scan. This technique is usually not feasible in this setting, however, because the necrotic parenchyma is often too thick to be drained in this manner. Such patients usually require surgical pancreatic debridement as described later.

On rare occasion, patients present with an ambiguous picture of diffuse abdominal pain and an elevated serum amylase and lipase. Although consistent with acute pancreatitis, the finding of diffuse abdominal pain should heighten suspicion of alternative intraabdominal pathology. Such patients may have an ischemic bowel or a perforated viscus. In this unusual setting, an exploratory laparotomy may be required to make a definitive diagnosis. In this context, the balance of morbidity from a negative exploration versus morbidity from a missed diagnosis must be weighed.

The management of pancreatitis and associated biliary tract disease has long been debated. Historically, delayed cholecystectomy had been advocated in patients with gallstone pancreatitis. At present, numerous studies have confirmed the safety of early operative intervention. It is now widely agreed that early laparoscopic cholecystectomy takes advantage of edematous tissue planes, which often makes dissection easier and safer. Therefore, patients presenting with gallstone pancreatitis most often undergo interval cholecystectomy during the index admission.

The role of ERCP in patients with gallstone pancreatitis has long been debated and remains controversial. Cholangiography is a vitally important step in the management of these patients and serves both diagnostic and potentially therapeutic functions. In general, preoperative ERCP is reserved for patients who have a high likelihood of persistent choledocholithiasis. This includes patients with obstructive jaundice, persistently elevated liver function tests, and persistent hyperamylasemia or hyperlipasemia. Patients whose biochemical parameters normalize are more likely to have spontaneously passed a stone. Such individuals are unlikely to need therapeutic biliary intervention and are best served with an intra-operative cholangiogram.

The finding of common bile duct stones intraoperatively is best handled on an institutional and individual basis. Centers that perform a high volume of ERCP can intervene postoperatively with little risk of failed stone extraction (<10%). Failed stone extraction usually mandates operative common bile duct exploration. Initial open or laparoscopic common bile duct exploration is probably a more reasonable approach in centers with less experience or in patients who have more than five stones or stones greater than 2 cm. Some authors favor elimination of preoperative ERCP in this algorithm, citing lower morbidity and cost associated with routine intra-operative cholangiography and laparoscopic common bile duct exploration. Although there is no widespread agreement on the sequence of treatment in these patients, the preceding algorithm represents a reasonable and safe approach.

## VII. CONDUCT OF OPERATION (PANCREATIC DÉBRIDEMENT)

The traditional approach to infected pancreatic necrosis includes extensive débridement followed by placement of suction drainage into the lesser sac with complete closure of the abdominal fascia. Closed suction drains have now been replaced with continuous lavage catheters that simultaneously ir-rigate and drain the lesser sac. Ongoing irrigation and suction of the lesser sac is effective, but reoperation is required for recurrent sepsis or intraab-dominal fluid collection.

An alternative approach to these patients is débridement and subse-quent packing and open drainage of the lesser sac. With this technique, the pancreas is débrided, and the lesser sac is packed and kept open. Re-operation is planned every 48 hours pending complete resolution of the necrosis accompanied by evidence of granulation tissue formation. There is no general agreement on which of these two techniques is the best form of treatment, and both are in widespread use. The following text describes the steps in pancreatic débridement that are common to both techniques.

The abdomen is prepped and draped in the usual sterile fashion. A bi-lateral subcostal incision is made and the peritoneum entered. The lesser sac is entered by dividing the gastrocolic ligament. The stomach is mobi-lized off the anterior surface of the pancreas. Finger dissection and bulb sy-ringe irrigation are used to evacuate necrotic debris.

Complete exposure of the pancreas is vital to successful débridement. The splenic flexure and left colon must be mobilized to fully expose the body and tail of the pancreas. It may be necessary to divide the middle colic vessels if necrosis extends to these vessels. The hepatic flexure is also mobi-lized. The right colon is only mobilized when necrosis extends to a retrocolic position. After mobilization of the colon, a generous Kocher maneuver should be performed. Extensive mobilization of the duodenum allows for bimanual inspection of the pancreatic head. Débridement in this region should be performed with extreme caution. It is vital to avoid unnecessary injury to the duodenum, jejunum, or superior mesenteric vessels.

Débridement should continue until bleeding is encountered. At this point, viable tissue is likely present and may be obscured by overlying necrosis and inflammation. It is important to remain conservative and plan return trips to the operating room if necessary rather than to extensively débride potentially viable parenchyma. Overaggressive débridement can result in diabetes or malabsorption syndromes, which may be avoided with a more cautious approach.

## POSTOPERATIVE ORDERS
**Admit to:** ICU
**Diagnosis:** pancreatitis
**Condition:** critical
**Vital signs:** q1h
**Activity:** bedrest
**Allergies:**
**Nursing:**
**Diet:** strict NPO
**IV fluids:** $D_5$/0.45% NS 20 mEq KCl/L at 125 ml/h (for 70-kg patient with no comorbidity)
**Medications:** Demerol PCA
Tylenol, 650 mg PR, q4h prn
Pepcid (or equivalent), 20 mg IV, q12h (if NPO)
Imipenem-cilastatin
**Laboratory tests:** CBC, BMP, ionized calcium, magnesium, phosphorus, amylase, lipase, LFTs, ABGs, PT, and PTT on arrival at ICU

### VIII. COMPLICATIONS

Morbidity after pancreatic débridement occurs in three major forms. The most common postoperative complication is bleeding. This can result from extensive débridement in the face of coagulopathy or poor surgical hemostasis. On other occasions, erosion of necrotic or inflamed tissue into an adjacent blood vessel can precipitate acute postoperative hemorrhage. When coagulopathy is present, fluid resuscitation and rapid correction of the coagulation deficit are the most important initial steps. In other cases, urgent return to the operating room may provide the safest and most definitive means of controlling postoperative bleeding. Angiography can also play a role in select cases.

Bowel ischemia or infarction can develop acutely or in delayed fashion after pancreatic débridement. This most often results from division of vital blood supply secondary to involvement of the mesocolon or mesentery by the inflammatory process. Such patients may require bowel resection or second-look procedures.

ACUTE PANCREATITIS    21

Small bowel fistulas can arise and may be more common in the setting of open packing of the lesser sac. Such fistulas tend to be proximal and high output, resulting in a low rate of spontaneous closure. Despite this, initial nonoperative management, including total parenteral nutrition, nasogastric suction, and possibly somatostatin, is advisable.

## IX. DISCHARGE ORDERS

Patients with acute pancreatitis are ready for discharge when they are tolerating a regular diet, without evidence of abdominal pain or tenderness, and their amylase and lipase levels have normalized. Patients with gallstone pancreatitis should have an interval laparoscopic cholecystectomy scheduled.

# CIRRHOSIS

*Justin S. Wu*
*Michael J. Henderson*

## I. INTRODUCTION

The aphorism "There is no such thing as a good cirrhotic patient" is particularly true when a patient with cirrhosis needs a general surgical procedure. This might equally be titled, "How to take a good-risk patient and convert him into a nightmare," with bleeding, ascites, fluid leak from the wound, infection, liver failure, and multisystem organ failure. These sequela can easily occur after general surgical interventions in patients with cirrhosis, but the risk of doing so can be minimized with careful management. Guidelines to the resident managing these patients focus on preoperative evaluation, assessing the necessity for surgery, the patient risk, and operative factors that can be optimized. In the perioperative period, attention to detail regarding coagulopathy, fluid management, and minimizing the risk of infection will improve outcomes. The important lesson for residents is that a good operation is not enough in such patients: the total care of the patient is essential for a good outcome.

## II. PATHOPHYSIOLOGY

The pathophysiology of cirrhosis as it affects general surgical care highlights two factors:

1. Development of portal hypertension
2. Liver function impairment

Portal hypertension, portal venous pressure exceeding 12 mm Hg often is associated with variceal bleeding and ascites. The pathophysiology of portal hypertension follows a well-defined sequence with (1) cirrhosis obstructing portal venous flow and raising portal pressure, (2) development of collaterals to allow splanchnic blood flow to drain around the high resistance in the liver, (3) expansion of plasma volume, and (4) development of a hyperdynamic systemic circulation. These factors all have potential implications in the management of a general surgical patient.

The collaterals, which from a purely practical point of view always flow from the high-pressure splanchnic circulation to a low-pressure systemic connection, can become the site of significant intraoperative bleeding. The bleeding occurs primarily at the natural locations around the gastroesophageal junction, in the retroperitoneum, or in the anterior abdominal wall but are also found at the sites of prior surgery. It is important to understand that any anastomosis of the high-pressure splanchnic venous system of the gut to the abdominal wall, such as with a stoma, invites the formation of collaterals (varices) at this site.

The systemic hemodynamic changes can also be misleading to the resident managing these patients. The characteristics of the hyperdynamic circulation are a high cardiac output, low total systemic vascular resistance, with a picture akin to sepsis. Of particular concern should be the patient with cirrhosis who has not developed this hyperdynamic circulation: this implies underlying cardiac disease and indicates an inability to respond to the stresses of a surgical intervention.

Impaired liver function is the most sinister component of cirrhosis with respect to prognosis. Cirrhosis is the end result of hepatocellular injury from any cause with necrosis, lobular collapse, an attempt at healing with irregular regenerative nodules, and the development of bridging fibrosis around these regenerative nodules. The liver failure component is a reflection of dysfunctional hepatocytes in a disorganized pattern that are unable to perform the normal functions of the liver. From a practical point of view, this means that coagulation may be impaired, as exhibited by a prolonged prothrombin time, and nutrition may be impaired, as exhibited by a low serum albumin. In addition, cirrhosis impairs the ability to metabolize drugs, such as narcotics and sedatives. Although patients with early cirrhosis may pass the "end of the bed test" by looking satisfactory, the above functions are impaired to some degree in all of them, and it is important at the time of evaluation to assess the severity.

## III. TYPICAL PRESENTATION

The patient with cirrhosis may present with any general surgical problem from a "simple" hernia through the full spectrum of gastrointestinal, endocrine, breast, and other general surgical problems. The evaluation of the general surgical pathology is the same for a patient with cirrhosis as for any patient: to reach an accurate diagnosis to allow planning of appropriate therapy.

The added component in these patients is asking the question as to the severity of their underlying liver disease and its likely impact on their long-term prognosis. The cirrhosis have an impact not only on the surgical decision but also on other disease-management decisions, such as chemotherapy or other medications indicated to manage the underlying diseases. It is these factors that form the focus of the workup from the cirrhosis perspective.

## IV. PREOPERATIVE WORKUP

Preoperative evaluation of cirrhosis is a combination of clinical assessment by history and physical examination, laboratory studies, and radiologic imaging. The goal of this evaluation is to accurately assess the severity of the underlying cirrhosis, assign a risk score, and define a treatment plan pertinent to the cirrhosis. The key ingredients of a preoperative workup in a patient with cirrhosis are to:

1. Assess liver function
2. Evaluate for ascites
3. Ascertain if there is portal hypertension

**Liver function** is assessed by a combination of clinical and laboratory data. The Child-Pugh classification given in Table 22-1 uses the clinical parameters of ascites and encephalopathy and the laboratory values of bilirubin, albumin, and prothrombin time to assign a risk score. Although this classification was developed to assess perioperative risk in patients with cirrhosis undergoing decompression surgery, it has proved useful for patients with cirrhosis having any surgical procedure. Ascites and encephalopathy are signs of liver decompensation and indicate an increased operative risk. A bilirubin in excess of 2 mg/dl indicates impaired liver function, and an albumin less than 3 g/dl is a warning sign of poor synthetic function. The most sensitive of the laboratory tests for evaluating liver function is prothrombin time; which if prolonged with an INR >1.3 indicates some impairment of liver function and with an INR >1.6 indicates significant impairment.

The Child-Pugh score assigns grades for assessing the perioperative mortality and morbidity risk for a patient with cirrhosis: (1) a patient graded A has only a minimally increased risk; (2) a patient graded B has a 5- to 10-fold increased operative risk; and (3) a patient graded C has a 10- to 20-fold increased risk. These broad guidelines apply to virtually any general surgical procedure.

**Is There Ascites?** Ascites initially is diagnosed clinically by abdominal examination and percussion looking for shifting dullness. When the diagnosis is in doubt, an abdominal ultrasound can be a useful adjunct in evaluating for ascites. The third limb of assessment is to determine whether the patient is on a strict salt-restriction diet and is taking significant

22

CIRRHOSIS

**TABLE 22-1**

**CHILD-PUGH SCORE**

|  | 1 Point | 2 Points | 3 Points |
|---|---|---|---|
| Bilirubin (mg/dl) | <2 | 2-3 | >3 |
| Albumin (g/dl) | >3.5 | 2.8-3.4 | <2.7 |
| Protime (INR) | <1.5 | 1.6-2.4 | >2.5 |
| Ascites | None | Mild | Moderate |
| Encephalopathy | None | 1-2 | 3-4 |
| Grade: | A = 5-6 points | B = 7-9 points | C = 10-15 points |

INR, international normalized ratio.

diuretics for control of ascites. A patient who is taking high-dose spirono-lactone (Aldactone) and furosemide (Lasix) to control ascites is at increased perioperative risk of developing significant ascites, which carries a high morbidity in abdominal operative procedures.

**Portal hypertension** as defined above is present in most patients with cirrhosis. This is important clinically if the patient has any of the sequela of portal hypertension, such as gastroesophageal varices, ascites, or hypersplenism. As a general guideline, a patient with cirrhosis should have an upper gastrointestinal endoscopy to look for varices. If moderate to large varices are present, the patient should be on a beta blocker to reduce the pressure in these varices and to reduce the risk of an initial variceal bleed. In addition, large gastroesophageal varices are harbingers of significant intra-abdominal portal hypertension and collaterals, which will play a significant role in any planned gastrointestinal procedure.

## PREOPERATIVE ORDERS

### Acute Variceal Bleeding

**Admit to:** general surgery service, ICU

**Diagnosis:** cirrhosis, esophagogastric acute variceal bleeding due to portal hypertension

**Condition:** guarded

**Vital signs:** q1h

**Activity:** bed rest

**Allergies:**

**Nursing:** intubation if indicated for airway; ventilator settings per ICU team; I&Os q1h; Foley to gravity; CVP q2h; arterial line; NGT to gravity after 1 L NS lavage

**Diet:** NPO

**IV fluids:** 2 large-bore IV access lines; $D_5$/0.45% NS + 20 mEq KCl at 100 ml/h

**Medications:** octreotide drip 50 $\mu$g/h
famotidine (Pepcid) 20 mg IV q12h
piperacillin-tazobactam (Zosyn) 3.375 g IV q6h

**Laboratory tests on admission:** CBC, PT-INR, PTT, CMP, GGT, hepatitis panel, ECG, CXR, T&C 6 units PRBCs

**Laboratory tests q6h:** CBC, PT-INR

**Consult:** GI service for upper endoscopy: possible banding and rule out peptic ulcer disease

**Consult:** alert interventional radiology for possible emergent TIPS

### Elective Distal Splenorenal Shunt

**Admit to:** general surgery service

**Diagnosis:** cirrhosis; preop distal splenorenal shunt

**Condition:** stable

**Vital signs:** per routine
**Activity:** ad lib
**Allergies:**
**Nursing:** I&Os per routine; prep weight; bowel prep: magnesium
    citrate 1 bottle PO at 2 PM day before surgery; hold all beta blockers
    48 hours before surgery and reserve SICU bed
**Diet:** 2 g Na restricted clear liquid diet; NPO after midnight
**IV fluids:** $D_5$/0.45% NS + 20 mEq KCl at 75 ml/h
**Medications:** dexamethasone 10 mg IV on call to OR
                ceftizoxime 1 g IV on call to OR
**Laboratory tests:** CBC, CMP, GGT, PT-INR, PTT, hepatitis panel, ECG,
    CXR, T&C 4 units PRBCs, galactose elimination capacity (if avail-
    able), angiogram: SMA and splenic artery to venous phase; hepatic
    venous pressure gradient and left renal vein
**Consult:** anesthesia

## V. OPERATIVE PROCEDURES

The key in perioperative management of patients with cirrhosis is for the surgeon to work in conjunction with the anesthesiologist. These patients not only
have impaired ability to metabolize anesthetic and narcotic drugs but also
require meticulous attention to detail in their perioperative fluid management
to minimize postoperative complications in the succeeding week.

Anesthetic drugs and narcotics, particularly those metabolized by the
liver, need to be used with caution in these patients. They may require
significant dose reduction, as these agents are potent precipitants to
encephalopathy. Being cautious with their medications to prevent
encephalopathy is better than having to treat them for it.

Perioperative fluid management starts with careful preoperative preparation and strives to minimize free sodium intake, thereby lessening the risk of
postoperative ascites. Avid sodium retention with a secondary hyperaldosteronism is the cause of fluid retention and ascites formation in the cirrhotic
patient. Thus, avoiding normal saline or Ringer's lactate, using 0.45% or
0.2% normal saline, and running the patient "dry" are the chief factors in
minimizing ascites. If the patient is truly intravascular-volume depleted, he or
she may require albumin, fresh-frozen plasma, or blood products: the goal in
this situation is to expand intravascular volume with fluid that will be
maintained in the circulation and not move into the tissue or become ascites.
When patients with cirrhosis have ascites, they should be on adequate doses
of spironolactone preoperatively to improve sodium excretion. A urine
sodium/potassium ratio >1.0 indicates improved sodium excretion.

Infection is the other major perioperative risk because of the impaired
immune response of the patient with cirrhosis. Increased translocation of
bacteria from the gastrointestinal tract occurs with portal hypertension.
Appropriate perioperative antibiotic prophylaxis should be used for any
abdominal procedure in patients with cirrhosis.

## POSTOPERATIVE ORDERS

**Admit to:** SICU, general surgery service

**Diagnosis:** s/p distal splenorenal shunt

**Condition:** stable

**Vital signs:** q1h

**Activity:** ad lib

**Allergies:**

**Nursing:** I&Os q1h; Foley to gravity; call house officer if urine output <15 ml/h; daily weights; PAS when in bed; IS 10 puffs q1h while awake; up in chair tid starting POD 1

**Diet:** NPO; NGT to gravity × 24 h, then ice chips; advance to 2 g Na, 30 g low fat diet

**IV fluids:** $D_5$/0.45% NS + 20 mEq KCl at 80 ml/h

**Medications:** ceftizoxime 1 g IV × 1 dose

famotidine (Pepcid) 20 mg IV q12h (change to PO when patient is able)

spironolactone 50 mg PO tid starting POD 1

**Laboratory tests on admission to SICU:** CBC, CMP, GGT, PT-INR, PTT, Mg, CXR

**Daily laboratory tests:** CBC, CMP, PT-INR, urine Na, urine K; angiogram on POD 6: shunt catheterization with pressures, SMA to portal phase

**Consult:** hepatology service regarding liver biopsy review and postshunt liver follow-up

## VI. COMPLICATIONS

The major postoperative complications encountered by patients with cirrhosis requiring general surgical procedures are:

1. Ascites
2. Liver failure
3. Infection

All of the above carry a significant morbidity and mortality risk. Ascites is frequently the initiating event that can lead to leaking of fluid through the wound, infection, and multisystem organ failure. Liver failure is the predominant cause of death. Management of these complications focuses on the priorities of:

1. Preoperative evaluation and risk assessment
2. Perioperative precautions
3. Postoperative diagnosis and therapy

For the high-risk patient with cirrhosis, Child-Pugh grade C preoperatively, every consideration must be given to not proceeding with a general surgical procedure. The only operation that will benefit this patient will be a liver transplant. If another operative procedure is unavoidable, the emphasis then is on minimizing the risks outlined above.

In the Child-Pugh grade B patient the perioperative risks are increased approximately 10-fold. Emphasis again must be on reducing these risks with careful fluid and electrolyte management and steps to minimize the risk of infection. The wisdom of proceeding with a general surgical procedure must be weighed against the risks of avoiding an operation.

A Child-Pugh grade A patient is a reasonable operative risk but again requires appropriate management precautions. An operation is one of the quickest ways to make a Child-Pugh grade A patient into a Child-Pugh grade C patient.

## VII. DISCHARGE INSTRUCTIONS

The management of a cirrhotic patient after a general surgical procedure is not completed at the time of discharge. It is necessary to continually emphasize to the patient and his or her family the risks associated with their liver disease. Continued careful fluid and electrolyte management with diuretics is important. Nutrition is another key factor, and the patient should be encouraged to maintain an adequate-protein, low-sodium (2 g) diet. Antibiotics are required for patients with persistent ascites to minimize the risk of translocation and bacterial peritonitis.

22

CIRRHOSIS

# LIVER CANCER AND RESECTION

*Eren Berber*

An appreciation of the hepatic segmental anatomy, a better understanding of liver physiology, use of intraoperative ultrasonography, improvements in surgical technique and postoperative care have resulted in a major advance in liver surgery. Meticulous preoperative preparation and perioperative management of these patients is essential for surgical outcome and requires an understanding of the multiple functions and complex pathophysiology of the liver.

## 23

## I. PATHOPHYSIOLOGY

Ninety percent of primary liver cancers are hepatocellular carcinomas. Approximately 10% are cholangiocarcinomas, hepatoblastomas, and sarcomas. Hepatocellular carcinoma is classified into several histologic types, with the fibrolamellar variant having a much better prognosis than the other types. The fibrolamellar variant usually is not associated with elevated serum alpha-fetoprotein levels, chronic hepatitis B infection, or cirrhosis and is more often resectable. Primary liver tumors generally exist as a large mass with or without satellite tumors. The tumor spreads initially to the hepatic veins and then to lung and bone. The average survival after diagnosis without treatment is 6 to 12 months.

The clinical behavior of hepatic colorectal metastases reflects the underlying biologic determinants of these tumors. The best survival is associated with resection of a solitary metastasis, clear surgical margins, and the absence of extrahepatic disease. Positive lymph nodes or dedifferentiation in the primary tumor are poor prognostic indicators. Extrahepatic metastases, even if they are resectable, virtually eliminate any survival value of hepatic resection. Metastases reach the liver by four routes: (1) direct invasion (stomach, colon, bile ducts, and gallbladder tumors), (2) lymphatics (breast and lung), (3) hepatic artery (lung, melanoma), and (4) portal vein. The portal vein is the most frequent route. Once established, metastases derive their entire blood supply from the hepatic artery.

Of the patients with colorectal liver metastases, only about 20% of the untreated patients are alive at 3 years, and very few live 5 years. Median survival is less than 1 year. The natural clinical course of neuroendocrine liver metastases is often slow, and survival of untreated patients may vary. The average survival of untreated metastatic carcinoid tumors has been reported to be 8 years. The 5-year survival of carcinoid and islet cell tumors ranges between 13% and 54%. For most other solid organ malignancies, the pattern of liver metastases is generally that of a generalized dissemination and carcinomatosis.

## II. TYPICAL PRESENTATION

Primary liver cancer is rare in the United States, with an incidence of 1 to 3 per 100,000 each year. The age range is usually between 40 and 60 years. The disease is more frequent in Asia and Africa, where it is associated with the presence of hepatitis B virus antigen in more than 70% of the cases; in contrast, the association in Western countries is 15% to 40%. The development of hepatocellular cancer (HCC) is also closely related to hepatitis C virus infection (75% to 80% of the patients with HCC in Spain and Japan). In Africa, aflatoxin from *Aspergillus flavus* is also etiologically related. In the United States, primary liver cancer is usually associated with cirrhosis or chronic hepatitis. Most of the patients are not candidates for surgical resection because of severe underlying disease, extrahepatic metastases, large tumor size, multicentricity, and major hepatic vascular involvement.

HCC is frequently silent in the early course of the disease. The most frequent complaint is general malaise, followed by anorexia, abdominal pain, abdominal fullness, and weight loss. Severe abdominal pain is associated with bleeding within the HCC nodule or tumor rupture into the peritoneal cavity. Liver failure or biliary system invasion may result in jaundice.

Liver metastases develop in as many of 50% of patients with a primary malignancy. However, isolated hepatic metastases most commonly develop from colorectal and neuroendocrine tumors. Colorectal cancer is responsible for two thirds to three fourths of liver metastases referred for resection. It is reported that between 10% and 30% of patients operated for primary colon cancer will have synchronous metastatic liver disease. However, only 25% of these patients have technically resectable liver metastases at the time of original surgery. In approximately 50% of patients, metachronous liver metastases will subsequently develop.

Patients with colorectal liver metastases do not generally have symptoms in the early course of the disease. The diagnosis may be made during routine preoperative or intraoperative evaluation of the primary tumor or during follow-up after resection of the primary cancer, where liver metastases are seen on computed tomography (CT) scans obtained for serial elevations of carcinoembryonic antigen (CEA).

Liver metastases develop in less than 5% of patients with a carcinoid tumor, 5% to 10% of the patients with insulinoma, in 23% to 90% of the patients with gastinoma, and in 70% to 75% of the patients with glucagonoma. Because of the limited efficacy of systemic therapies, the slow growth of tumor, and the presence of significant symptoms related to hormone production, both aggressive, complete surgical resection and cytoreductive surgery have been advocated for neuroendocrine liver metastases.

In patients with neuroendocrine liver metastases, symptoms are usually related to hormone oversecretion. Metastatic carcinoid tumors, most commonly originating from the gastrointestinal tract, can result in the carcinoid syndrome with flushing and diarrhea.

## III. PREOPERATIVE WORKUP

Routine liver function tests are obtained to detect underlying liver disease. A more specific test, such as measurement of the indocyanine green retention rate, can be useful to select the type of treatment for HCC patients with associated chronic liver disease. Alpha-fetoprotein (AFP) is used as a tumor marker for HCC; however, it may be normal in 75% of the patients and is meaningful if it is found to be elevated. Other blood tests including albumin level, coagulation studies (prothrombin time/partial thromboplastin time [PT/PTT]), and hemogram are also obtained. Liver volume can be calculated radiographically (by CT and magnetic resonance imaging [MRI]) and may be used as an approximate guide to hepatic resection.

Actual diagnosis of HCC is made by histology of tissue obtained by a percutaneous biopsy. Ultrasonography, CT, MRI, and angiography are the radiologic studies available to determine the anatomic location of the tumor and to differentiate it from other mass lesions of the liver. For most tumors, MRI offers no significant advantage over a contrast CT scan. It may have an advantage in detecting lesions smaller than 2 cm, however. CT scanning 2 to 3 weeks after injection of iodized poppy seed oil through the hepatic artery (Lipiodol CT) has also been advocated to detect small intrahepatic metastases of HCC. Metastatic disease, most commonly to the lungs and bone, is a contraindication for resection. A CT scan of the chest and a bone scan should be a part of the workup for a patient considered for surgery. Poor liver function and cirrhosis are contraindications for a major liver resection.

Plasma CEA levels are elevated in 89% to 95% of the patients with colorectal liver metastases. Radiologic imaging with CT or MRI should be obtained to establish the extent of hepatic and extrahepatic disease. CT arterioportography (CTAP) is a sensitive imaging technique, however, it requires the placement of a catheter in the superior mesenteric artery. It is also hindered by the flow artifacts within the liver that appear as defects, increasing the false-positive rate. MRI has a lower incidence of false positive results than CT or CTAP, and also when the nature of a lesion is unclear, MRI can characterize it more accurately. Chest CT and colonoscopy should also be performed before resection to rule out pulmonary metastasis and metachronous colon cancer.

### PREOPERATIVE ORDERS

**Nursing:** bowel preparation not necessary
**Diet:** NPO after midnight before surgery
**Laboratory tests:** LFTs, CBC, PT, PTT, AFP and CEA levels, and T&C for 4 U PRBCs.

## IV. SURGICAL ANATOMY

The ligaments of the liver include the falciform ligament, the right and left posterior coronary ligaments, and the right and left triangular ligaments. The hepatoduodenal ligament contains the extrahepatic bile duct system, the hepatic artery, and the portal vein. The portal vein is formed behind the pancreatic head by the confluence of the splenic vein, the superior mesenteric vein, and in a minority of the cases, the inferior mesenteric vein. The portal vein divides into a left and right branch in the liver. The three major hepatic veins—the right, left, and the middle—are formed by the hepatic venous system that begins from the central vein. The hepatic veins are intersegmental· the middle hepatic vein lies in the main lobar fissure, the left hepatic vein in the left segmental fissure, and the right hepatic vein in the right segmental fissure (Figs. 23-1 and 23-2).

The liver is divided into two lobes by the main portal fissure, which extends from the gallbladder fossa to the left side of the inferior vena cava. The right portal fissure divides the right lobe into an anteromedial and posteriomedial sector. The falciform ligament divides the left lobe into a medial and lateral segment. The liver is further divided into eight Couinaud segments, which are the smallest anatomic hepatic units. In this system, segment I, the caudate lobe, is autonomous in that it receives branches from both the right and left portal vein and hepatic artery branches, and its hepatic venous drainage is independent and may drain directly into the inferior vena cava (Figs. 23-1 and 23-2).

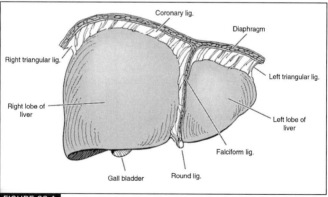

**FIGURE 23-1**

The lobes and ligaments of the liver. The liver is divided into the right and left lobes by a line extending from the gallbladder fossa to the inferior vena cava. The lower free border of the falciform ligament is termed the "round ligament" and contains the obliterated left umbilical vein.

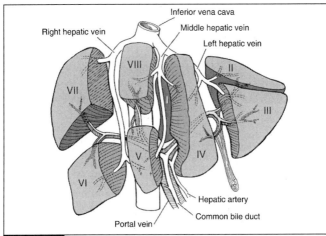

#### FIGURE 23-2

Segmental and vascular anatomy of the liver. The liver is divided into eight Couinaud segments. The hepatoduodenal ligament includes the portal vein, hepatic artery, and the extrahepatic bile ducts. The bile duct descends along the right margin of the ligament to the right of the hepatic artery and anterior to the portal vein. The hepatic veins are intersegmental. The right hepatic vein usually drains directly into the vena cava, whereas the middle and the left hepatic veins coalesce 60% of the time to drain into the inferior vena cava.

Resection along the main portal fissure is termed a right or left lobectomy (or hepatectomy). Resection of the entire right lobe and the medial segment of the left lobe is termed a right extended lobectomy (trisegmentectomy). Left lateral segmentectomy includes removal of segments II and III. Unisegmentectomy refers to removal of a single segment (Fig. 23-3).

#### V. CONDUCT OF OPERATION

A first-generation cephalosporin is used for surgical prophylaxis and if significant blood loss is anticipated, autologous blood should be available for intraoperative use.

Before considering resection, exploration of the extent of hepatic and extrahepatic disease is critical. Two important diagnostic tools in the operating room include laparoscopy and intraoperative ultrasonography. Laparoscopic evaluation of the liver and the abdominal cavity may identify unresectable metastatic disease and cirrhosis in the nontumor-bearing portion. Intraoperative ultrasonography aids in defining the location of vascular

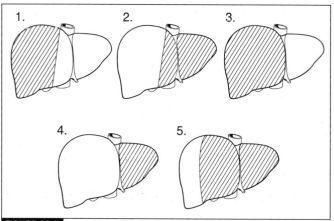

**FIGURE 23-3**

Schematic drawing showing the major resections: (1) right hepatectomy, (2) left hepatectomy, (3) extended right hepatectomy, (4) left lateral segmentectomy, and (5) extended left hepatectomy.

structures, the extent of resection for adequate margins, and the presence of occult intrahepatic or extrahepatic metastases.

For right hepatic lobectomy, a right subcostal incision is made, either with a left subcostal extension in a chevron fashion or with an extension craniad over the xiphoid. Ligamentum teres, the falciform, right triangular, and right coronary ligaments to the inferior vena cava are transected to facilitate the delivery of the right lobe into the wound. The cystic artery and duct are ligated and divided before dissection of the hepatoduodenal structures. The right hepatic artery, the right portal vein, and the right main hepatic duct are dissected free, and tapes are passed around them. These structures may then be doubly ligated in continuity and divided, or the vascular tapes may be tightened for temporary occlusion. After this step, hepatectomy can be completed in one of two approaches. In the first one, hepatic veins are secured outside the liver as they drain into the cava. Then the capsule of the liver is incised, and the parenchyma is transected by clamping, dividing, and ligating vessels and ducts in the interlobar plane. In the second approach, which is safer than the former, the hepatic parenchyma is transected in the interlobar plane. The parenchyma is transected using the ultrasonic aspirator (CUSA) or the digital dissection technique, which involves disrupting liver tissue but not vascular or biliary tissues in the interlobar plane. These structures are then ligated and divided. The dissection is continued posterosuperiorly until the right hepatic vein is encountered. The hepatic vein is isolated within the liver parenchyma, doubly clamped, and then divided with the caval side being closed with continuous sutures. After transection of the parenchyma, the specimen is removed, and the vascular and ductal tapes are released to determine the presence of bleeding or biliary leak. The raw surface of the liver is coagulated with argon beam and may be covered with a pedicle of omentum, although it is not necessary. Local hemostatic agents may also be applied to the raw surface of the liver. The remaining Glisson's capsule may sometimes be approximated with interrupted catgut sutures to reduce the raw area and provide a tamponade effect. Usually two Jackson Pratt drains are used to drain the subphrenic space.

If the remaining parenchyma is normal (ie, no fatty change, fibrosis), intermittent clamping of the porta hepatis (Pringle's maneuver) might be used during resection to control intraparenchymal bleeding. Pringle's maneuver may be safely maintained for up to 60 minutes at ambient temperature. Resection of large central tumors close to the vena cava or the hepatic veins might be performed using total vascular exclusion, which involves simultaneous clamping of the hepatic pedicle and vena cava above and below the liver.

Major hepatic resections are not indicated for patients with advanced cirrhosis, because the risks of intraoperative bleeding from parenchymal vessels and collaterals are significantly increased. Because of lack of reserve and impaired hepatic regeneration, the incidence of liver failure is also increased in these patients.

## VARIATIONS OF OPERATION

Left hepatectomy is essentially the mirror image of a right hepatectomy. It is performed by first identifying and securing the left hepatic artery, left portal vein, and the left hepatic bile duct with hilar dissection. The left and middle hepatic veins are exposed by mobilizing the left lobe of the liver. The liver tissue is divided in the interlobar plane using the same principles.

## POSTOPERATIVE ORDERS

**Admit to:** ICU
**Diagnosis:** s/p liver resection
**Condition:** stable
**Vital signs:** per routine
**Activity:** bed rest, OOB to chair with assistance
**Allergies:**
**Nursing:** strict I&Os, NGT to LCWS overnight, Foley catheter to gravity and remove after epidural discontinued, Pneumoboots, and IS; drains are removed after 4 to 5 days if the drainage is not bilious
**Diet:** NPO then clear fluids POD 1 if bowel function returns
**IV fluids:** $D_5/0.45\%$ NS with 20 mEq KCl at 150 ml/h; albumin infusions generally not necessary
**Medications:** antibiotics for one or two doses postoperatively vitamin K if persistently elevated PT

**Laboratory tests:** a full set of liver enzymes (AST, ALT, ALP, $\gamma$-glutaryl transpeptidase, bilirubin), PT, CBC, and renal function are obtained daily at least for the first 3 days; subsequent studies are obtained according to the patient's course

## VI. COMPLICATIONS

Bleeding in the immediate postoperative period is generally due to ineffective hemostasis and thus usually warrants reexploration. Pleural effusion is the most frequent complication observed. Development of a subphrenic abscess can be managed with catheter drainage under ultrasonographic guidance. Other reported complications include wound infection, intraabdominal infection, bile leak, pulmonary embolism, pneumonia, and liver failure.

## VII. DISCHARGE ORDERS

Follow-up after hepatic resection for cancer should include frequent visits (every 3 months in the first year) with routine blood tests and tumor markers. Although additional studies may be required depending on the primary tumor of the patient, abdominal CT scans are generally obtained every 6 to 9 months to follow the liver.

# PANCREATIC CANCER

*Martin Goodman*

There are approximately 27,000 new cases of pancreatic cancer each year. It is the fifth leading cause of cancer deaths in the United States behind lung, colorectal, breast, and prostate cancer. Ten percent of patients only live 1 year, and less than 4%, 5 years. Age of onset is usually in the fifth decade of life.

## I. PATHOPHYSIOLOGY

Pancreatic cancer is three times more common in smokers than in non-smokers. It is more frequent in men than women, and African-Americans than whites. There may be a link to diabetes mellitus and chronic pancreatitis; however, these might be complications of the disease rather than etiologic factors. Chromosomal abnormalities in tumor suppresser genes *P53, DPC4,* and *MTS1* have been linked to an increased risk of pancreatic cancer and other gastrointestinal malignancies.

Histologically, pancreatic malignancies can be broken down into two groups, exocrine or endocrine in origin. Eighty-five percent of all primary pancreatic malignancies are derived from exocrine cells, with ductal adenocarcinoma being the most common. Histologic variants of ductal adenocarcinoma include giant cell, adenosquamous, microcystic, mucinous, and cystadenocarcinoma. Tumors of endocrine origin include insulinomas, gastrinomas, vasoactive intestinal polypeptide–secreting tumor (VIPomas), all of which are islet cell tumors. Other tumors can metastasize to the pancreas such as breast, lung, melanoma, gastric, colon, and renal cell cancers. Lymphoma can also occur in the pancreas.

The following staging is from the American Joint Committee on Cancer Staging (AJCC).

| | | | |
|---|---|---|---|
| Tis | Carcinoma in situ | | |
| T1 | Tumor limited to the pancreas ≤2 cm in diameter | | |
| T2 | Tumor limited to the pancreas >2 cm in diameter | | |
| T3 | Tumor extends directly into duodenum, bile duct, or peripancreatic tissue | | |
| T4 | Tumor extends to stomach, colon, large vessels | | |
| N0 | No regional nodes | | |
| N1 | Regional nodes | | |
| M0 | No distant metastasis | | |
| M1 | Distant metastasis | | |
| Stage I | T1-T2 | N0 | M0 |
| Stage II | T3 | N0 | M0 |
| Stage III | T1-T3 | N1 | M0 |
| Stage IVA | T4 | Any N | M0 |
| Stage IVB | Any T | Any N | M1 |

## II. TYPICAL PRESENTATION

The most common presentation of pancreatic malignancy to the head or uncinate process includes weight loss, pain, and jaundice. Weight loss may be caused by anorexia and malabsorption from gland dysfunction giving rise to steatorrhea. Pain, which is initially visceral in origin, starts in the midepigastric region and is sometimes confused with peptic ulcer disease or gallbladder disease. Some patients will present with pain similar to that of chronic pancreatitis because of pancreatic duct obstruction from the tumor. Pain that radiates to the back is somatic in origin and is indicative of invasion to the celiac plexus.

Painless jaundice can represent an obstruction of the common bile duct either intrinsically from a gallstone or stricture or extrinsically from a mass. Approximately 75% of patients with adenocarcinoma of the head or uncinate process present with painless jaundice, which is frequently associated with pruritus. Other clinical signs and symptoms include gastric outlet obstruction, adult-onset diabetes, chronic fatigue, and malaise.

## III. PREOPERATIVE WORKUP

As with any presentation, a through history and physical examination must be done. Laboratory studies needed include CBC, BMP, LFTs, PT, PTT, amylase, lipase, carbohydrate antigen 19-9 (CA 19-9), and CEA. Patients with or without jaundice and an elevated total bilirubin should raise the suspicion of a mass obstructing the common bile duct. Elevated alkaline phosphatase, $\gamma$-glutamyl transferase, and other transaminases could also be slightly elevated. Serum markers are not reliable for diagnosing pancreatic malignancies; however, preoperative levels of CEA and CA 19-9 can be followed after treatment to evaluate response and follow for recurrent disease.

Radiographic imaging is essential. Patients who present with jaundice or an elevated bilirubin will require a right upper quadrant ultrasonogram to evaluate the gallbladder, common bile duct, and liver. Patients with a suspected pancreatic mass will need a dynamic CT scan with intravenous and oral contrast with thin cuts through the pancreas. This gives the most information to evaluate the extent of the disease and resectability. Unresectability is determined by extrapancreatic disease, especially hepatic metastasis and the local extension involving the superior mesenteric artery (SMA) or celiac axis and its branches. Portal vein thrombosis is also a deemed an unresectable sign. Lesions abutting the superior mesenteric vein (SMV) or portal vein can still be resected with vein resection and reconstruction.

Newer techniques such as endoscopic ultrasonography (EUS) provide evidence for enlarged celiac nodes and can determine the dimensions of the mass. Fine-needle aspiration (FNA) can also be performed with EUS in an attempt to get a tissue diagnosis.

Endoscopic retrograde cholangiopancreatography (ERCP) is often used to evaluate patients with jaundice and dilated intrahepatic and extrahepatic ducts. Biopsies and brushings are performed if any stricture or narrowing is found. A double duct sign is pathognomonic of a mass at the head of the pancreas. A stent can be placed for biliary drainage and help with symptoms of pruritus. There is no evidence that this improves or increases morbidity or mortality.

Preoperative angiography is rarely needed to evaluate for aberrant vascular anatomy, especially looking for a replaced right hepatic artery. It can be assessed with careful inspection intraoperatively.

The algorithm in the evaluation of a suspected mass at the head of the pancreas should be as follows: (1) right upper quadrant ultrasonography, (2) dynamic CT scan, and (3) ERCP. Dynamic CT scan should be performed before ERCP to prevent distortion of the images if a biliary drainage stent is placed.

Patients with neoplasms of the body and tail of the pancreas usually present late in their disease course. Symptoms could include weight loss, anorexia, vague abdominal pain, or obstruction. These patients are usually diagnosed inadvertently by a CT scan usually looking for other pathology.

All patients with a pancreatic mass will need a chest x-ray looking for metastatic disease or any other underlying pulmonary pathology. A preoperative electrocardiogram is also required. Many patients will require a full cardiac and pulmonary evaluation.

**PREOPERATIVE ORDERS**

1. Reservation of an ICU bed
2. Clear liquid diet 24 hours before surgery and NPO 8 hours before surgery
3. Antibiotics
4. Heparin 5000 units SC
5. PAS
6. A consult to anesthesia to place an epidural catheter to control postoperative pain
7. CXR and ECG if studies are greater than 1 month old
8. CBC, electrolytes, BUN, creatinine, PT, and PTT
9. T&C for 4 units of blood for OR
10. Bowel preparation

Before the induction of anesthesia, compression stockings should be placed and turned on. Subcutaneous heparin and antibiotics are administered. Some patients might require central venous access.

**IV. CONDUCT OF OPERATION**

Laparoscopy is used first to look for metastatic disease not revealed by the CT scan. A careful exploration of the liver and peritoneal surfaces can be performed easily without the need for a large incision. Any suspicious areas

24

PANCREATIC CANCER

are biopsied and sent for frozen sections. If laparoscopy identifies metastatic disease, the operation is stopped, and medical oncology is consulted either in the hospital or on an outpatient basis. Most patients can leave the day of surgery or postoperative day 1.

Tumors of the head and uncinate process are resected with a standard pancreaticoduodenectomy, which is modified from Whipple's initial procedure. The incision can be either a midline or chevron type. Once the incision is made, a through exploration is again performed to look for metastatic disease. If the tumor is deemed unresectable, a bypass procedure can be performed in the presence of biliary or gastric obstruction. A choledochojejunostomy and gastrojejunostomy are both performed. If the patient was having pain preoperatively, a celiac block can be done by injecting 10 ml of 95% ethanol in the paraaortic adventia on each side of the celiac axis. This can give relief for 3 to 6 months, which is usually longer than their life expectancy.

The resection is divided into five steps in a clockwise fashion.

1. A Cattell-Braasch maneuver is performed by mobilizing the right colon to the ligament of Treitz. The lesser sac is then entered through a plane between the greater omentum and transverse colon. The SMV can be identified at this time by following the middle colic vein to its drainage into the SMV or as it enters under the neck of the pancreas. Adherence of the tumor to the SMV or SMA can be evaluated at this time.

2. A Kocher maneuver is performed by mobilizing the duodenum to the left lateral edge of the aorta. The surgeon should not completely mobilize it to the ligament of Treitz, or the small bowel will slip through the defect and make the operation more difficult.

3. The portal dissection starts by palpating the posterolateral aspect of the common bile duct looking for a replaced right hepatic artery. If it is present, great care must be used to preserve the artery. The common hepatic artery is identified and dissected to find the right gastric and gastroduodenal artery. Both the gastroduodenal artery and right gastric artery are ligated and divided. A cholecystectomy is performed with the common hepatic duct divided just cephalad to the cystic duct. The portal vein is also identified and controlled with vessel loops. The posterior pancreatic duodenal vein is a branch of the portal vein found supralateral near the neck of the pancreas and can cause difficult bleeding if care is not taken.

4. The stomach is transected at the third or fourth transverse vein on the lesser curvature to the confluence of the gastroepiploic veins on the greater curvature. The omentum is also divided at the greater curvature transection. The jejunum is transected 10 cm distal from the ligament of Treitz. The duodenal and jejunal mesenteries are ligated and divided to the level of the aorta.

5. Until this point no bridges have been burned. The posterior neck of the pancreas is bluntly dissected if not done so in step 1 or 2. There are no vessels in this area. If adherence to the portal vein or SMV is noted, the resection can proceed more distal in preparation for venous resection. Traction sutures are placed inferior and superior on the neck of the pancreas. The pancreas is then transected proximal to the traction stitches with electrocautery. Once the pancreas is divided, the specimen is dissected free from the retroperitoneum by ligating and dividing venous tributaries and the inferior pancreaticoduodenal artery with complete exposure of the SMA to its origin.

Reconstruction is performed with four steps in a counterclockwise fashion.

1. The pancreatic remnant is mobilized approximately 2 to 3 cm in preparation for the anastomosis. The transected jejunum is brought up retrocolic with enough length so there is no tension on the anastomosis. A neoduodenum should not be made by bringing out the jejunum through the defect in the mesentery where the duodenum was. A neoduodenum can obstruct early if there is a recurrence in this area. The pancreaticojejunostomy can be performed in one of two ways: duct to mucosa or invaginated. This depends on the surgeon and the size of the pancreatic duct. A fibrotic pancreas is better to hold stitches. With larger ducts, greater than 3 mm, a duct-to-mucosa anastomosis can be performed. A small enterotomy is made on the antimesenteric border of the jejunum. Using absorbable 4.0 or 5.0 monofilament suture, the duct of the pancreas to full-thickness jejunum is anastomosed in an interrupted fashion. A silicone elastomer (Silastic) stent is placed across the anastomosis before tying down the sutures. A second layer of nonabsorbable 3.0 monofilament suture is then placed. There should be no tension on this anastomosis. If the duct is small or not visualized, the pancreatic remnant is invaginated into the side of the jejunum in a similar fashion, taking care not to occlude the duct. This is done by placing the pancreas into the jejunum itself.
2. The hepaticojejunostomy is now performed in a single layer, again using an absorbable 4.0 or 5.0 monofilament suture in an interrupted fashion. The placement should be tension free, as well as avoiding placing a kink between it and the pancreaticojejunostomy. Some surgeons will place a stent across this anastomosis.
3. Gastrointestinal continuity is established at this point. A one- or two-layer anastomosis is made, depending on the surgeon's preference. The afferent limb should be approximately 25 to 30 cm, and it can be retrocolic or antecolic. For a retrocolic anastomosis the gastric side should be tacked down to the inferior aspect of the transverse mesocolon.
4. A gastrostomy, feeding jejunostomy, and closed drains are placed.

**24**

**PANCREATIC CANCER**

## VARIATIONS OF OPERATION

The reason for performing a pylorus-sparing versus the modified Whipple procedure is to prevent postgastrectomy syndromes such as early and late dumping. There is, however, an increased risk of prolonged gastric stasis. If a pylorus-sparing pancreaticoduodenectomy is being performed, the duodenum is transected 2 cm distal to the pylorus. Preservation of the right gastroepiploic artery is required in a pylorus-sparing pancreaticoduodenectomy.

The SMV or portal vein reconstruction is performed using an interposition graft of internal jugular or internal iliac vein.

Contrary to tumors of the pancreatic head, tumors of the body and tail are treated with a distal pancreatectomy and splenectomy. Most patients present with metastatic disease because of the late onset of symptoms.

Once again, laparoscopy is performed initially to look for metastatic disease. A midline or chevron incision is made, and a thorough exploration is performed. The splenic flexure is mobilized and the lesser sac entered. The Aird maneuver is performed by mobilizing the spleen from its bed and rolling the pancreas medially and elevating it through a posterior plane.

The SMV is approached much in the fashion previously described. The posterior aspect of the neck is mobilized bluntly just enough to get a stapling device under and across the neck. Once the splenic artery is divided it is ligated at its origin from the celiac axis followed by the splenic vein where it joins the SMV. The retroperitoneal attachments to the pancreas can be bluntly dissected. The remaining venous and arterial tributaries found on the superior and inferior aspect of the pancreas are ligated and transected. The specimen is then removed.

If the pancreatic duct is identified on the transected pancreas, it should be oversewn. Some surgeons will oversew the entire stump. Drains are placed, as well as a feeding jejunostomy tube.

## POSTOPERATIVE ORDERS

**Admit to:** ICU or step-down unit
**Diagnosis:** pancreatic cancer s/p resection
**Condition:** guarded
**Vital signs:** pulse and BP, recorded q1-q2h
**Activity:** bed rest
**Allergies:**
**Nursing:** Foley to gravity, NGT to LCWS, PAS, flush G-tube and J-tube with 30 ml $H_2O$ q6h, gastrostomy tube to gravity, IS qh while awake, ETT placement, ventilator orders if needed
**Diet:** NPO
**IV fluids:** Any solution of choice at 125 ml/h
**Medications:**
    heparin 5000 units SC q8h
    antibiotic of choice × 48 h

epidural as per anesthesia or PCA

octreotide 150 mg SC, q8h

any other medications recommended by consultants

**Laboratory tests:** CBC, BMP, calcium, magnesium, phosphorus, PT, PTT, ABGs, ECG, CXR to look for line placement, CBC, and BMC in AM

Consult: physical therapy

Consult: nutrition

Consult: home care for tube feedings

Consult: medical oncology

Octreotide may be used for 7 days to help prevent a pancreatic leak; however, its use is controversial. Both compression boots and heparin are needed, because these patients are at high risk for deep vein thrombosis and pulmonary embolism.

Patients who needed to go to the intensive care unit postoperatively can usually be transferred to the floor within 48 hours. Tube feedings usually can be started between 24 to 48 hours. The nasogastric tube is removed once there is decreased output and the G-tube is functioning well. A clear liquid diet can be started as soon as bowel function returns while clamping the G-tube during the day and unclamping at night.

## V. COMPLICATIONS

The mortality of this procedure is 2% to 3%. Morbidity ranges from 10% to 40%. Postoperative bleeding can be medical or surgical as in any procedure. The divided gastroduodenal artery should be the first place investigated if the patient returns to the operating room. Pancreatic fistulas can occur up to 10% of the time and can be difficult to manage. Other complications include sepsis, biliary fistula, renal failure, pancreatitis, pulmonary and cardiac events, and prolonged return of gastrointestinal function.

## VI. DISCHARGE INSTRUCTIONS

The 5-year survival after resection is 25%, with most patients having a recurrence within 2 years. Patients usually can be discharged home or to a rehabilitation center in 10 days to 2 weeks. Patients and families should be taught drain care. Drains will be left in at least to the first postoperative office visit. Pain medications should be given. Patients are instructed to do no lifting greater than 10 pounds, no driving, and continue using the incentive spirometer. Patients will go home with tube feedings, usually cycled at night until they are able to take enough calories to maintain themselves. Patients need to call their surgeon if they have a fever, nausea or vomiting, the wound gets painful and red or drains fluid, or there is increased output from the drains. A follow-up visit should be scheduled within 2 weeks after discharge. An appointment with a medical oncologist should also be arranged.

# ENDOSCOPIC RETROGRADE CHOLANGIOPANCREATOGRAPHY

*Jeffrey Hazey*

A number of techniques have been established to image the biliary tract and pancreatic duct. These include percutaneous transhepatic cholangiography (PTHC), magnetic resonance cholangiopancreatography (MRCP), and endoscopic retrograde cholangiopancreatography (ERCP). Each has a unique ability to diagnose and potentially treat disease of the common bile duct (CBD) or pancreatic duct (PD).

PTHC can both image and provide drainage for the biliary tree transhepatically. This drain can provide external and internal drainage into the duodenum to treat bile duct injuries. It can decompress obstructive lesions whether they be neoplastic or benign as with choledocholithiasis. PTHC requires a dilated biliary tract to cannulate the bile ducts percutaneously and is more likely to fail in patients with small or normal size bile ducts.

MRCP possesses the ability to image the biliary tract and pancreatic duct as a diagnostic tool but has no potential for therapeutic intervention.

The most widely accepted technique to image the biliary tract and pancreatic duct and to provide a route for therapeutic intervention is ERCP. It is considered the "gold standard" because of its ability to visualize lesions and conditions affecting any locale in the biliary tree or ampulla of Vater. It is effective in diagnosing and treating lesions of the pancreas and PD. ERCP is the only procedure that provides therapeutic intervention to stent, brush, biopsy, cut, and extract stones or foreign bodies from the CBD or PD.

## I. PATHOPHYSIOLOGY

Diagnostic and therapeutic ERCP must be considered together. There are essentially five fundamental clinical indications.

**Diagnosis and Treatment of Jaundice.** A wide range of disease processes and conditions can cause obstructive jaundice. Obstructive lesions include benign and malignant tumors of the bile ducts, pancreatic head, ampulla of Vater, and duodenum. Chronic or acute pancreatitis involving the pancreatic head can mimic an obstructive neoplasm presenting as a mass or distal biliary stricture. Primary disease processes of the liver including ascending cholangitis, primary biliary cirrhosis, and primary sclerosing cholangitis can be diagnosed with ERCP imaging of the biliary tree.

**Postcholecystectomy Pain and Complications.** A number of complications as a result of cholecystectomy are best diagnosed and treated by ERCP. Biliary strictures, cystic duct stump leak, CBD injuries and retained common bile duct stones can be diagnosed and managed by ERCP.

Typically, stenting for strictures, CBD injuries, and cystic duct leaks prevents the need for reoperation. Stent management includes repeat ERCP and removal or change of a stent as dictated by resolution of the complication. Stents typically last approximately 3 months and require changing if prolonged stenting is required. Should the patient experience fever/chills, right upper quadrant pain, or jaundice typical of ascending cholangitis, urgent evaluation of the stent is necessary with replacement with a new stent if indicated.

**Abdominal Pain of Unknown Cause.** A number of conditions cause abdominal pain in the absence of abnormal imaging studies (ie, ultrasonography), liver function tests, or amylase. Subtle duct abnormalities indicative of early mass lesions not detected by CT scan can be diagnosed.

**Pancreatitis of Unknown Cause.** Patients with acute or chronic pancreatitis in the absence of cholelithiasis, a history of alcoholism, or serum abnormalities can be successfully diagnosed and managed with ERCP. Causes include pancreatic divisum diagnosed by the lack of communication between the duct of Wirsung and Santorini and the main pancreatic duct draining by way of the minor duodenal papilla can cause acute and chronic pancreatitis. Sphincter of Oddi dysfunction diagnosed by obtaining sphincter of Oddi manometry can cause the equivalent of biliary colic in the absence of cholelithiasis. Pancreatic pseudocysts have long been thought to be an absolute contraindication to ERCP for fear of seeding the pseudocyst with bacteria and turning a sterile pseudocyst into an infection of the pancreas. With careful technique and gentle injection of contrast, if it is necessary to define PD ductal anatomy to plan a surgical procedure, ERCP can be performed safely in the face of a pancreatic pseudocyst.

**Postorthotopic Liver Transplantation.** Postoperative bile duct strictures as a result of anastomosis or dissection during orthotopic liver transplantation can be successfully diagnosed and managed with ERCP with or without biliary stenting.

## II. TYPICAL PRESENTATION

The typical presentation leading a patient to ERCP is jaundice. This is obstructive jaundice with elevation of direct or conjugated bilirubin. This may be "painless jaundice" seen in masses involving the bile duct, pancreatic head, ampulla, or duodenum. Postcholecystectomy pain may indicate a bile leak from the cystic duct or a CBD injury necessitating ERCP and stenting. Epigastric pain and an elevation in the serum bilirubin as a result of gallstone pancreatitis may indicate a retained CBD stone. Active acute pancreatitis is a relative contraindication to ERCP, and evaluation of potentially retained stones should be delayed until the pain resolves and the serum amylase is clearly trending downward. Gallstone pancreatitis is not in and of itself an indication for ERCP, because 75% to 80% of these CBD stones pass without any intervention. Evaluation of the biliary tree may be delayed until cholecystectomy in the form of an intraoperative cholangiogram given a clinically improving patient preoperatively.

## III. PREOPERATIVE WORKUP

A number of studies assist the surgeon in the decision to perform ERCP. Elevation of serum bilirubin (conjugated) implies obstruction of the biliary tree. Serum amylase will rise with pancreatitis. Charcot's triad of fever/chills, right upper quadrant pain, and elevation of serum bilirubin (jaundice) is the classic finding in patients with cholangitis. Right upper quadrant ultrasonography is used to diagnose cholelithiasis or choledo-cholithiasis and can delineate the size of the CBD. A dilated CBD implies downstream obstruction, whereas a CBD of normal caliber can frequently rule out a significant obstructive process. A hepato-iminodiacetic acid (HIDA) scan may aid in the diagnosis of bile leak, and the newer cholecystokinin-HIDA is a provocative test to quantify the ejection fraction of the gallbladder. Patients may present with right upper quadrant pain and biliary colic in the absence of cholelithiasis. An ejection fraction below 35% to 40% is diagnostic for biliary dyskinesia. The newest approach to imaging the biliary tree and pancreatic duct is MRCP. As mentioned, this is a diagnostic test without therapeutic potential.

### PREOPERATIVE ORDERS

Before undergoing ERCP, the patient should have a baseline set of liver function tests including bilirubin, amylase, hemoglobin, and coagulation studies (PT and PTT). Should the patient need a sphincterotomy to aid in stone retrieval or placement of a stent, a baseline hemoglobin and normal coagulation studies are essential. Therapeutic ERCP will often require pre-operative antibiotics to prevent cholangitis if the biliary tree needs to be manipulated or instrumented. In addition, the patient should be NPO for at least 6 hours before the procedure with a functioning IV line necessary for intravenous sedation. This IV line is best placed in the right hand or arm to ensure easy access to the site during the procedure.

## IV. SURGICAL ANATOMY

The main duodenal papilla lies on the medial wall of the distal second portion of the duodenum. It has a common channel and orifice through which the CBD and the main PD of Wirsung drain. For approximately 2 to 3 cm proximal to the ampulla of Vater, the CBD runs in the intramural duodenum, and the bulge can be seen protruding on the duodenal mucosa. Proximal to this is the minor duodenal papilla, which drains the accessory pancreatic duct of Santorini. Pancreatic divisum or ventral pancreas occurs when the main pancreatic duct drains by way of the minor duodenal papilla, and there is no communication with the ampulla of Vater.

To perform ERCP, a side-viewing duodenoscope is used to facilitate visualization and cannulation of the ampulla. The common channel of the CBD and PD varies. Typically, the orifice to cannulate the CBD is in the 11 o'clock position and proximal to the PD when the ampulla is viewed "en-face." This anatomic knowledge is necessary for selective cannulation of the CBD or PD.

## V. CONDUCT OF OPERATION

ERCP requires an endoscopist and two assistants. One to monitor the patient and medicate, with a second to directly assist the endoscopist with passage of cannulas, guidewires, dilators, baskets, balloons, or stents. Fluoroscopy in the form of a C-arm or built-in fluoroscopy unit are necessary to image the biliary tree and PD. This procedure may be performed in radiology or an endoscopy suite suited for continuous radiographic assessment. The patient is brought to the endoscopy suite and placed on the fluoroscope table in the left side-down position rolled over to nearly prone with his or her left arm behind the back. Blood pressure monitoring and continuous pulse oximetry are used, and nasal cannula oxygen is placed to ensure oxygenation during intravenous sedation. The patient's throat is anesthetized with cetacaine spray, and the patient is asked to swallow the local anesthetic to suppress the tendency to gag during passage of the scope and when pressure is placed on the oropharynx. Intravenous sedation is used typically with meperidine (Demerol) and diazepam (Valium) or midazolam (Versed) to affect a deep conscious sedation. Atropine can be used to paralyze the stomach and Buscopan or glucagon is used to suppress duodenal and sphincter muscle activity.

The scope is passed blindly into the esophagus and stomach. The stomach is insufflated, and visualization of the pylorus is obtained. Once located, the scope is passed through the pylorus and into the duodenum. The scope is rotated into the retroperitoneal duodenum and passed into the third portion of the duodenum. The scope is pulled back and positioned with an "en-face" visualization of the major duodenal papilla. With this view, selective cannulation of the ampulla with injection of contrast into the CBD or PD can be performed. Once fluoroscopic confirmation of successful cannulation is established, a guidewire is passed and threaded distally into the system in preparation for therapeutic maneuvering. Over this wire, endoscopic sphincterotomy, balloon extraction of CBD stones, brush biopsy, dilators, or stents can be passed as required. The entire process is dynamic with constant repositioning of the scope, catheters, and repeat injections of contrast for frequent fluoroscopic confirmation of position and assessment of therapeutic procedures.

Once the diagnostic or therapeutic ERCP is completed, the scope is withdrawn and the patient recovered in a monitored setting for approximately 1 hour.

## POSTOPERATIVE ORDERS

After the procedure, patients are monitored with blood pressure, continuous pulse oximetry, and periodic "checks" for about an hour. Once the patient is awake, liquids are introduced to ensure his or her ability to tolerate a diet.

## VI. COMPLICATIONS

As with any invasive procedure, ERCP has complications common to other procedures and those unique to this technique. Medication reactions and cardiopulmonary complications can be significant in patients with multiple comorbidities. Complications unique to ERCP include bleeding, infection, perforation, and pancreatitis.

1. Bleeding after ERCP can be the result of an overaggresive sphincter-otomy with transection of a commonly encountered vessel at the top of the "transverse fold" of duodenal mucosa. This anatomic landmark is located proximal to the ampulla. This fold overlies the CBD as it courses through the intramural portion of the duodenum. This complication is further aggravated by a patient with long-standing liver disease who is coagulopathic, taking coumadin, or taking heparin.
2. Infection can be the result of strictures or infected bile during instrumentation of the CBD. This can be further exacerbated by placement of a prosthetic stent, but adequate biliary drainage will often offset this risk. Infection can occur soon after the procedure with seeding of the biliary system at the time of manipulation or weeks to months later. These infections can present as cholangitis or sepsis and commonly occur when a stent malfunctions or fails to drain appropriately (ie, clogs). Treatment is antibiotic coverage of biliary or pancreatic pathogens with removal and replacement of the stent as necessary.
3. Perforation of the esophagus, stomach, or duodenum is uncommon. The blind passage of the endoscope puts the esophagus at risk; thus it is imperative that the scope not be advanced against resistance. The stomach is a rare site of perforation, but previous upper abdominal surgery with associated adhesions and tethering of the stomach or duodenum can place these at risk. Narrowing of the duodenum secondary to mass lesions, pancreatitis, or pseudocyst formation can put the duodenum at risk for perforation as well.
4. Post-ERCP pancreatitis occurs in about 3% of patients undergoing ERCP. This can result from a single injection of the pancreatic duct with contrast but more commonly occurs with repeat overzealous injections during a difficult bile duct cannulation. Acinarization, characterized as visualization of terminal pancreatic ducts in the periphery of the gland, is clearly associated with postprocedural development of pancreatitis. The severity of pancreatitis can be variable. Abdominal pain and elevations in serum amylase can run a

**25**

CHOLANGIOPANCREATOGRAPHY

spectrum from relatively benign lasting only a few hours to complicated or life threatening. Pseudocyst formation or pancreatic necrosis
can be seen after ERCP, thus hospitalization, serial examinations,
and monitoring are occasionally necessary for managing these
patients with abdominal pain.

## VII. DISCHARGE INSTRUCTIONS

Patients are frequently sent home with no specific orders and told to return
should they experience increased abdominal pain, persistent vomiting, fever
or chills, or jaundice. Patients may be given postprocedure antibiotics at
the discretion of the endoscopist, depending on their condition and the procedure. Postprocedure pain medication is again at the discretion of the
treating endoscopist.

# PART VII

## Hernia

# INGUINAL HERNIA

*Keith Zuccala*

Approximately 700,000 inguinal hernia repairs are performed annually; 75% of all hernias are of the inguinal type. Most hernias occur in men (25% of men vs 2% of women will have hernias during their entire lifetime). The natural history of this disease is one of progressively worsening symptoms, which can eventually lead to visceral strangulation, ischemia, and ultimately perforation. Patients often have these hernias for years without progression, but, with certainty, none of them resolve spontaneously. Operative intervention is the "gold standard" for treatment of inguinal hernias, although the proper technique and approach continue to be debated, most likely because the perfect repair has yet to be discovered.

**26**

## I. PATHOPHYSIOLOGY

The pathophysiology of inguinal hernias depends on the type of hernia. Indirect hernias (the most common type in either gender) are due to an "escape" of the peritoneal or intraabdominal contents through the internal ring along the pathway (processus vaginalis) created by passage of the spermatic cord or round ligament. In most people the processus obliterates after testicular descent, but in those with indirect hernias, it remains open or "patent," or in the case of pediatric hernias, the abdominal contents escape before the processus vaginalis has a chance to close. Prematurity and low birth weight are contributing factors to inguinal hernias in the pediatric population.

Direct hernias are thought to be due to a weakening of the abdominal wall musculature. Chronic straining to urinate, defecate, coughing, and heavy lifting are all thought to be causative factors. They are believed to eventually cause trauma and weakness to the inguinal floor, and thereby predispose to the formation of direct hernias. Several interesting histologic factors have also been noted including the decrease in content of hydroxyproline (a major component of collagen) in patients with groin hernias. Patients who smoke are also at an increased risk for groin hernias. Smokers are noted to have elevated serum neutrophil elastase activity that contributes to the breakdown of connective tissue. Smokers have a higher incidence of groin hernias than nonsmokers do, especially women.

Patients present with a groin mass that may be constant or intermittent. It is often, but not always, accompanied by discomfort, which may be "burning" and can radiate down to the genitalia or along the medial thigh. A hernia is considered *reducible* if it can be pushed back up the inguinal canal and the sac/contents can be "reduced" back into the peritoneal cavity. If a hernia cannot be "reduced," it is considered *incarcerated,* and if the content's vascular supply is compromised, then it is considered *strangulated.*

Almost without exception, the indications for herniorrhaphy (direct suture repair) or hernioplasty (repair incorporating prosthetic material) are the presence of an inguinal hernia in all but the rarest of circumstances. Only patients with otherwise terminal conditions should not be considered for operative repair. Mechanical trusses and other nonoperative treatments universally fail to relieve symptoms or arrest the progression of this disease. Trusses may even cause scar formation if used for the long term. Patients who are at great risk because of poor cardiopulmonary status can have this repair done under "local" anesthesia with good results and minimal risk. The repair can be performed on an elective basis, unless the hernia is acutely incarcerated and unreducible or if there is any question of strangulation. Strangulation (and acute incarceration) represents a surgical emergency and requires prompt operative intervention after timely but adequate resuscitation.

## II. TYPICAL PRESENTATION

Most patients present with a groin mass, which usually, but not always, causes pain and discomfort. Sometimes patients present with a history of inguinal pain but no obvious mass. If the hernia has spontaneously reduced, a mass may not be present, but with proper examination in the standing and supine positions, while the patient is relaxed and while performing a Valsalva maneuver, the hernia should be palpable. One of the most reliable ways to palpate a hernia is to have the patient perform the Valsalva maneuver or cough while standing and palpate the pubic tubercle on the affected side. The only structure passing over the tubercle (through the external ring) should be the spermatic cord or round ligament. Other structures palpated are almost universally hernia components. The index finger can also be inserted into the inguinal canal through the external ring and with a Valsalva maneuver; oftentimes a hernia can be palpated. If the bulge pushes down the canal against the examiner's fingertip, the patient most likely has an indirect hernia. If the bulge pushes from the floor of the canal out toward the skin against the side of the examiner's finger, the patient most likely has a direct hernia. The distinction preoperatively is more academic than practically useful, because the approach for repair of either type of inguinal hernia is the same. Of note, however, is that occasionally (3% of all hernias) patients may have a femoral hernia (more common in women), which can be difficult to differentiate from an inguinal hernia on examination. A femoral hernia protrudes through the femoral canal medial to the femoral vein and below the ilioinguinal ligament. The hernia sac may emerge from below the ligament and turn cephalad, lying over the external oblique fascia however, creating a groin mass that may be difficult to distinguish from an inguinal hernia preoperatively.

## III. SURGICAL ANATOMY

Inguinal hernias can be divided into two types on the basis of their anatomic location, direct and indirect. The first branch off of the external iliac artery is the inferior epigastric artery, which supplies the inferior rectus sheath musculature. This artery and its two accompanying veins bisect the myopectineal orifice and establish whether the hernia is considered indirect or direct. Hernias along the spermatic cord, or round ligament in women, that pass through the internal ring by way of a patent processus vaginalis *lateral* to the inferior epigastric vessels are considered *indirect* inguinal hernias. Conversely, hernias *medial* to the inferior epigastric vessels, within the Hesselbach triangle, are *direct* hernias. The Hesselbach triangle is defined as the space within the anterior abdominal wall bordered by the inferior epigastric artery, the ilioinguinal ligament, and the lateral border of the rectus sheath.

In adults the inguinal canal is approximately 4 cm long and 2 to 4 cm superior to the ilioinguinal ligament running parallel to the ligament. The canal is the space through which the spermatic cord or round ligament runs between the internal and external rings. The cord is made up of cremasteric muscle, a venous pampiniform plexus, the testicular artery, the genital branch of the genitofemoral nerve, the vas deferens, cremasteric artery, lymphatics, and the processus vaginalis. The "walls" of the inguinal canal must be viewed in the anatomic context of the groin region. The canal passes obliquely from a deep, superior and lateral internal ring, to a more superficial, inferior, and medial external ring. Remember, the canal runs parallel to the ilioinguinal ligament and is passing from deep (preperitoneal) to superficial (the cord ends at the testicle). The superficial border of the canal is the *external oblique aponeurosis.* The opposite wall or deep border, most commonly known as the *floor,* is formed by the transversalis fascia and the aponeurosis of the transversus abdominis muscle. It is a weakness in the *floor* through which direct hernias occur and through the internal ring (located in the *floor* of the canal) through which indirect hernias occur. As can be seen, the floor is the most important structure of the inguinal canal. The inferolateral border of the canal is created from the ilioinguinal ligament and the lacunar ligament, whereas the superomedial border is formed from a coalescence of the internal oblique muscle, the transversus abdominus muscle, and their respective aponeuroses.

## IV. CONDUCT OF OPERATION

Open hernia repair can be performed under multiple different types of anesthesia, from general to spinal to local. Oftentimes, the type of anesthesia may be determined by the clinical condition of the patient and any comorbid factors. Patients at higher risk from general anesthesia because of cardiopulmonary dysfunction can have their hernia repairs done under local anesthesia with almost no compromise to the operation or repair. Once the patient is anesthetized, the skin should be prepped and draped aseptically. Patients are shaved immediately before the prep, if at all. Patients should receive 1 g cefazolin (Ancef) intravenously before, or on induction, but in either case preceding the incision, unless there is a significant allergic contraindication. Prophylactic antibiotics need to be given before the incision is made, so that drug serum levels are adequate before the start of the procedure. "Remembering" to give the antibiotic just before the mesh is inserted is a waste of money and constitutes poor patient care.

The patient's abdomen may be gently palpated once he or she is adequately anesthetized to document final location of the hernia. One must be careful, however, not to reduce incarcerated or potentially strangulated hernias, because compromised abdominal viscera may unknowingly be reduced back into the peritoneal cavity without the surgeons knowledge and will be unable to be closely examined before their controlled reduction. The incision is begun after the anterior superior iliac spine and the pubic tubercle have been palpated superficially. These two landmarks, along with the ilioinguinal ligament, are used for placement of the incision and possibly local anesthetic if an ilioinguinal nerve block is to be performed. The block is placed 2 cm medial and 2 cm inferior to the anterior superior iliac spine just at the exterior oblique fascia level. The incision is made to follow the Langer lines and should be therefore somewhat curvilinear in nature. The incision should run from the tubercle out laterally for approximately 5 to 6 cm, staying parallel and 2 cm superior to the ilioinguinal ligament. Dissection is then carried through the subcutaneous tissue, including Camper's fascia and Scarpa's fascia, which can be initially mistaken for the external oblique in some well-developed individuals. There are several subcutaneous superficial epigastric vessels that will be encountered and should be ligated. Once the external oblique is encountered, it should be cleaned off from the internal to the external ring. The rings may be difficult to find, especially in obese individuals, and the easiest method for finding the external ring is to clean the fascia inferiolaterally down to the ilioinguinal ligament. The ligament may then be followed medially toward the tubercle. The fibers of the ligament will form the inferior crus of the external ring, so that the ring may be easily located.

Once the ring is identified, an incision is made in the external oblique fascia, parallel to its fibers midway between the internal and external rings. The fascia is then opened from one ring to the other, taking care to identify and preserve the ilioinguinal nerve, which usually lies just under the external oblique fascial layer. The ilioinguinal and iliohypogastric nerves that course through this area supply sensory innervation to the skin of the lower abdomen, penis, and scrotum, and their injury can cause considerable discomfort to both the patient and the surgeon.

The cord itself is then bluntly dissected off of the floor of the canal at the level of the pubic tubercle. Once the cord has been mobilized, a Penrose drain is loosely looped around it to give the surgeon further control during dissection. Mobilization of the cord anywhere but at the level of the tubercle can cause mistaken dissection and obliteration of tissue planes, causing incomplete repair or injury to cord structures.

The canal's floor is checked for any laxity or obvious direct hernias, and then the cord is dissected using mostly blunt and sharp dissection to avoid injury to important cord structures. Electrocautery may be used judiciously for hemostatsis. The cremasteric fibers are cut and released from the cord, and then gentle teasing and careful dissection should allow the surgeon to identify and separate the indirect hernia sac from the cord itself. Occasionally a cord lipoma may be encountered, which should be removed along with separation of the hernia sac from the cord. The end of the hernia sac should be identified, and then the dissection should be carried back to the level of the internal ring. The hernia sac in adults should be opened very carefully with a sharp dissection technique, and the sac should be checked for visceral contents. A *sliding* hernia contains intraabdominal organs in the sac. (Of note, the most common organ encountered in a right-sided sliding hernia is the cecum, and the sigmoid colon on the left.) The presence of both a direct and an indirect hernia is often referred to as a "pantaloon" hernia. Once the sac has been opened and any visceral contents reduced, the sac is twisted along its axis and then suture ligated just superficial to the internal ring. The excess sac is excised, and the cut edge is thoroughly checked for bleeding before being allowed to fall back into the peritoneal cavity. The options for reconstruction of the inguinal floor are legion and mostly of a historical footnote at present. The currently accepted "best repair" at most centers is a Lichtenstein, tension-free repair. A synthetic mesh (usually polypropylene) is measured and cut to the appropriate size and then sutured (with a nonabsorbable, monofilament suture) along the inguinal canal in an effort to reconstruct the floor. Sometimes a mesh "plug" may be placed to reduce a direct hernia or partially "fill" an enlarged internal ring before the mesh overlay used to repair the floor is sutured in place (the so called "plug and patch" technique). The mesh overlay is sutured from the aponeurotic tissue overlying the pubic tubercle to the shelving portion of the ilioinguinal ligament (Poupart's ligament) all the way to a point lateral to the internal ring. The first sutures placed over the tubercle are especially critical, because it is at this point that most hernias recur. If too exuberant a suture is placed, however, and periosteum is pierced, the patient may have chronic pain here. Equally important is to take care not to "bite" too deep when suturing to Poupart's ligament, because the femoral vessels lie just deep to this structure. (NOTE: Femoral hernias occur through the femoral canal and may emerge from under Poupart's ligament.) The superomedial edge of the mesh is sutured to the conjoined tendon superiorly beyond the internal ring. A slit is made in the mesh to allow the cord structures to pass easily without strangulation.

The canal should be thoroughly irrigated and checked for hemostasis before closure of the external oblique fascia. The fascia is closed with a running, absorbable suture (ie, Vicryl 3-0) along the lateral half of the incision, taking care not to entrap or injure the nerves. Scarpa's fascia should be closed with similar sutures, the subcutaneous tissue irrigated

**26**

**INGUINAL HERNIA**

one final time, and then the skin closed with a subcuticular absorbable (ie, Vicryl 4-0) suture, with a dry, sterile dressing finally applied.

## LAPAROSCOPIC HERNIA REPAIRS

A recent alternative to the traditional open Lichtenstein repair is a laparoscopic repair of inguinal hernias. There is much controversy about the merits and problems with laparoscopic vs open techniques, which is beyond the scope of this text, but suffice it to say that more and more laparoscopic repairs are being performed with improved results.

There are primarily two types of laparoscopic approaches the totally extraperitoneal approach (TEPA) and thc transabdominal preperitoneal approach (TAPP). The repairs are fairly similar, with the actual divergence lying in the laparoscopic approach used to access the preperitoneal space. Mesh is used in either case, with tension-free principles applied, making these two repairs variations on the Lichtenstein theme of hernioplasty.

The TEPA repair stays all extraperitoneal. The initial port is placed just inferior to the umbilicus, and a special balloon dissector is passed along the posterior rectus sheath down to the pubic symphysis. The balloon is then used to dissect the preperitoneal space exposing the entire myopectineal orifice (this may also be done bluntly sans balloon, which is less costly but more temporally demanding), allowing visualization of all types of groin hernias. With either type of laparoscopic approach, both sides may be attacked from the same working ports, thereby lending some ammunition to the arguments of laparoscopic proponents, who claim that bilateral hernia sufferers avoid two groin incisions with the laparoscopic technique. Once the preperitoneal space is adequately dissected with the "dissecting" balloon, it is exchanged for a "working" balloon, and $CO_2$ insufflation is used to maintain adequate visualization. Two 5-mm ports are then inserted under direct visualization, using a Safe-Track technique, and these are used for instrument placement. The safe-track technique involves using a 25-gauge needle on a syringe to localize the port site by means of direct visualization with the laparoscope, before making any port site incisions. The cord is skeletonized, the hernia sac and contents are reduced, and there is some limited dissection to expose "safe" structures into which small corkscrew-shaped tacks are inserted to hold the mesh in place. Medial to the inferior epigastric vessels the mesh is tacked to Cooper's ligament, the lacunar ligament, the posterior rectus muscle, and the transverse abdominis aponeurosis. Laterally the mesh is tacked to the lateral aspect of the transversus abdominis aponeurosis and to the iliopubic tract. Care must be taken not to tack too laterally, because this is where several nerves course, which may be easily injured or entrapped. These nerves include the femoral cutaneous, ilioinguinal, and iliohypogastric. Medially, greater danger lies in the *triangle of doom.* The triangle's apex is the internal ring, and its two borders are the ductus deferens and the spermatic vessels. Within this space runs the external iliac artery, vein, and femoral nerve. Just medial to this area, near Cooper's ligament, is the obturator artery, which also should be avoided for obvious reasons.

The TAPP actually involves placement of trocars and ports intraperitoneally, similar to a diagnostic laparoscopy, for example. The peritoneum is then incised and a flap created lateral to the medial umbilical ligament, taking care not to injure the inferior epigastric vessels during the dissection. Once the preperitoneal space is entered, the dissection and conduct of the operation is similar to the TEPA. In either type of laparoscopic approach, general anesthesia is required, and the cost is significantly higher (especially with TEPA because of the specialized balloons) than with an open repair; however, visualization is improved, there is less pain, and a more rapid recovery time for the patient. Certainly in patients with bilateral hernias, or those with recurrent hernias, a laparoscopic repair seems to show some advantage to open technique. Long-term follow-up and randomized, prospective, controlled trials should eventually give us a more complete picture regarding the efficacy of laparoscopic hernia repair.

## POSTOPERATIVE/DISCHARGE ORDERS

Most inguinal hernia repairs will be done on an outpatient basis. These patients will go home the same day after adequate recovery from the anesthesia. All patients will need a prescription for postoperative analgesia. Narcotic-acetaminophen combinations are usually prescribed (eg, Percocet, Vicodin, Darvocet N-100), but with recent COX-2 inhibitor NSAIDs (eg, Vioxx) on the market, these may be better suited for many patients. Their complication profile is less than the narcotics, and they negate the need for stool softeners or laxatives for narcotic-associated constipation.

Immediate postoperative orders should include the following:

**Admission or discharge status:** discharge after recovery from anesthesia when criteria met

**Discharge criteria:** tolerating PO without N/V, voiding without difficulty, ambulating without difficulty, normal vital signs

**Activity:** no heavy lifting, straining, or bending for 4 to 6 weeks; OK to walk and use stairs tonight, shower after 24 hours is OK, no baths, pools

**Follow-up appointment:** 7 to 14 days

Physician's phone number for questions or concerns: call immediately for signs of infection (erythema, purulent drainage, increasing pain, opened wound) or any generalized worsening of overall condition (eg, fever, chills, N/V, inability to void)

**Medications:** OK to take all home medications (check for drug interactions with analgesics)

Give the recovery nurses postoperative pain orders including one-time IV or IM route in addition to PO (eg, meperidine [Demerol] 25 mg IV × 1 prn, hydrocodone [Vicodin] 1 PO q4h prn)

Recovery room antiemetic order (eg, compazine 5 mg IV × 1 prn)

## V. POTENTIAL COMPLICATIONS

As with any surgery, there are always the basic complications including but not limited to recurrence, bleeding, infection, and reaction to the medications or anesthetics used. Recurrence rates for inguinal hernias range from 1% to 10% for primary repairs and 5% to 35% for recurrent hernias. Potential bleeding may require blood transfusions and should be discussed preoperatively. Infections are an obvious potential problem that can run from a minor stitch abscess at the skin to a full-blown fasciitis requiring mesh debridement and wide resection. Wound infection rates run from 0.1% to 3%. When a laparoscopic repair is to be performed, the inherent dangers of laparoscopy need to be outlined, including risk of trocar or needle injury to organs, vessels, and nerves, potential bowel obstruction with TAPP if the peritoneal flap fails and small bowel adheres to the mesh. Possible complications from the Foley catheter and NGT placement also need to be addressed. Specific complications of hernias include injury to the spermatic cord structures, any of which can decrease fertility in men. The specific nerves that may be injured and entrapped also need to be addressed, including the ilioinguinal, iliohypogastric (both of which are more commonly injured in open repairs), and the genitofemoral and femoral cutaneous nerves (which are in greater danger during laparoscopic repairs). *Meralgia paresthetica* is pain and paresthesias in the anterolateral thigh caused by injury or entrapment of the femoral cutaneous nerve. Many patients recover from neuralgias with conservative therapy, but occasionally entrapped nerves may cause chronic pain requiring operative intervention. Suturing of the mesh may endanger surrounding structures, including vessels, nerves, bladder, and bowel.

One of the most common complications of hernia repairs is the accumulation of a seroma or hematoma postoperatively (0.5% to 5% incidence). Most patients have some form of transient scrotal enlargement as a result of $CO_2$ dissection, hematoma, seroma, or combinations of these that can be marked in a small percentage (2% to 3%) but usually resolve spontaneously.

Systemic postoperative complications, including myocardial infarction, congestive heart failure, atelectasis, pulmonary embolism, and pneumonia are fortunately rare but have been reported. Death related to hernia repair is extremely unusual but has occurred, especially in patients with advanced age and comorbid conditions.

# UMBILICAL/ ABDOMINAL HERNIA

*Conrad Simfendorfer*

Umbilical hernias result from an abdominal wall defect at the umbilicus. A weak area of the abdominal wall fascia is created by the attachment of the round ligament at the inferior border of the umbilicus along with remnants of the urachus and umbilical arteries. Umbilical hernias in children are thought to be congenital, whereas those in adults are generally acquired and are called paraumbilical hernias, most often occurring in multiparous women, and patients with increased intraabdominal pressure and concomitant chronic abdominal distention, as from ascites.

**27**

## I. PATHOPHYSIOLOGY

**Uncomplicated Hernia.** Typical symptoms are a dull ache and a bulge at the umbilicus. The ache may be described as a burning or a pain, which is exacerbated by activity or with coughing or sneezing. This is often relieved by recumbency and relaxation of the abdominal muscles.

**Incarcerated Hernia.** In an incarcerated hernia the viscera are contained within the hernia sac and cannot be disgorged from the sac. This occurs under the following conditions: (1) adhesions form between the interior of the sac and the viscus; (2) adhesions form between the neck of the sac at several sites, such that the viscera cannot exit; and (3) contortion and adhesion between viscera or development of edema in the hernia contents. Typically, patients are asymptomatic, except for the presence of a persistent bulge.

**Strangulated Hernia.** In a strangulated hernia the blood supply to a viscus, usually the small bowel, is compromised. It may be of acute onset, with torsion of the hernia contents, or a less acute onset from bowel obstruction, venous outflow obstruction, or lymphatic obstruction, leading to increasing edema. Strangulation is typically accompanied by pain at a known hernia site. Often, there is concomitant bowel obstruction. There is a 10% mortality and major morbidity associated with strangulation. Urgent operation is indicated for patients with strangulated hernia.

**Obstruction.** Hernias are the leading cause of intestinal obstruction worldwide. In the United States, it is the third most common cause for obstruction after intraabdominal adhesions and abdominal cancer. Symptoms are generally those associated with bowel obstruction, mainly abdominal pain, bloating, nausea, vomiting, and obstipation. Therefore, it is mandatory to examine the patient for hernia with a suspected bowel obstruction.

Urgent operation with repair of the hernia and relief of the bowel obstruction is indicated, given the increased concern for strangulation.

## II. TYPICAL PRESENTATION

Umbilical hernias constitute about 14% of hernias in the United States, with a female dominance of 1.7:1. They also have a bimodal age distribution, with peaks in the pediatric population and then in the 40- to 60-year-old group. Typical presentation, as previously described, is of a dull ache or bulge at the umbilicus, with sensations of burning or pain. Many times patients may describe a specific episode of muscular straining during which a sudden discomfort occurred, followed by symptoms of discomfort and/or bulge. Over time these symptoms may increase in duration, intensity, and frequency, as well as complaints of increasing size of the hernia. Occasionally, patients may be seen with acute symptoms of strangulation or obstruction.

## III. PREOPERATIVE WORKUP

Diagnosis of umbilical hernia is typically made on the basis of history and physical examination. Questions should be made of any bowel complaints, particularly symptoms of intermittent bowel obstruction. On physical examination, care should be taken to evaluate the patient for any other abdominal or inguinal hernias, as well as previous scars. The reducibility of the hernia, size of the abdominal wall defect, and amount of abdominal contents in the hernia are important factors during examination.

Further testing is usually not required for the diagnosis of umbilical hernia, occasionally computed tomography (CT) or ultrasonography may allow delineation of hernia from abdominal wall mass in a patient with significant adipose tissue.

Occasionally, the factors that may have contributed to the development of the hernia need to be addressed, including causes for increased intraabdominal pressures from ascites, obstructive uropathy, partially obstructive cancers, and severe chronic obstructive pulmonary disease. These contributing elements need to be nullified or alleviated as much as possible before repair of the hernia.

### PREOPERATIVE ORDERS

The preoperative workup generally includes standard preoperative preparations for abdominal surgery, including basic laboratory examinations, and preoperative antibiotics.

## IV. SURGICAL ANATOMY

An umbilical hernia results from an abdominal wall defect at the umbilicus, at the site of the attachment of the round ligament, and remnants of the urachus and umbilical arteries, at the inferior rim of the umbilicus. Eighty percent of umbilical hernias in adults occur in patients with single midline aponeurotic decussation, whereas 20% occur in those with triple midline aponeurotic decussation. The hernia is composed generally of a peritoneal sac and intraabdominal contents.

## V. CONDUCT OF OPERATION

The patient is placed in the supine position and either general anesthesia with endotracheal intubation or monitored intravenous sedation with local anesthetic are induced, depending on patient comorbidities and surgeon preference. The abdomen is prepped and draped sterilely. Typically, a semi-lunar incision is made either above or below the umbilicus, depending on the hernia protrusion. If the hernia is very large and the umbilicus is to be removed, an elliptical incision is made around the hernia and umbilicus. After the incision, the dissection is extended to anterior abdominal fascia, raising flaps inferiorly and superiorly. The hernia sac is identified circumferentially, incised carefully, and then opened. If possible, the intraabdominal contents are reduced. Occasionally, omentum may be incarcerated in the hernia, necessitating amputation and careful control of bleeding by individual ligature.

In case strangulated small intestine is encountered within the hernia, the apex of the sac is incised and the strangulated bowel identified. The hernia sac is enlarged transversely by dividing the fascia of the anterior abdominal wall, the posterior fascia, and peritoneum with retraction of the rectus muscle laterally. A small bowel resection is then carried out in the usual fashion.

When closing, first, the edges of the hernia sac are grasped, and the peritoneum is closed transversely with a continuous suture. Then, the anterior rectus sheath is closed, either by imbrication or figure-of-eight interrupted sutures in a single layer, depending on the laxity of the fascial layer. If the defect is large or the rectus sheath is difficult to reapproximate, a Prolene mesh is placed to close the defect. The subcutaneous tissues are closed with interrupted 3-0 Vicryl sutures, and the skin is reapproximated with a running subcuticular 4-0 Vicryl suture. Benzoin, Steri-Strips, and sterile dressing are applied.

Occasionally, subcutaneous drains are placed if there has been extensive subcutaneous dissection and the risk of seroma exists.

### VARIATIONS OF OPERATION

Laparoscopic umbilical hernia repair, although not the standard approach, has been performed by many centers. The laparoscopic approach often enhances visualization of the hernia. Preparation and positioning of the patient is similar to the open repair. General anesthesia is induced. Trocar placement is variable, depending on the size of the hernia. Because the hernia is located at the umbilicus, ports need to be placed either inferiorly, superiorly, or lateral to the umbilicus. The hernia is then reduced internally, and a Prolene mesh is stapled to the abdominal wall.

An umbilical hernia in a child is not the same defect as in an adult; therefore, an expectant approach can be taken, and the hernia may be observed until the child reaches 4 years, with the expectation of spontaneous closure. If it does not close, surgical repair is warrented.

## POSTOPERATIVE ORDERS

In cases of uncomplicated umbilical hernia repair, surgery may be performed as an outpatient procedure, with discharge to home a few hours after recovery from anesthesia. If the surgery is complicated by strangulation, bowel resection, or bowel perforation, the patient is admitted to hospital and managed accordingly, including NPO, bowel rest, nasogastric tube, and intravenous antibiotics.

## VI. POTENTIAL COMPLICATIONS

Strangulation is associated with a mortality of 10% and major morbidity. Surgery may also be complicated by bowel perforation, bowel ischemia, wound infection, bleeding, and recurrence.

Factors responsible for hernia recurrence include closure under excessive tension, failure to use adequate musculoaponeurotic margins, wound infections, inadequate collagen formation from either malnutrition or administration of corticosteroids, and, finally, chronically high intraabdominal pressures.

## VII. DISCHARGE ORDERS

Patients are normally discharged to home the same day of surgery. They are given no dietary restrictions. They are instructed not to drive while taking narcotics. Activity is restricted to no heavy lifting or strenuous activity for 4 to 6 weeks. Patients are seen in follow-up 1 to 2 weeks after their operation.

# PART VIII

## Endocrine

# THYROIDECTOMY

*Jitendra V. Singh*

Thyroid disease is a common disorder affecting 5% to 10% of adults in the United States. Patients typically present with symptoms of hyperthyroidism, hypothyroidism, diffuse or nodular thyroid enlargements, or some combination of the preceding. Careful evaluation is necessary when choosing medical vs surgical therapy. Major indications for surgical therapy include cosmetic complaints, enlargements compromising the trachea or esophagus, malignancy, and in some instances hyperthyroidism (ie, hyperthyroidism in pregnancy in which radioactive iodine is contraindicated).

**28**

## I. PATHOPHYSIOLOGY

### GOITERS

Enlargements of the thyroid, collectively known as goiters, can be diffuse or focal and smooth or nodular. They may be associated with an underactive, overactive, or normal functioning thyroid. Generally, hypothyroid or euthyroid diffuse nonnodular goiters are secondary to a benign process, whereas euthyroid nodular goiters may be due to a malignancy.

Causes of diffuse thyroid enlargements include iodine deficiency and thyroiditis. Clinically they present as large, bulky, smooth, and soft enlargements, which may grow to sizable proportions. Goiters secondary to iodine deficiency are uncommon in the United States as a result of supplemented salt. Thyroiditis, a more common occurrence, may be acute, subacute, or chronic. Acute thyroiditis is secondary to hematogenous spread of infectious microorganisms such as staphylococcus and streptococcus. Subacute thyroiditis is thought to be of viral origin and is often preceded by an upper respiratory infection. Major forms of subacute thyroiditis include giant cell, de Quervain's thyroiditis, and granulomatous thyroiditis. Chronic thyroiditis occurs in two major forms, Hashimoto's and Riedels. Hashimoto's thyroiditis is a relatively common autoimmune disorder occurring predominantly in women. It usually coexists with other autoimmune disorders such as type 1 diabetes mellitus and rheumatoid arthritis. Antithyroid antibodies are commonly present in the serum. Riedel's thyroiditis is a rare form of thyroiditis in which the thyroid parenchyma is completely replaced with dense fibrous connective tissue.

Diffuse multinodular goiters are by far the most common form of thyroid enlargement. Most nodules are hypoplastic and do not take up radioactive iodine ("cold" nodules). Occasionally, nodules are hyperplastic and actively produce thyroid hormone. These nodules take up radioactive iodine and are termed "hot" nodules.

### HYPERTHYROIDISM/THYROTOXICOSIS

Common hyperthyroid conditions requiring surgical intervention include Graves' disease (diffuse toxic nonnodular goiter) and Plummer's syndrome (nodular goiter). Graves' disease occurs more frequently in women, with an increased incidence in HLA-DR3- and HLAB8-positive individuals. In these individuals thyrotoxicosis is due to overproduction of thyroid-stimulating immunoglobins, which bind the thyroid-stimulating hormone (TSH) receptor, stimulating the thyroid to produce massive amounts of hormone. Classic ophthalmopathy in Graves' patients is secondary to infiltration of the extraocular muscles by lymphocytes causing diffuse inflammation. In Plummer's disease, thyrotoxicosis is due to overproduction of thyroid hormone by hyperplastic nodules. The combination of hyperthyroidism, nodular goiter, and the absence of exopthalmos characterize this syndrome.

## THYROID CANCER

Thyroid cancer accounts for 1% of all cancers in adults with an incidence of 4/100,000 in the United States. Most thyroid cancers are asymptomatic and are commonly discovered incidentally on routine physical examination. Thyroid surgery is most commonly performed to either diagnose or treat a suspected malignancy. There are four basic types of thyroid cancer, which differ in behavior and response to therapy. The various types are discussed below.

**Papillary Carcinoma.** Papillary carcinoma accounts for 70% of all thyroid cancers. Women are more commonly affected than men. There is an increased incidence in patients with a prior history of radiation exposure. It is characterized by a slow rate of growth and sizes ranging from 1.5 cm to tumors that involve the entire gland. Disease spread is through the lymphatics in 50% of cases and rarely hematogenously. Distant metastasis is infrequent. Surgical options include total lobectomy with isthmusectomy, near-total thyroidectomy, or total thyroidectomy. Ten-year survival rate is greater than 80%. Subtotal or partial lobectomy is contraindicated because of the increased incidence of tumor recurrence.

**Follicular Carcinoma.** Follicular carcinoma accounts for 10% of all thyroid cancers. Women are more commonly affected than men. It is characteristically more aggressive, with occasional lymphogenous spread to regional lymph nodes. There is a greater tendency for hematogenous spread to lung, bone, and liver. Metastases can be identified with radioactive iodine. Metastases to bone may appear 10 to 20 years after resection of the primary lesion. Total thyroidectomy is the surgical treatment of choice. The 10-year survival rate is approximately 40%.

**Hurthel Cell Cancer.** Hurthel cell cancer is a clinically distinct subgroup of follicular carcinomas that represents approximately 5% of all thyroid cancers. Men are affected more commonly than women. Total thyroidectomy is the treatment of choice, with a 10-year survival rate of 60%.

**Medullary Carcinoma of Thyroid.** Medullary carcinoma of the thyroid (MCT) accounts for 7% of all thyroid malignancies. Men and women are affected equally. An aggressive tumor of specific calcitonin-producing cells (C cells) of the thyroid, 90% are sporadic occurrences typically presenting as a solitary nodule. Less commonly, MCT is associated with MEN-II or Sipple's syndrome, which is a familial occurrence of MCT associated with bilateral pheochromocytoma and hyperparathyroidism. It is usually mutifocal and carries a better prognosis than sporadic MCT. The treatment of choice in both cases is total thyroidectomy. Of note is the high incidence of nodal involvement in MCT. Therefore all central compartment lymph nodes must be resected. Prognosis is highly dependent on completeness of tumor resection and degree of spread.

**Lymphoma of the Thyroid.** Lymphoma of the thyroid is rare, usually occurring in association with Hashimoto's thyroiditis. Women are more commonly affected. Patients usually present with a history of rapidly enlarging neck mass with compressive symptoms. The tumor is sensitive to chemotherapy and radiation therapy. Surgical intervention is indicated for diagnosis and relief of compression.

**Anaplastic Carcinoma.** Anaplastic carcinoma is rare, accounting for 3% of all thyroid cancers. It is a highly aggressive tumor with a dismal outcome. The tumor extensively infiltrates local lymph nodes, the trachea, larynx, esophagus, carotid arteries, and jugular veins. Surgical intervention should only be considered in patients with tumor confined to the thyroid. Mean survival is 2 to 4 months.

## II. TYPICAL PRESENTATION

### THYROID GOITERS

Iodine deficiency goiters typically present as large, bulky, and smooth enlargements of varying sizes. When large enough, they can produce compressive symptoms of dysphagia, dyspnea, hoarseness, and tracheal or esophageal deviation. Such compressive symptoms suggest substernal extension of the gland. In some instances, emergency surgical intervention is required for severe respiratory distress. Patients with thyroiditis may present with hyperthyroid or hypothyroid symptoms, sore throat pain, and tenderness and swelling over one or both lobes. On physical examination the gland is indurated, enlarged, and tender. Occasionally, subacute thyroiditis is painless. Postpartum thyroiditis is also painless. A nodular thyroid with elevated TSH and low thyroxine ($T_4$) and positive antithyroid antibodies is suggestive of Hashimoto's thyroiditis.

### HYPERTHYROIDISM/THYROTOXICOSIS

Patients with Graves' disease typically present with hyperthyroid symptoms, including palpitations, diaphoresis, heat intolerance, irritability, weight loss, anxiety, and fatigue. Physical signs include an audible bruit over the gland, hand tremors, and cardiac dysrhythmia. Other physical findings include exopthalmos, pretibial edema, and eyelid edema. Elevated free $T_4$ and suppressed TSH confirm the diagnosis of thyrotoxicosis. Plummer's disease usually presents with palpitations and muscle weakness. Typical symptoms of thyrotoxicosis are uncommon in Plummer's disease. Physical signs include multinodular goiter, muscle wasting, and dysrhythmias.

## III. PREOPERATIVE WORKUP

A thyroid function test is part of the initial workup for all patients with suspected thyroid disease. Serum TSH and $T_4$ will give an accurate indication of thyroid function. In patients with solitary or multiple nodules, fine-needle aspiration (FNA) biopsy should be performed to assess benign or malignant features of the nodule. If suspicious or frankly malignant cells are seen, thyroidectomy is indicated.

Other studies that may be indicated preoperatively include ultrasonography and nuclear scintigraphy. Ultrasonography provides a noninvasive method for determining size and density of a thyroid lesion. Generally, a partially cystic and partially solid mass may indicate a papillary carcinoma, whereas a solid mass with a surrounding halo indicates a benign process. Nuclear scintigraphy with technetium-99 or iodine-131 is used to further assess the nature of thyroid disease. Nodules showing uptake of radiolabel are "hot" and generally tend to be benign in nature, whereas those that do not take up radiolabel are "cold" and nodules may be malignant or benign.

Hyperthyroid patients undergoing subtotal thyroidectomy require special preoperative preparation to avoid the fatal complications of thyroid storm and to technically facilitate the surgery. A euthyroid state should be achieved before surgery, with the use of antithyroid medications such as propylthiouracil. In addition 2 to 5 drops of potassium iodide solution or Lugol's iodine solution should be administered 2 weeks before surgery to decrease the friability and vascularity of the thyroid gland. Hyperthyroid patients requiring emergency surgery for unrelated problems (ie, acute appendicitis) should receive potassium iodide in conjuction with a beta-blocker to antagonize the peripheral manifestations of thyrotoxicosis. This combination has been shown to significantly lower serum thyroid hormone levels.

### PREOPERATIVE ORDERS

**Diet:** NPO after midnight
**Laboratory tests:** CBC, BMP, calcium, thyroid function tests, INR
and PTT, CXR, ECG if age >35 years or significant cardiac disease
**Medications:** antibiotic on call to OR
PAS on call to OR

## IV. SURGICAL ANATOMY

The normal thyroid weighs 15 to 20 g and lies directly on the anterolateral aspects of the trachea attached by loose connective tissue. It consists of a right and left lobe attached by the isthmus and an ascending pyramidal lobe. The thyroid gland is surrounded by a connective tissue capsule that is continuous with the substance of the organ. Blood supply to the gland is principally by means of the superior and inferior thyroid arteries, which arise from the external carotid artery and the thyrocervical trunk, respectively. Occasionally, the thyroid internal mammary artery is present, which may arise from either the aorta or the inominate artery. Venous drainage is by way of the superior, middle, and inferior thyroid veins.

Understanding relational anatomy of the parathyroids and laryngeal nerves is crucial in avoiding postoperative complications. The right recurrent laryngeal nerve loops around the right subclavian artery and ascends in the tracheoesophageal groove passing behind the right lobe of the thyroid gland. The left recurrent laryngeal nerve passes beneath the aorta and ascends in the tracheoesophageal groove toward the larynx. Both nerves enter the larynx at the level of the cricoid cartilage passing under or through the posterior superior suspensory ligament of the thyroid (Berry's ligament) before entering the cricothyroid muscle. Approximately 15% of patients have anomalous anatomy in which the nerves may be embedded in the substance of the thyroid.

There are four parathyroid glands, two superior and two inferior, each located on the posterior surface of the thyroid gland. The superior parathyroids are located at the level of the cricothyroid cartilage. The inferior parathyroids are commonly found just below the junction of the inferior thyroid artery and the recurrent laryngeal nerve. Each gland is surrounded by its own capsule. Occasionally, the parathyroids are found in the capsule of the thyroid gland or embedded deep into the substance of the thyroid.

## V. CONDUCT OF OPERATION

Positioning the patient properly is essential for adequate exposure of the thyroid gland. The neck is hyperextended by placing a small pillow or rolled towels between the scapulae. A 5-cm symmetric skin incision is made across the anterior neck, two fingerbreadths above the sternal notch. A longer incision may be required in patients with large or low-lying glands. The incision is extended through the subcutaneous tissue and the platysma muscle under which lies an avascular plane. In this plane, the superior and inferior skin flaps can be raised, exposing the strap muscles, sternohyoid and sternothyroid muscles. Dissection of the strap muscles is carried out carefully by lifting them anteriorly avoiding the inferior thyroid vein, which courses longitudinally over the trachea. The sternohyoid muscle is then bluntly dissected away from the sternothyroid. With the sternohyoid muscle retracted, the sternothyroid muscle is carefully dissected from the underlying thyroid lobes. Once the thyroid is completely exposed, the gland is elevated anteriorly and medially, opening a plane exposing the carotid artery and one or more middle thyroid veins. The middle thyroid veins are ligated at this time. In cases of large goiters or tumors, the strap muscles must be divided for improved access to the gland.

After the gland is fully exposed, the upper pole of the thyroid is mobilized caudally and laterally, avoiding injury to the superior laryngeal nerve. After careful dissection, other superior pole vessels are identified and doubly ligated with silk. At this point the superior parathyroid glands are also identified. The thyroid is then mobilized by sweeping dorsally all tissue along the posterolateral border of the thyroid. The inferior thyroid artery and vein are identified and ligated. At this time, a curved Kelly clamp is gently passed under the isthmus, which is divided. The recurrent laryngeal nerves are identified by following their appropriate course on their respective sides. Careful identification of the nerve passing through Berry's ligament on each side is crucial for avoiding the complication of nerve damage. Care must also be taken to avoid injury to the superior laryngeal nerve as well. Once each side is dissected, the thyroid gland can be safely removed. Once the gland is completely removed, the strap muscles are loosely approximated, the skin is closed, and a drain is placed.

## VARIATIONS OF OPERATION

The preceding describes a total thyroidectomy. Subtotal thyroidectomy and lobectomy are performed with the same basic principles as described earlier. In a subtotal thyroidectomy, a total lobectomy is performed on one side and a partial lobectomy is performed on the contralateral side. Dividing the isthmus flush with the contralateral gland performs a simple lobectomy or subtotal lobectomy. In cases of substernal goiters, a neck incision may be too small, therefore a sternotomy is performed.

## POSTOPERATIVE ORDERS

**Admit to:** surgical ward
**Diagnosis:**
**Condition:**
**Vital signs:** q4h
**Activity:** bed rest; ambulate in 6 to 8 h if tolerated; IS q1h when awake
**Allergies:**
**Diet:** NPO × 8 h; advance from clear liquids to regular diet as tolerated
**Nursing:** I&Os q4h × 24 h, then I&Os per routine, tracheostomy tray to bedside, remove drains on POD 1; every other skin suture can be removed on POD 2, and the rest on POD 4
**IV fluids:** $D_5$/LR or $D_5$/NS at 100 ml/h with 20 mEq of KCl
**Medications:** cefazolin (Ancef) 1 g IVPB q8h × 3 doses
meperidine (Demerol) 50 mg IV/IM q3-4h prn for pain

hydroxyzine (Vistaril) 25-50 mg IV/IM q3-4h prn for
nausea
**Laboratory tests:** CBC, BMP, serum calcium, $PO_4$

## VI. POTENTIAL COMPLICATIONS

Complications of thyroidectomy include recurrent laryngeal nerve damage, hypoparathyroidism, superior laryngeal nerve injury, bleeding with hematoma formation, wound infection, keloid formation, and, infrequently, intraoperative or postoperative thyroid storm.

Recurrent laryngeal nerve injury occurs with an incidence of about 1%. Unilateral recurrent laryngeal nerve injury or damage results in vocal cord paralysis, causing symptoms of voice hoarseness, dysphagia, and cough. Furthermore, the vocal cords may be displaced to the paramedian region. If nerve damage occurs bilaterally, the vocal cords may cause airway obstruction, leading to acute respiratory distress necessitating emergency tracheostomy. Injury can be avoided or minimized by carefully identifying the nerves. Identification itself damages the nerve, causing temporary voice disturbance; however, the incidence of permanent damage is decreased. Precise dissection of Berry's ligament and good hemostasis significantly decrease the risk of nerve injury or damage.

The risk of hypoparathyroidism varies with the degree of thyroid pathology. As expected, there is an increased incidence of hypoparathyroidism in patients undergoing total thyroidectomy as opposed to a subtotal thyroidectomy. The incidence of hypoparathyroidism is also higher in patients undergoing central neck compartment clearance for medullary carcinoma. Most of the time postthyroidectomy hypoparathyroidism is transient and results from temporary insults to the parathyroid glands from nonmeticulous operative technique. Serum calcium and signs and symptoms of hypocalcemia must be monitored carefully and treated appropriately.

Hemorrhage into the wound is an important complication that requires immediate attention. An expanding hematoma may compress the airway, causing sudden respiratory distress. If hemorrhage is suspected, the wound is opened and drained at the bedside, and the patient is promptly returned to the operating room.

Thyroid storm is a rare and fatal complication with features of high fever, diaphoresis, tachycardia, restlessness, vomiting, diarrhea, and delirium. Oxygen and antipyretics should be administered immediately. Propranolol is administered for tachycardia and sodium iodide to calm the "storm."

## VII. DISCHARGE INSTRUCTIONS

Patients can resume normal activity after discharge from the hospital. All patients having undergone a total thyroidectomy must be on thyroid hormone replacement therapy. Of patients having undergone a subtotal thyroidectomy, 20% to 30% will require thyroid hormone replacement.

**28**

**THYROIDECTOMY**

# PARATHYROIDECTOMY

*Lee Akst*

Hyperparathyroidism is the most common cause of hypercalcemia in the out-patient population. Other causes include malignancies, with or without bone metastases, granulomatous diseases such as sarcoidosis, endocrine disorders, and renal disease. Although hypercalcemia itself can be managed medically through aggressive hydration, loop diuretics, and calcitonin, surgery is the definitive therapy and is successful in curing hypercalcemia caused by hyperparathyroidism in 95% of patients. Hyperparathyroidism can be divided into three categories: primary, secondary, and tertiary. Each of these categories presents differently and may require a different treatment plan.

## I. PATHOPHYSIOLOGY

### PRIMARY HYPERPARATHYROIDISM

Primary hyperparathyroidism occurs when one or more of the parathyroid glands produce excess parathyroid hormone. This form of hyperparathyroidism occurs roughly in 1/1000 people, although its reported incidence will increase as routine serum calcium levels make diagnosis more frequent. Ninety percent of cases of primary hyperparathyroidism are found to be due to a solitary adenoma. The remaining 10% are caused by four-gland hyperplasia. Surgery is indicated in asymptomatic patients with persistent calcium elevation 1 to 1.6 mg/dl above normal, calciuria greater than 400 mg/d, or bone density 2 or more standard deviations less than the mean for age- and sex-matched controls. Surgery is also indicated for patients with symptomatic disease.

### SECONDARY HYPERPARATHYROIDISM

Secondary hyperparathyroidism occurs when increased parathyroid activity results from dysfunction of another organ system. The most common cause of secondary hyperparathyroidism is renal insufficiency. Decreased serum calcium in these patients stimulates parathyroid hormone production. Decreased serum calcium levels in patients with renal insufficiency is due to several mechanisms. Impaired phosphorus excretion leads to decreased serum calcium, because the two ions precipitate out of the serum as calcium stones. Renal insufficiency also decreases the 1-hydroxylation of vitamin D, limiting calcium absorption from the gut. Parathyroid hyperplasia results from an effort by the parathyroid to raise the calcium level. Although treatment of secondary hyperparathyroidism is often aimed at treating the underlying disease, parathyroidectomy is indicated for uncontrolled symptoms such as pathologic fractures, bone pain, or soft tissue calcifications. In these cases there is almost always diffuse hyperplasia of all four parathyroid glands. The goal of surgery is to remove $3\frac{1}{2}$ glands or to remove all four glands and autotransplant a portion of one of the glands.

## TERTIARY HYPERPARATHYROIDISM

Tertiary hyperparathyroidism is the name for the clinical entity in which hyperparathyroidism and hypercalcemia persist after resolution of the underlying disorder that caused secondary hyperparathyroidism. In the case of renal failure, successful renal transplant removes the driving force for increased parathyroid hormone production, and parathyroid hyperplasia should resolve. If the reactive hyperplasia is irreversible in any or all of the parathyroid glands, tertiary hyperparathyroidism results. Persistent, diffuse, four-gland hyperplasia is the most common form of tertiary hyperparathyroidism and occurs in up to 30% of patients who have pretransplant hyperparathyroidism. As with primary hyperplasia, removal of either $3\frac{1}{2}$ glands or removal of all four glands with autotransplantation is indicated.

## PARATHYROID CARCINOMA

Parathyroid carcinoma technically falls within the classification of primary hyperparathyroidism but occurs in less than 1% of cases. Suspicion for carcinoma should be raised by the presence of extremely elevated calcium levels or a palpable neck mass. In cases of parathyroid carcinoma, excision of the cancer should also include a thyroid lobectomy. The local recurrence rate is approximately 30%, and radical neck dissection should occur in these instances. In another 30% of cases the disease will be metastatic to lung, liver, or bone.

## II. TYPICAL PRESENTATION

Most patients (70%) with hyperparathyroidism are asymptomatic. Their hyperparathyroidism is diagnosed only after hypercalcemia is noted on routine blood work. Symptomatic patients complain of "stones, bones, groans, and psychic overtones." "Stones" refers to the nephrolithiasis or nephrocalcinosis that results from the development of calcium stones. Calcium phosphate stones are more common than calcium oxalate. "Bones" is a reference to the bone pain, arthralgias, and muscle aches that accompany the extra resorption of bone driven by excess parathyroid hormone. "Groans" refers to the peptic ulcer disease and pancreatitis found in patients with hyperparathyroidism. These symptoms occur in approximately 20% of patients with hyperparathyroidism. "Psychic overtones," referring to fatigue, depression, anxiety, or irritability, is seen in approximately 40% of this group.

Few of these symptoms are visible, and parathyroid adenomas are rarely palpable. If a mass is palpated, parathyroid carcinoma or associated thyroid pathology may be present. Therefore the diagnosis of hyperparathyroidism is often suspected on the basis of history rather than physical examination.

## III. PREOPERATIVE WORKUP

The diagnosis of hyperparathyroidism is confirmed by laboratory measurement of parathyroid hormone levels (Table 29-1). In primary, secondary, and tertiary hyperparathyroidism, parathyroid hormone (PTH) levels should

## TABLE 29-1
### PARATHYROID HORMONE LEVELS CONFIRMING HYPERPARATHYROIDISM

|  | Parathyroid Hormone | Calcium | Phosphorus |
|---|---|---|---|
| Primary | ↑↑ | ↑ | ↓ |
| Secondary | ↑ | ↓ | ↑ |
| Tertiary | ↑ | ↑ | ↓ |

be elevated above normal. Calcium and phosphorus levels will vary according to the pathophysiology involved, and these levels help to classify hyperparathyroidism. Laboratory tests to evaluate renal function (blood urea nitrogen [BUN] and creatinine) are also ordered as part of a hyperparathyroidism workup, given the relationship between kidney disease and parathyroid function.

Radiographically, hyperparathyroidism is often associated with varying degrees of osteoporosis, because PTH leaches calcium from bones. Radiologic findings of hyperparathyroidism include solitary bone cysts called Brown tumors, subperiosteal resorption seen on the radial aspects of the second and third phalanges, nephrolithiaisis, and diffuse systemic calcifications. Despite these associations, radiographs are not routinely obtained to diagnose hyperparathyroidism.

Once the diagnosis of hyperparathyroidism is established, the preoperative workup often includes localization studies. These tests, when successful, can decrease operating room time and expenses and reduce morbidity by directing the surgeon to the affected gland or glands. Options for preoperative localization include sestamibi scanning, ultrasonography, computed tomography (CT), or magnetic resonance imaging (MRI) scanning, and selective venous sampling. Sestamibi scans are the test of choice for first-time parathyroidectomy patients. They are the least expensive option, are 85% to 90% accurate in identifying single adenomas, and are useful in identifying ectopic parathyroid glands. Sestamibi scans are less useful, though, in patients with multiple adenomas, diffuse parathyroid hyperplasia, or associated thyroid disease. Although ultrasonography can accurately localize adenomas, it cannot locate ectopic parathyroid glands hidden behind the trachea or sternum. Ultrasonography is also more expensive than sestamibi scans. Likewise, CT and MRI are both more expensive than radionuclide studies, and CT provides poor resolution of glands smaller than 1 cm. Venous sampling, although effective, is expensive and invasive, so it is often reserved for reoperative patients in whom abnormal parathyroid tissue could not be found in the first dissection.

### PREOPERATIVE ORDERS
**Diet:** NPO after midnight
**Medications:** antibiotic on call to OR
            PAS on call to OR
**Laboratory tests:** BMP, CBC, PTH, calcium, phosphorus, and ALP levels, CXR, ECG

## IV. SURGICAL ANATOMY

Most patients have four parathyroid glands, two upper and two lower. These paired glands are closely related to the thyroid, normally lying along its posterior surface. Visualization of the parathyroids requires medial rotation of each thyroid lobe. The superior parathyroid glands are located near the point at which the recurrent laryngeal nerve crosses the cricothyroid muscle. The inferior parathyroids are more variable in position and are normally found within 1 to 2 cm of the point at which the inferior thyroid artery enters the thyroid gland. Both the inferior and superior parathyroid arteries usually branch from the inferior thyroid artery. Variations have been described in which the superior parathyroid artery branches form the superior thyroid artery instead.

The parathyroids form during the fifth week of gestation from the dorsal third and fourth branchial pouches. The third arch also forms the thymus gland, and the descent of the thymus carries the third pouch parathyroid tissue inferiorly. Meanwhile, the fourth pouch parathyroid tissue does not migrate. Paradoxically, then, the third pouch parathyroid tissue becomes the inferior parathyroid glands, whereas the fourth pouch tissue becomes the superior glands. Knowledge of this embryologic development may aid the surgeon to locate ectopic parathyroid tissue. For instance, a common ectopic location for an inferior gland is in the thymus, also a third arch derivative, whereas ectopic superior glands may be found in the posterior mediastinum, a fourth arch derivative. Ectopic parathyroid tissue may also be found buried within a thyroid lobe.

## V. CONDUCT OF OPERATION

The patient is placed supine on the operating table, and a shoulder roll is placed so that the neck is extended. A transverse incision is made two fingerbreadths above the clavicular heads. This incision should parallel the natural skin lines of the neck to yield a cosmetically satisfactory result. The incision is carried through the platysma muscle and its associated fascial planes until the strap muscles are identified. These strap muscles are the sternohyoid anteriorly and the sternothyroid posteriorly. These paired muscles are divided in the midline and retracted laterally to expose the thyroid. Careful palpation of structures such as the hyoid bone, laryngeal prominence, and trachea can help to identify midline. With a thyroid lobe exposed, the middle thyroid vein can be divided and ligated. At this point the thyroid lobe is carefully mobilized with a combination of blunt and sharp dissection. Particular attention should be paid to hemostasis, because the parathyroid glands are more easily located in a dry field. The division of the middle thyroid vein, along with superior and inferior mobilization of the thyroid lobe, allows the undersurface of the thyroid lobe to be exposed by medial retraction.

With the thyroid lobe retracted medially, the inferior thyroid artery and recurrent laryngeal nerve are isolated and carefully protected. In most patients, the recurrent laryngeal nerve passes posterior to the inferior thyroid artery. The parathyroid glands are normally tan in color, whereas fat and lymph nodes appear more yellow. The upper gland is normally found in the fatty tissue adjacent to the thyroid gland just superior to the entrance of the inferior thyroid artery. The lower parathyroid glands are more variable in position. If a lower gland cannot be visualized, the thyrothymic ligament and the thymus itself should be searched, because these are common locations for ectopic lower parathyroid glands. If an upper gland cannot be found, it may be hidden behind the inferior thyroid artery or its branches.

If an adenoma is identified, it is removed by carefully dissecting it free of other tissues and dividing the vascular pedicle at its base. All excised adenomas should be sent to pathology for frozen section, so that their cell type can be confirmed histologically. Similarly, frozen sections are often obtained on sliver biopsies of normal glands, to ensure that normal parathyroid tissue is being left with the patient. Confirmation that all adenomatous tissue has been excised can be obtained through preexcision and postexcision intraoperative PTH levels: if the PTH levels fall by more than 50%, it is assumed that the diseased gland has been removed. The postexcision blood sample must be taken at least 10 minutes after the removal of the pathologic gland or glands, so that the level has time to fall to its new baseline state. If two or three of the parathyroid glands are abnormal, the abnormal glands are removed and the normal gland biopsied as described previously. In cases of four-gland hyperplasia (such as occur in secondary hyperparathyroidism), $3\frac{1}{2}$ glands are removed, preserving half a gland to ensure that the patient does not become hypoparathyroid postoperatively. If an adenoma is excised and the pathologist reports hyperplasia within the surrounding parathyroid tissue, $3\frac{1}{2}$ glands are removed and the other half gland is preserved.

When parathyroid tissue that is not resected has a compromised blood supply after dissection, it can be autotransplanted. The tissue is minced and inserted into a pocket located either within the ipsilateral sternocleidomastoid muscle or the brachioradialis muscle of the nondominant forearm. The pocket is closed with nonabsorbable suture, and its position is marked with a clip. Should the transplanted parathyroid tissue every hypertrophy, it can easily be accessed within these superficial muscles. Transplanted parathyroid tissue will develop new blood vessels and resume function within several weeks.

Hemostasis is assured before closure. The strap muscles and the platysma are reapproximated with absorbable suture. The skin itself is closed with Michelle clips, providing hemostasis of the skin edges. These clips are replaced by Steri-Strips on postoperative day 1.

## VARIATIONS OF OPERATION

Because of the high percentage of solitary adenomas accounting for cases of primary hyperparathyroidism (90%), a preoperative sestamibi scan may be used to direct dissection to only one side of the neck. In these cases,

**29**

**PARATHYROIDECTOMY**

histologic evaluation of both the adenoma and one normal gland is required. Any hyperplastic tissue mandates a bilateral exploration and a $3\frac{1}{2}$ gland parathyroidectomy. When only one side of the neck is dissected, intraoperative PTH levels can confirm the absence of other pathologic tissue.

Parathyroidectomy for parathyroid carcinoma requires a more aggressive approach. Because local recurrence of parathyroid carcinoma occurs in about 30% of patients, wide local excision and ipsilateral thyroid lobectomy are performed. Intact tumor removal prevents seeding of the operative field. Skeletonizing the tracheoesophageal groove and excising paratracheal lymph nodes improve survival. Formal neck dissection is reserved for patients with palpable lymphadenopathy. After surgery, radiation therapy may help to control localized microscopic disease.

## POSTOPERATIVE ORDERS

Parathyroidectomy is considered a "clean" case, and patients need not be maintained on antibiotics postoperatively. A regular diet may be resumed when the patient is awake and alert. Hypocalcemia is a concern in all patients after parathyroidectomy, so calcium levels are routinely checked the evening of the operative day and the next morning. Patients with hypocalcemia might complain of perioral or digital numbness and tingling, so these complaints should prompt evaluation of calcium levels. Excess bone demineralization due to excess parathyroid hormone preoperatively may be manifested by an elevated alkaline phosphatase level. These patients should receive calcium and vitamin D supplementation postoperatively.

**Admit to:** surgery
**Diagnosis:** s/p parathyroidectomy
**Condition:** stable
**Vital signs:** q4h x 4, then per routine
**Activity:** as tolerated
**Allergies:**
**Nursing:** strict I&Os, IS, PAS
**Diet:** clear liquid when awake and alert; advance as tolerated
**IV fluids:** lactated Ringer's at 100 ml/h
**Medications:** Percocet, ondansetron (Zofran), Os-Cal, vitamin D
**Laboratory tests:** Ca level this PM, Ca and PTH levels in AM

## VI. POTENTIAL COMPLICATIONS

### HEMATOMA

Hematoma may occur if proper hemostasis is not obtained before closing or if a tie slips off of a vessel. In the closed compartment of the neck a hematoma can rapidly displace the trachea and compromise the airway. In patients in whom respiratory distress develops as a consequence of neck surgery, the wound is immediately reopened to decompress the airway. Light pressure is held over the operative field until the patient can be returned to the operating room for definitive control of the bleeding.

## PERSISTENT HYPERPARATHYROIDISM

Recurrent or persistent hyperparathyroidism is seen in about 5% of patients after parathyroid surgery. These patients require reoperation. Recurrent hyperparathyroidism generally occurs in patients with renal failure, with hypertrophy of the remaining 0.5 gland. Persistent hyperparathyroidism occurs when hyperplastic or adenomatous parathyroid tissue is not found during the original exploration. This is more common in patients with ectopic parathyroid tissue. Ectopic parathyroid tissue may be located within the mediastinum or behind the sternum. As in thyroidectomy, reoperation is technically difficult, with an increased risk of injury to nerves or other vital structures. Therefore, localization studies are used to help guide dissection.

## HYPOCALCEMIA

In as many as 20% to 30% of patients, temporary hypocalcemia may develop after parathyroid surgery. In these patients the lowest levels are usually reached 1 to 3 days postoperatively, although an asymptomatic low level may develop within hours. Patients may complain of perioral or digital numbness and tingling or demonstrate Chvostek's sign (facial grimace after tapping of the facial nerve as it exits the stylomastoid foramen) or Trousseau's sign (carpopedal spasm when a blood pressure cuff is maintained above systolic pressure for 3 to 4 minutes). In patients with symptomatic hypocalcemia, calcium can be replaced orally or intravenously. Simultaneous vitamin D supplementation aids in the uptake of this calcium. Although supplementation is usually tapered as stunned or autotransplanted parathyroid tissue resumes normal function, patients with permanent hypocalcemia after total parathyroidectomy require lifelong calcium replacement.

## NERVE DAMAGE

The recurrent laryngeal nerves are damaged in 1% to 3% of parathyroidectomies. Ten percent of these injuries are permanent. Unilateral nerve palsy causes hoarseness, which may improve over time as the damaged nerve regenerates. The degree of hoarseness depends on the position in which the vocal cord is paralyzed. If a cord is paralyzed in its midline position, apposition of the contralateral cord minimizes symptoms. Conversely, if the cord is paralyzed in its lateral position, apposition does not occur, and vocal difficulties are more severe. If hoarseness does not improve within 6 months after the original surgery, permanent nerve injury is likely. In this case, surgical repositioning of the paralyzed cord to the midline improves voice.

29

PARATHYROIDECTOMY

## VII. DISCHARGE INSTRUCTIONS

Patients normally are discharged on postoperative day 1 after parathyroid surgery. At discharge, patients should be ambulating, tolerating a regular diet, and have adequate calcium levels. There should be no signs of wound infection or hematoma. Pain is ordinarily controlled through low-potency narcotics or nonprescription antiinflammatory medicines. Specific discharge instructions include calcium supplementation should the patient experience hypocalcemia, which may not develop until after the patient has returned home. Patients are normally seen in follow-up within 2 to 3 weeks. Calcium and parathyroid hormone levels are repeated at that time.

# NEOPLASMS OF THE ENDOCRINE PANCREAS

*Eric E. Roselli*

Neoplasms of the endocrine pancreas are rare tumors with an incidence of approximately 5 per million per year. These can either be functional tumors, and thus classified by a characteristic syndrome resulting from the secreted product, or nonfunctional and classified as such. Malignancy is determined only by local nodal invasion or distal spread and not by histologic examination. There are four general treatment principles: recognize the syndrome; detect hormone elevations by radioimmunoassay; localize and stage; operative intervention is the mainstay of treatment.

## I. PATHOPHYSIOLOGY

These tumors originate from neural crest cells and manifest as symptoms attributable to the secreted product. The hormones secreted by these tumors all have physiologic functions that are normally kept in check by a feedback mechanism. This normal regulatory process is no longer in effect once spontaneous production by the tumor occurs.

Insulinoma is the most common endocrine neoplasm of the pancreas. Autonomous insulin production from the tumor leads to spontaneous hypoglycemia. Subsequently, central nervous system dysfunction results, and the compensatory release of glucagon and epinephrine occurs.

The pathophysiology of gastrinoma was first described by Zollinger and Ellison in 1955. In addition to acetylcholine and histamine, gastrin stimulates the secretion of hydrochloric acid from the parietal cells of the stomach by means of calcium-induced stimulation of the $K^+$-$H^+$-ATPase pump. Gastrin normally is released from the chief cells of the stomach and inhibited by a low pH and somatostatin. In gastrinoma the resulting hypersecretion of acid overwhelms the normal mucosal defenses. Repeated cellular damage from hydrochloric acid exposure leads to ulceration.

Vasoactive intestinal polypeptide–secreting tumor (VIPoma) was first reported by Verner and Morrison in 1958. Vasoactive intestinal peptide is a widely distributed neurotransmitter inhibitory to vascular and nonvascular smooth muscle and excitatory to glandular epithelium. As such, it affects multiple organs, and its characteristic syndrome is described later.

Glucagon acts counter to insulin in almost all respects. It promotes mobilization of fuels, especially glucose, by means of the activation of several enzymes predominantly in the liver. The subsequent effects are therefore related to the catabolic action of this hormone. The increased gluconeogenesis leads to an overall reduction in plasma amino acids and increased urinary nitrogen.

Somatostatinoma is the least common of the pancreatic endocrine neoplasms occurring in 1 in 40 million people. Somatostatin is a profound inhibitor of both insulin and glucagon. It acts throughout the gastrointestinal system to inhibit motility, secretions, and the digestion and absorption of nutrients.

Some other described functional neoplasms include the exceptionally rare calcitoninoma, parathyrinoma, gastrin–releasing factor tumor (GRFoma), adenosine-triphosphate hormone–secreting tumor (ADTHoma), and neurotensinoma. Unlike all of the aforementioned tumors, nonfunctional islet cell tumors have no specific syndrome, because they lack the typical hormones. The pathology inflicted by these tumors is related to the physical presence of the tumor and their malignant characteristics.

Multiple endocrine neoplasia type 1 (MEN 1) is characterized by hyperparathyroidism, pituitary tumors, and pancreatic endocrine tumors. The most common islet cell tumor in MEN 1 is the gastrinoma, followed by the insulinoma. Unlike sporadic gastrinomas, these patients often have multiple tumors. MEN 1 patients account for 30% of gastrinoma patients.

## II. TYPICAL PRESENTATION

Insulinoma presents as Whipple's triad: (1) symptoms of hypoglycemia with fasting, (2) documented serum glucose <50 mg/dl, and (3) relief of symptoms with exogenous glucose administration. Neuroglycopenic symptoms are those due to dysfunction of the central nervous system, including confusion, seizure, obtundation, personality change, and coma. The compensatory catecholamine surge leads to symptoms including palpitations, trembling, diaphoresis, and tachycardia. Ninety percent of tumors are amenable to surgical cure; 10% are metastatic to the liver or peripancreatic nodes, and 10% are associated with MEN 1. These tumors are usually multiple.

Gastrinoma patients present with abdominal pain and peptic ulceration (90%), diarrhea (50%), reflux (50%), and often esophagitis. For 1 in 1000 patients, gastrinomas are the cause of primary duodenal ulcer, and for 1 in 2000 patients, they are the cause of recurrent ulcers after surgery.

Because of its effects on smooth muscle and glandular epithelium, VIPoma is seen as the syndrome known as WDHA: watery diarrhea of up to 5 L per day, hypokalemia secondary to fecal losses, and achlorhydria.

The wide-ranging catabolic effects of glucagonoma are manifest by its syndrome, which includes a pathognomonic dermatitis (necrolytic migratory erythema), diabetes, stomatitis, anemia, and weight loss.

The secretory-inhibiting characteristics of somatostatin lead to the typical presentation of a somatostatinoma, including steatorrhea, diabetes, hypochlorhydria, and cholelithiasis.

The symptoms typical of the mass effect of nonfunctional tumors include abdominal pain, weight loss, and jaundice.

## III. PREOPERATIVE WORKUP

Because of the characteristic syndromes associated with most of these neoplasms, a likely diagnosis is often made after a thorough history and physical examination. Specific studies for each specific tumor can then confirm the diagnosis.

### INSULINOMA

To confirm the presence of Whipple's triad, the patient must undergo a monitored fast in which the blood sugar is checked every 4 to 6 hours. The diagnosis is confirmed by a blood sugar less than 50 mg/dl, a serum insulin level greater than 25 $\mu$U/ml, and an insulin/glucose ratio greater than 0.4. The differential diagnosis includes surreptitious insulin administration. Elevated C-peptide (>1.5 ng/ml) and proinsulin levels help to rule this out. Similarly, sulfonylureas levels are assessed. On localization studies, these tumors are evenly distributed throughout the pancreas.

### GASTRINOMA

Screening is indicated in patients with recurrent ulcers, failed medical therapy, postoperative ulcers, a family history of peptic ulcer disease, and prolonged diarrhea and in MEN 1 kindred. A serum gastrin level greater than 200 pg/ml suggests gastrinoma, and a level greater than 1000 pg/ml strongly suggests gastrinoma. These findings of hypergastrinemia require further testing. Gastric acid analysis helps to differentiate ulcerogenic from nonulcerogenic hypergastrinemia. Basal acid output (BAO) greater than 15 mg/h and a BAO to a maximal acid output ratio of greater than 0.6 is indicative of ulcerogenic hypergastrinemia. The diagnosis can be confirmed by the secretin stimulation test to further differentiate gastinoma from antral G cell hyperplasia. With the patient in a fasting state, check the serum gastrin level every 5 minutes for 30 minutes after administering 2 U/kg of intravenous secretin. A positive test result shows an increase in gastrin of greater than 200 pg/ml from the basal level. Localization techniques find most of these tumors within the gastrinoma triangle: to the right of the superior mesenteric vessels in the pancreatic head or duodenum. Furthermore, patients with a gastrinoma should be screened for possible MEN 1 with a serum calcium and prolactin level.

### VIPOMA

Because these patients present with the WDHA syndrome, a diarrhea workup, including endoscopy, radiographic bowel studies, and blood and stool analysis, should first be performed to rule out more common causes like villous adenoma, laxative abuse, celiac disease, infection, inflammatory bowel disease, and carcinoid. In addition to the usual localization strategy mentioned later, a computed tomography (CT) scan of the chest should be included, because 10% of these tumors are extrapancreatic.

### GLUCAGONOMA

An elevated fasting glucagon level is greater than 150 pg/ml. Localization studies find most of these tumors in the body or tail of the pancreas.

### SOMATOSTATINOMA

An elevated fasting level of somatostatin is greater than 100 pg/ml. Most of these tumors are localized in the head or uncinate process of the pancreas.

### NONFUNCTIONAL ISLET CELL TUMORS

Without a characteristic hormonal syndrome, these tumors are usually found on CT. If the patient has obstructive jaundice, a preoperative cholangiogram may be needed.

### LOCALIZATION STUDIES

CT scan is the initial study recommended for evaluation of endocrine pancreas neoplasms. If performed as a focused dynamic scan with thin cuts through the pancreas and intravenous and oral contrast, it is 35% to 85% accurate in localizing tumors. Furthermore, it allows for assessment of peripancreatic nodal enlargement and hepatic metastases.

Visceral angiography has traditionally been the next step in localizing these neoplasms, ranging from 45% to 85% accuracy.

In recent years endoscopic ultrasonography (EUS) has mostly replaced angiography for localizing tumors not visualized on the initial CT. In one study, EUS localized 32 of 39 tumors not seen on CT.

Selective transhepatic portal venous hormone sampling is still occasionally used for occult tumors with an accuracy of 70% to 95%.

The selective arterial secretin stimulation test is another option for localizing occult gastrinomas. It is performed by means of serial injections through the splenic, gastroduodenal, and inferior pancreatic duodenal arteries. It is a more sensitive technique than portal sampling.

Finally, intraoperative ultrasonography combined with surgical exploration is the only localization necessary for insulinomas. No preoperative localizing studies are required.

### PREOPERATIVE ORDERS

Neoplasm-specific measures should be performed before surgery. Insulinoma patients may require preoperative admission and intravenous fluids while NPO preoperatively. For gastrinomas, acid suppression should achieve a gastric pH greater than 4 using omeprazole doses of 20 to 200 mg/d. VIPomas require vigorous preoperative fluid resuscitation. To counteract its catabolic effects, preoperative total parenteral nutrition (TPN) should be administered to glucagonoma patients. Similarly, because of the impaired absorption and secretory functions seen in somatostatinoma, preoperative TPN and control of hyperglycemia should be emphasized. Also, in patients in whom distal pancreatectomy is the proposed operation, one must remember to administer preoperative pneumococcal vaccinations to help prevent overwhelming postsplenectomy sepsis.

**Nursing:** Accuchecks q6h for insulinoma, somatostatinoma, and glucagonoma; IS teaching
**Diet:** NPO after midnight
**IV fluids or TPN:** as above
**Laboratory tests:** T&C, CBC, BMP, PT, and PTT
**Medications:** cefazolin (Ancef) 1 g on call to OR
PAS on call to OR

## IV. SURGICAL ANATOMY

Gastrinomas and somatostatinomas are found to the right of the superior mesenteric artery (SMA) 75% of the time, and insulinomas and glucagonomas are found to the left of the SMA about 75% of the time. The gastrinoma triangle is bound superiorly by the junction of the cystic duct and common bile duct, inferiorly by the junction of the second and third portions of the duodenum, and medially by the junction of the neck and body of the pancreas. The pancreas is a retroperitoneal structure with no serosa. Its full exploration requires extensive dissection and evaluation of surrounding lymph nodes.

## V. CONDUCT OF OPERATION

The operative objectives universal to all of these tumors are to either cure or safely debulk maximal tumor mass and thus control hormone excess while simultaneously preserving maximum functional pancreatic parenchyma.

Surgery is indicated in patients with symptoms, those whose tumors are believed to be resectable, and for palliative debulking, except for nonfunctional tumors and in some metastatic gastrinomas that can be controlled with high-dose omeprazole.

The patient is positioned supine. After the induction of general anesthesia, including paralysis, a Foley catheter is placed, and the abdomen is shaved, prepped, and draped in usual sterile fashion.

The abdomen may be entered either through a midline upper abdominal incision or a chevron incision. The peritoneal cavity is carefully entered, and a brief exploratory laparotomy is performed to assess for metastatic disease, paying special attention to the liver.

Attention is then turned to performing a thorough exploration of the pancreas to localize the tumor. The gastrocolic ligament is divided to expose the body and tail of the pancreas. A full Kocher maneuver is performed to mobilize the duodenum, head, and uncinate process of the

30

NEOPLASMS OF THE ENDOCRINE PANCREAS

pancreas. Longitudinal dissection is then continued along the superior and inferior borders of the pancreas to allow for careful bimanual examination of the entire pancreas. The pancreatic tail in the splenic hilum is very difficult to assess.

The liver is assessed for metastases. The extrapancreatic sites, including the duodenum (by means of duodenotomy for gastrinoma if necessary, and always in MEN 1 patients), are examined. Other important extrapancreatic sites include the splenic hilum, small bowel, and mesentery. Any suspicious peripancreatic lymph nodes should be sent for frozen section, and the pelvis should be carefully evaluated in women.

Another important aspect of the initial exploration is intraoperative ultrasonography for tumor localization and to evaluate the pancreatic duct. This is especially important for MEN 1 patients and insulinomas, which commonly have multiple lesions.

Intraoperative esophagogastroduodenoscopy (EGD) with duodenal illumination is sometimes used for gastrinomas to help localize duodenal lesions. Retroperitoneal and adrenal exploration is necessary to thoroughly evaluate patients with VIPomas, because they can often be found here. A cholecystectomy should be performed in patients with somatostatinomas because of the risk of cholelithiasis.

Once the tumor is localized and the full abdomen has been thoroughly assessed for metastases, attention is turned to resection of the tumor. This can be achieved with various approaches.

*Enucleation* is the favored technique for insulinomas and some other tumors, especially if the lesion is less than 2 cm and does not involve the duct. Once the tumor is shelled out of the pancreas, the cavity is left open and a 10-mm closed suction drain is placed at the site.

*Distal pancreatectomy* is the most commonly used procedure for VIPomas and glucagonomas. This operation in combination with enucleation is also recommended for MEN 1 patients. Some important details of the operation include the Aird maneuver, in which the spleen and tail of the pancreas are mobilized anteriorly and to the right. Then the splenic artery and vein are suture ligated and divided 1 cm to the right of the area of proposed resection. Pancreatic tissue can next be resected, either sharply with subsequent suture ligature of the duct or with a gastrointestinal anastomosis (GIA) stapler. Drain the transected end with closed-suction Jackson-Pratt drains.

Finally, a *pancreaticoduodenectomy* may be indicated for some gastrinomas and nonfunctional islet cell tumors. It is rarely necessary for insulinomas. Important details of this operation include performing the Cattell-Braasch maneuver, mobilizing the ascending colon to the midline. This is followed by a Kocher maneuver extended to the left lateral edge of the aorta. Proceed with the portal dissection by dividing the gastroduodenal artery, mobilizing the gallbladder, and dividing the common bile duct just proximal to the cystic duct. The stomach is then transected with a stapler. The jejunum is likewise transected with a stapler, 10 cm distal to the ligament of Treitz. Its mesentery is sequentially divided and ligated. Traction sutures are placed on the superior and inferior portions of the pancreas at the level of the portal vein. It is then divided, and the specimen is handed off the table. Reconstruction then proceeds by way of an end-to-side pancreaticojejunostomy, followed by performance of an end-to-side choledochojejunostomy, and finally an end-to-side gastrojejunostomy. Before closing, closed suction drains should be placed at the pancreatic anastomosis, and a feeding jejunostomy to provide enteral nutrition to patients in whom delayed gastric emptying develops. Refer to the section on exocrine pancreas tumors for further details of this complex operation.

## VARIATIONS OF OPERATION

Blind pancreaticoduodenectomy is deferred in unlocalized insulinoma. If the tumor is not found, one should close and perform an angiographic localization procedure (peripheral vesicular system or intraarterial $Ca^{2+}$). This operation is controversial in gastrinoma. If preoperative studies localize the tumor to the "gastrinoma triangle" without a palpable tumor, some recommend performing a classic Whipple procedure so as to include all of the duodenum in the resection.

A longitudinal duodenotomy with tumor excision and primary repair should be performed for gastrinomas in MEN I kindred.

Biliary-enteric bypass is indicated for palliation in nonfunctional islet cell tumors. Another palliative option for metastatic disease includes laparoscopic thermal ablation of liver lesions.

## POSTOPERATIVE ORDERS

**Admit to:**
**Diagnosis:** s/p enucleation or distal pancreatectomy or pancreaticoduodenectomy
**Condition:** stable
**Vital signs:** per routine
**Activity:** bed rest then ambulate with assist in AM
**Allergies:**
**Nursing:** strict I&Os, NGT to LCWS, Foley to gravity, PAS until ambulating, IS × 10/h while awake, Jackson-Pratt drains to self–bulb suction
**Diet:** NPO until return of bowel function, then advance to regular diet
**IV fluids:** $D_5$/LR at 125 ml/h initially as patient will have third space losses, discontinue drains when output is less than 50 ml/d or drain amylase is less than serum amylase
**Medications:** IV PCA while NPO then oral analgesics once tolerable
**Laboratory tests:**

For metastatic or unresectable disease, consults should be placed to oncology.

Insulinoma patients should have debulking, as it is helpful because of the indolent course of these tumors. Nutrition should be consulted to teach dietary manipulations with high carbohydrates, frequent meals, and night-time snacks. Diazoxide and octreotide may also offer some symptomatic relief.

Metastatic or unresectable gastrinoma patients should be placed on omeprazole, which has nearly replaced total gastrectomy for palliation—except in noncompliant patients.

Palliative debulking is indicated for patients with VIPoma, and octreotide offers excellent symptomatic relief. Likewise, for glucagonoma, debulking should be considered, and octreotide often controls the hyperglycemia and dermatitis.

Somatostatinoma is most often metastatic at diagnosis, and debulking is indicated.

Combination chemotherapy with streptozocin, 5-fluorouracil, and doxorubicin has shown a 50% response in gastrinoma, 69% response in nonfunctional islet cell tumors, and marginal results in other tumors.

## VI. COMPLICATIONS

Pancreatic leak is the most common major morbidity associated with these operations. It is usually amenable to conservative therapy such as bowel rest with octreotide, TPN, and drainage.

## VII. DISCHARGE INSTRUCTIONS

Diet is unrestricted. No heavy lifting for 6 weeks. No driving while taking narcotic pain medications. Follow-up is in 1 to 2 weeks for a routine post-operative wound check. Gastrin levels should be checked in 1 month and repeated in 6 to 12 months to evaluate for tumor recurrence.

# ADRENAL DISEASE

*Lee E. Ponsky*

The adrenal glands are bilateral endocrine organs located at the superior and medial aspect of each kidney in the retroperitoneum. Historically adrenal pathology was discovered as a result of the signs and symptoms of adrenal dysfunction. However, with the introduction of computed tomography (CT) scans, the discovery of asymptomatic adrenal masses has increased significantly. The identification of these incidental masses has placed the responsibility on the physician to accurately diagnose these masses and commence the appropriate management. Since the 1990s the evolution and advancement of minimally invasive surgery has allowed laparoscopy to become the technique of choice for most surgical adrenal disease.

**31**

## I. PATHOPHYSIOLOGY

The adrenal gland consists of the cortex and the medulla, each of which behaves functionally as a distinct organ. The adrenal cortex is made up of three zones, each of which produces specific hormones. The zona glomerulosa is the outer zone and is the only source of the mineralocorticoid aldosterone. Aldosterone stimulates sodium retention and potassium secretion in the kidney, therefore promoting volume expansion. Aldosterone release is under the primary control of angiotensin II. Angiotensin II is a part of the renin-angiotensin-aldosterone system. The zona fasiculata is the middle zone, which produces and secretes cortisol, the major glucocorticoid found in the body. Cortisol is essential for cellular metabolism. The regulation of cortisol release involves the hypothalamus, pituitary gland, and adrenal gland intercommunication. Corticotropin-releasing hormone (CRH) is synthesized in the hypothalamus and delivered to the anterior pituitary by means of the portal system. CRH in turn stimulates adrenocorticotropic hormone (ACTH) release from the anterior pituitary. ACTH directly stimulates cortisol release from the zona fasiculata of the adrenal gland. The release of cortisol then has a feedback inhibition of ACTH secretion. The zona reticularis is the inner zone, adjacent to the medulla, which produces and secretes the principal androgens dehydroepiandrosterone (DHEA) and androstenedione. Adrenal androgens are significantly less active than testosterone; however, they can play a significant role in pathologic states of excess production. Adrenal androgen release is under some control of ACTH, but other mechanisms are also involved.

The deficiency or excess of these hormones results in the various pathologies associated with the adrenal cortex. For example, deficiency of one of the five enzymes necessary to convert cholesterol to cortisol can lead to congenital adrenal hyperplasia (CAH). The various signs and symptoms that may present depend on the deficiency of each specific enzyme, the associated lack of pituitary feedback, the subsequent adrenal

213

hyperplasia, and excess of the proximal precursors. With a proper understanding of the enzymatic pathways it is now possible to stimulate the system to demonstrate a more pronounced deficiency of a specific enzyme or hormone to assist with a diagnosis. ACTH, also known as corticotropin, can be administered to help uncover adrenal insufficiency (Addison's disease).

The excess of one or more of these hormones can result in the signs and symptoms of Cushing's syndrome, primary hyperaldosteronism (Conn's syndrome), or adrenal carcinoma. To help explain a specific diagnosis, the hormones or enzymes or both can be suppressed with synthetic compounds or drugs such as dexamethasone or metyrapone to identify the different types of Cushing's syndrome.

The adrenal medulla is located in the center of the adrenal gland. It is made up of chromaffin cells, which secrete catecholamines, primarily epinephrine; however, norepinephrine and dopamine are also secreted to a lesser degree. The enzyme that allows for the methylation of norepinephrine to form epinephrine is almost exclusively located in the adrenal medulla. An elevation of both norepinephrine and epinephrine highly suggests an abnormality in the adrenal medulla. The catecholamines bind to an adrenoreceptor, which then stimulates an organ specific response.

Systemic catecholamines, which are secreted by the adrenal medulla, have a short half-life of less than 20 seconds. The primary measurable metabolite of the catecholamines is vanillylmandelic acid (VMA), which is found in the urine. Metanephrine and normetanephrine are also metabolites of the catecholamines, which can be measured when evaluating patients for catecholamine-secreting tumors (pheochromocytomas).

## II. TYPICAL PRESENTATION

### CUSHING'S SYNDROME

Cushing's syndrome describes the signs and symptoms associated with elevated levels of glucocorticoids. The most common manifestations are found in young adults, more commonly in women, and include the following:

| | |
|---|---|
| Obesity | Osteoporosis |
| Hypertension | Easy bruising |
| Diabetes | Acne |
| Muscle weakness | Pigmentation |
| Hirsutism | Mental changes |
| Menstrual abnormalities | Edema |
| Sexual dysfunction | Headache |
| Purple striae | Poor healing |
| Moon facies | |

It is important to properly distinguish the terms Cushing's syndrome from Cushing's disease. Cushing's syndrome refers to the constellation of signs and symptoms resulting from excess systemic cortisol, whereas Cushing's disease refers to those patients with elevated cortisol as a result of excessive *pituitary* secretion of ACTH. Cushing's disease accounts for most patients with an endogenous cause of Cushing's syndrome. The most common cause of Cushing's syndrome is an exogenous source of cortisol (ie, therapeutic steroids). Patients are often not aware that they are taking steroid-containing medications, or often will not consider steroid-containing creams, ointments, and lotions as medications, when the physician obtains their history.

## HYPERALDOSTERONISM (CONN'S SYNDROME)

Hyperaldosteronism is characterized by hypertension, hypokalemia, and sodium retention. These factors often result in volume expansion, suppressed plasma renin activity, and alkalosis. The hypokalemia can lead to muscle weakness, periodic paralysis, or both. Other symptoms include nocturia, urinary frequency, headaches, polydypsia, parasthesias, visual disturbances, and cramps. On CT scan benign adenomas are rarely larger than 3 cm; however, most aldosterone-secreting carcinomas are larger than 3 cm.

## PHEOCHROMOCYTOMA

Pheochromocytoma manifests itself by means of the physiologic effects of epinephrine and norepinephrine. The signs and symptoms are extremely variable. The most consistent sign is hypertension. Additional symptoms include headache, excessive sweating, palpitations with or without tachycardia, anxiety, tremors, chest or abdominal pain, nausea, vomiting, weakness, fatigue, weight loss, dyspnea, visual disturbances, vertigo, constipation, seizures, bradycardia, paresthesia, and warmth with or without heat intolerance. Approximately 10% of patients with a pheochromocytoma do not have hypertension.

## III. PREOPERATIVE WORKUP

A detailed history and physical examination are essential. Also, an accurate list of all medications, lotions, creams, and so on needs to be elicited.

It is imperative to use the appropriate imaging techniques to correctly localize the adrenal pathology before surgery. Although ultrasonography will often detect adrenal lesions incidentally or as a screening test, CT or magnetic resonance imaging (MRI) are the examinations of choice to adequately evaluate the lesions. Radionuclide imaging such as

$^{131}$I-metaiodobenzylguanidine ($^{131}$I-MIBG) can be used to assist in the diagnosis, particularly for small lesions.

## CUSHING'S SYNDROME

For patients with Cushing's syndrome, cortisol hypersecretion must be confirmed. The determination of the 24-hour excretion of cortisol in the urine is the most direct and reliable index of cortisol secretion at this time. For those patients with equivocal 24-hour urinary cortisol excretion, the dexamethasone suppression test can be used to confirm hypersecretion of cortisol and distinguish the pituitary from adrenal or extraadrenal source. Dexamethasone is a synthetic steroid 30 times more potent than cortisol. Pituitary ACTH secretion is normally regulated by means of a negative feedback inhibition by cortisol. In normal individuals, 0.5 mg of dexamethasone given orally every 6 hours for 2 days causes a significant fall in 17-hydroxycorticosteroid, urinary free cortisol, or plasma cortisol. A less reliable alternative method is to administer 1 mg between 11 PM and 12 AM, and then measure the plasma cortisol level between 8 and 9 AM. Patients with Cushing's syndrome do not demonstrate suppression in response to the low-dose dexamethasone. The high-dose dexamethasone suppression test is used to help distinguish pituitary from adrenal Cushing's syndrome. For the high-dose test the patient is given 2 mg of dexamethasone every 6 hours for 2 days. The plasma cortisol and urinary free cortisol levels are than measured on day 2. In patients with pituitary-dependent Cushing's syndrome (Cushing's disease), there should be at least a 50% suppression of cortisol. Those with adrenal-dependent Cushing's syndrome or ectopic ACTH production will not demonstrate suppression.

## HYPERALDOSTERONISM (CONN'S SYNDROME)

The laboratory evaluation of these patients should include plasma potassium, aldosterone, renin, and bicarbonate levels. A 24-hour urinary excretion of aldosterone, sodium, and potassium is also useful. The plasma renin level would be decreased and aldosterone increased. Expected laboratory values would include hypokalemia, increased plasma bicarbonate, and increased urinary excretion of potassium. These patients should have their hypokalemia, alkalosis, and hypertension treated before surgery.

## PHEOCHROMOCYTOMA

The preoperative evaluation of these patients must include measurement of urinary epinephrine, norepinephrine, metanephrine, normetanephrine, and VMA. Plasma catecholamines can also be measured. Some patients with essential hypertension may demonstrate signs or symptoms of pheochromocytoma, as well as slightly elevated plasma catecholamine levels. These patients can be distinguished by use of the clonidine suppression test. The patients are given a single 0.3-mg dose of clonidine orally. Patients with neurogenic hypertension demonstrate a fall in plasma norepinephrine and epinephrine to a level below 500 pg/ml 2 to 3 hours after the medication is taken. In patients with pheochromocytoma, these catecholamines will not decrease.

MRI should be the imaging modality of choice in patients with biochemical findings of a pheochromocytoma. These lesions have a characteristic bright appearance on T2-weighted studies. The patient's blood pressure must be controlled preoperatively. Preoperative treatments are often initiated in these patients to avoid intraoperative hypertension and postexcisional hypotension. Many surgeons use alpha-adrenergic blockade preoperatively; if the patient remains tachycardic after the alpha blockade, beta-adrenergic blockade can be given after the alpha blockade. It is absolutely essential that the beta-blocker be given after the alpha-blocker to avoid acute right heart failure. The patient should also be well hydrated preoperatively to allow for adequate volume restoration. Alpha-blockade is often achieved with oral phenoxybenzamine for approximately 5 to 7 days before surgery. If beta-blockade is necessary, propanolol is often used for 2 to 4 days before surgery. There are others who use only calcium channel blockers and intravenous hydration preoperatively.

## PREOPERATIVE ORDERS

### Cushing's Syndrome
**Diet:** NPO after midnight
**Medications:** cefazolin (Ancef) 1 g IV on call to OR
PAS on call to OR

### Hyperaldosteronism (Conn's Syndrome)
**Diet:** NPO after midnight
**Medications:** cefazolin (Ancef) 1 g IV on call to OR
PAS on call to OR

### Pheochromocytoma
**Admit to:** hospital the night before surgery
**Diet:** NPO after midnight
**IV fluids:** $D_5$/0.45% NS + 20 mEq KCl at 150 ml/h (to maximize volume expansion preoperatively)
**Medications:** allow patient to take his or her normal antihypertensive medications
cefazolin (Ancef) 1 g IV on call to OR
PAS on call to OR

## IV. SURGICAL ANATOMY

The adrenal glands are paired organs in the retroperitoneum. They are located superior, medial, and slightly anterior to the corresponding kidneys. They are

ADRENAL DISEASE

31

usually approximately 5 cm in length by 3 cm in width and 1 cm thick. In the normal adult the gland usually weighs about 5 g. Grossly, the adrenals have a golden appearance. The blood supply from the numerous peripheral arterial branches enters primarily from the medial aspect. The main sources of arterial blood supply are from the inferior phrenic artery, the corresponding renal artery, and the aorta. The venous drainage differs between the right and the left. The right adrenal vein is very short and empties directly into the vena cava; the left adrenal vein empties into the left renal vein.

## V. CONDUCT OF OPERATION

### TRANSABDOMINAL LAPAROSCOPIC ADRENALECTOMY

**Left Adrenalectomy.** The patient is securely positioned in the right lateral decubitus position, the kidney rest is raised, and the table is flexed. It is important that the patient be padded appropriately. The surgeon and assistants stand facing the anterior aspect of the abdomen. The monitor is positioned on the opposite side of the operating table. The table is flexed, and the kidney bridge is raised. The patient is than prepped and draped. Pneumoperitoneum is obtained by either the Veress needle or open technique. A 3-4 trocar approach is most often used. A trocar is placed below the costal margin 2 to 3 fingerbreadths lateral to the lateral border of the left rectus muscle and is used for dissection in the left hand. A second port is placed at the lateral border of the left rectus, midway between the xiphoid and the umbilicus, functioning as the camera port. A third port is placed 3 to 4 fingerbreadths below the costal margin at the midclavicular line for the right hand. An additional trocar may be necessary for retraction. Initially the spleen, splenic flexure, and descending colon are mobilized. The left renal vein can be dissected to assist with identification and control of the main adrenal vein at its origin. The inferior phrenic, aortic, and renal hilar branches are ligated/clipped and divided as they are encountered throughout the dissection. Once the gland is completely free, hemostasis should be confirmed. The gland should be extracted intact within an impermeable bag.

**Right Adrenalectomy.** The patient is securely positioned in the left lateral decubitus position, the kidney rest is raised, and the table is flexed. The trocar placement is the same as for a left adrenalectomy, except an additional trocar is placed immediately below the xiphoid process. This additional port is used for retraction of the liver. The liver is retracted anteriorly and superiorly. The hepatic flexure does not need to be mobilized. The peritoneum overlying the lateral aspect of the superior pole of the right kidney is incised and reflected medially. The incision is extended from the line of Toldt laterally to the inferior vena cava medially, allowing access to the retroperitoneum and facilitating the exposure of the adrenal gland. The dissection is initiated between the medial border of the adrenal gland and the right lateral edge of the inferior vena cava. The main adrenal vein is short, and one must be careful during this part of the dissection. Once the vein is identified, it is ligated and divided. The dissection continues superiorly and inferiorly while clipping and dividing all arterial branches as they are encountered. The dissection continues meticulously until the gland is completely mobilized and free. The specimen should then be placed in an impermeable bag and removed through a port site.

## RETROPERITONEAL LAPAROSCOPIC ADRENALECTOMY

**Left Adrenalectomy.** Left adrenalectomy can be performed from either the lateral approach (most common) or posterior approach. The patient is positioned securely in the right lateral decubitus position, the kidney rest is raised, and the table is flexed. The camera port is placed just above the lateral border of the psoas. The left-handed port is placed approximately 2 fingerbreadths above the iliac crest. The right-handed port is placed just off the tip of the twelfth rib. The balloon dilator is used to develop the working space in the retroperitoneum. Gerota's fascia is incised. The area between the aorta and the adrenal gland is dissected to identify and control adrenal branches arising from the aorta. The plane between the upper pole of the kidney and the adrenal is developed. The main adrenal vein is then identified, clipped, and divided at its origin from the left renal vein. The adrenal gland is then dissected from its surrounding attachments, controlling the branches from the inferior phrenic artery and aorta as they are encountered. Once the gland is dissected free, it is placed in an extraction bag and removed through a port site.

**Right Adrenalectomy.** The important distinction between the left and right retroperitoneoscopic adrenalectomy is the steps in controlling the main adrenal vein. The right adrenal vein is short and drains directly into the vena cava. It is important to be cognizant of the location of the duodenum to avoid inadvertent injury. The remainder of the dissection does not differ significantly from the left retroperitoneal adrenalectomy.

Open adrenalectomy is always an option, particularly for patients in whom laparoscopy may be contraindicated.

## POSTOPERATIVE ORDERS

**Admit to:** nursing floor
**Diagnosis:** s/p laparoscopic adrenalectomy
**Condition:** stable
**Vital signs:** per routine
**Activity:** OOB and ambulate
**Allergies:**
**Nursing:** I&Os, PAS, IS × 10/h while awake, trocar site care per routine

**Diet:** (transabdominal) sips of clear liquids in AM, advance as tolerated; (retroperitoneal) clear liquids evening of surgery, advance as tolerated
**IV fluids:** $D_5$/LR at 125 ml/h
**Medications:** ketorolac tromethamine (Toradol) 30 mg IV × 1 in recovery room

        Percocet, 5/325 mg PO q4h prn for pain
        meperidine (Demerol) 25 to 50 mg IV/IM q4-6h prn for breakthrough pain
        prochlorperazine (Compazine) 10 mg IV q6h prn for N/V
**Laboratory tests:** Hb and HCT in AM

## VI. COMPLICATIONS

Hemorrhage is a potential complication of any surgical procedure. The anatomy of the adrenal vascular supply limits the ability to obtain vascular control during the dissection. The right adrenal vein is short and drains directly into the vena cava; it is therefore imperative to be cautious when manipulating the gland to avoid injury or avulsion of the renal vein. The adrenal arteries are often small and short. Care must be taken not to injure or avulse the adrenal arteries. In addition, the vessels must be properly identified and controlled as the dissection proceeds. Adequate vascular control and decreased oozing will also help improve visualization. If major bleeding occurs, a vascular clamp or forceps can be used to temporarily control the bleeding with pressure. Once the source of bleeding is identified, it can be controlled with surgical clips or sutures. It may be necessary to place an additional port if one of the existing ports is being used for temporary vascular control. Of course, it is never wrong to convert to an open laparotomy.

The close proximity of the adrenal gland to the spleen and pancreas on the left predisposes these organs to injury during dissection or retraction. One must also be aware of the potential for injury to the colon, stomach, and left kidney. During dissection of the right adrenal gland, there is potential for injury to the liver, duodenum, and right kidney. If one suspects an injury to the liver or pancreas, it may be necessary to leave a drain. If the injured organ cannot be adequately controlled or repaired laparoscopically, conversion to open laparotomy is necessary.

In patients with pheochromocytoma there is a risk of intraoperative hypertension during tumor manipulation. Minimizing tumor manipulation and ligating the adrenal vein at the onset of the procedure is imperative. After the excision of a pheochromocytoma the patient is predisposed to hypotension. It is important that these patients are well hydrated preoperatively to ensure they have adequate intravascular volume expansion.

Other potential complications that may be less common or less severe include pneumothorax, wound dehiscence, subcutaneous emphysema, and infection.

## VII. DISCHARGE ORDERS

Discharge home
Standard wound care
No heavy lifting, no strenuous activity for 4 to 6 wk
Regular diet
Pain medication as needed
No driving while taking narcotics
Resume home medications
Follow-up in 4 wk

# BREAST CANCER

*Michael Rosen*
*Emad Zakhary*

Breast cancer is the second most common malignancy in U.S. women. There is a 1 in 8 lifetime risk of diagnosis and a 1 in 28 chance of dying from breast cancer.

## I. PATHOPHYSIOLOGY

Several risk factors are associated with breast cancer. These include family history, early menarche, late menopause, obesity, alcohol use, estrogen replacement therapy, and radiation exposure. Specific genes linked to inheritance of breast cancer are *BRCA1, BRCA2, P53* (Li Fraumeni syndrome, and the gene *ca4s5ng* Cowden syndrome). Another theory poses an increased expression of oncogenes (*c-erbB-2, c-ras, c-myc*), of cell cycle proteins (cyclins, Ki-67), and of proteases (cathepsin D) as increasing the risk of breast cancer.

### DUCTAL CARCINOMA IN SITU

Ductal carcinoma in situ (DCIS) is a preinvasive lesion that should be treated as a malignancy. The management is controversial, because DCIS shows marked biologic and behavioral variability. Mastectomy has a cure rate of 98% to 99% and remains the "gold standard." The indications for considering mastectomy in the treatment of DCIS include a palpable or large mass (>2 cm), comedo histopathology, high grade, involved tumor margins after local excision, segmental or multicentric disease, young age, and genetic factors. The lifetime risk of recurrent carcinoma is 2%. There is no indication to proceed with axillary dissection because the chance of nodal involvement is only 1% to 2%.

Excision alone may have a recurrence rate of 18%. In general, 50% of recurrences are seen as invasive carcinoma. However, selected cases of nonpalpable or small (<1 cm) low-grade, noncomedo DCIS may be suitable for local excision with adequate margins (5-10 mm) and close surveillance. Excision and radiation therapy is another alternative. Studies suggest that breast irradiation after excision significantly reduced invasive recurrence. Lesions 1 to 2 cm in size of low or intermediate grade may be suitable for this option. Finally, the addition of tamoxifen after excision and radiation reduced recurrence from 13% to 8% (National Surgical Adjuvant Breast and Bowel Project [NSABP] B-24).

### LOBULAR CARCINOMA IN SITU

Lobular carcinoma in situ (LCIS) is a risk factor for cancer development rather than a precursor. It is an incidental finding in a breast biopsy performed for another indication. Most occur in premenopausal women. The risk of breast cancer development in both breasts is equal and is approximately 1% per year or 20% to 25% lifetime risk. The lesion is usually multicentric and bilateral. Subsequent malignancies may be either infiltrating, lobular, or more commonly ductal carcinoma.

At present, the consensus for treatment is lifelong close surveillance with clinical follow-up involving monthly breast self-examination, clinical examination two to four times yearly, and an annual mammography. Bilateral mastectomy may be a consideration for cases with a family history of breast cancer consistent with *BRCA1* or *BRCA2* hereditary patterns. There is no role for radiation.

## INVASIVE BREAST CANCER

There are two main options for the treatment of early-stage invasive cancer [Stage I (T1, N0, M0) and Stage II (T1, N1, M0 or T2, N0-1, M0)]. The first option is modified radical mastectomy with or without breast reconstruction. Second, breast-conserving therapy (BCT) can be performed, consisting of lumpectomy, axillary dissection, and subsequent breast irradiation. There is no survival difference for patients treated with mastectomy or BCT.

Locally advanced breast cancer (LABC) comprises large primary tumors (T3), skin changes as peau d'orange, satellite nodules, ulceration (T4b), fixation to chest wall (T4ba), fixed axillary nodes (N2), or ipsilateral internal mammary nodes (N3), and inflammatory breast cancer (T4d). LABC comprises noninflammatory LABC and inflammatory locally advanced breast cancer (IBC).

## INFLAMMATORY BREAST CANCER

Inflammatory breast cancer (IBC) is rare (1%-4% of all breast cancers) but carries a poor prognosis. Characteristic clinical features are erythema, peau d'orange, and skin ridges. The breast is diffusely swollen, with or without a palpable mass, which may be diffuse and nondefinable. The disease progresses rapidly, because more than three quarters have palpable axillary metastases at presentation. Delayed diagnosis is common and is usually the result of confusion with bacterial infection. A breast biopsy, including a portion of skin, will demonstrate tumor emboli in subdermal lymphatics.

The management of LABC involves a complete metastatic workup. Patients receive neoadjuvant chemotherapy until maximum tumor response (usually three to four courses). Generally, there is a high response rate (30%-40%). Then a modified radical mastectomy is performed. Finally, patients undergo radiotherapy to the chest wall, axilla, and supraclavicular regions and further chemotherapy; hormone therapy may be added as needed.

In some centers, patients with T3 tumors and large T2 tumors who respond to neoadjuvant chemotherapy can be converted to breast conservation surgery. In cases of IBC, if the inflammatory skin changes do not resolve completely with induction chemotherapy, the breast is irradiated before mastectomy. In cases of IIIA disease, no clear benefit for preoperative versus postoperative chemotherapy has been demonstrated. Because these cases are technically resectable, modified radical mastectomy with adjuvant therapy given postoperatively is appropriate.

## BREAST CANCER DURING PREGNANCY

Recent data indicate that stage-for-stage carcinoma of the breast in pregnancy is associated with a prognosis similar to that of nonpregnant women. There are, however, proportionately more cases with stage II and stage III cancers diagnosed during pregnancy.

Diagnosis is more difficult because of the low level of suspicion, the nodularity of the breast, and the decreased accuracy of mammography because of breast density. Thus, any dominant masses should be biopsied.

The treatment of breast cancer is somewhat different during pregnancy. For instance, no radiotherapy should be given during the entire pregnancy, and chemotherapy should be avoided during the first trimester. Modified radical mastectomy is indicated for stage I and II disease. For cases requiring adjuvant systemic treatment, chemotherapy can be given after the first trimester. Segmental mastectomy is contraindicated except in the third trimester, when radiotherapy could be reasonably delayed (4 to 6 weeks) until delivery. Termination of pregnancy has no role in stage I or II. There is no evidence that abortion benefits control or survival rate.

In stage III disease, treatment is combined multimodality therapy. Abortion may be indicated in early-stage pregnancy because of the need to administer chemotherapy and radiotherapy. Abortion can be avoided if chemotherapy can be delayed until after the first trimester and if radiation can be delayed until after delivery. Cesarean section may be considered in the third trimester to minimize delay in initiating cytotoxic therapy for stage II and III disease.

There is no proof that subsequent pregnancy has a detrimental effect on cases treated for breast cancer. Childbearing or estrogen-containing compounds must be considered cautiously in patients at high risk for recurrent disease (eg, stage II, III, and inflammatory cancer). Finally, lactation should be suppressed promptly in the postpartum period.

## MALE BREAST CANCER

Less than 1% of all breast cancer occurs in men. The incidence peaks at 60 to 69 years (ie, 5-10 years older than that in women). Several risk factors, including exogenous estrogen exposure, Klinefelter syndrome, irradiation, gynecomastia, orchitis, and high endogenous estrogen levels, have been associated with male breast cancer. However, there is no evidence of progression from gynecomastia to cancer. Thirty percent of patients have a family history of breast cancer. Linkage to the *BRCA2* locus on chromosome 13q in men, as opposed to linkage to *BRCA1* genes on chromosome 17q in women, is reported. There is also an increased incidence in Jewish and African-American men.

Lesions typically present as a hard, eccentric, nontender mass, with skin and nipple retraction, and occasionally patients will have nipple discharge. The diagnosis is usually delayed. In previous reports, 50% to 60% of patients presented with palpable axillary adenopathy. Infiltrating ductal carcinoma constitutes 85% of the cases. Paget's disease occurs rarely. Eighty percent of the tumors are estrogen receptor positive.

Mammography helps to differentiate gynecomastia from cancer. Gynecomastia is smooth and extends backwards from the nipple, forming a symmetrical cone; whereas cancer is eccentric with irregular margins and often with microcalcifications. Tissue diagnosis through a biopsy is essential. Men should undergo a similar staging workup as in women.

Modified radical mastectomy is currently the standard treatment. Radical mastectomy, which was done in the past, still has a role in patients who are seen with advanced disease. Adjuvant radiotherapy and chemotherapy carry the same indications as in women. In addition, tamoxifen is appropriate for estrogen receptor–positive cases. Orchiectomy and estrogenic steroids may induce remission in patients with metastatic disease.

The overall survival is worse than that for women, but when it is corrected for disease stage, survival is similar. Those with node-negative disease have an 80% survival rate at 10 years; this reduces to 40% for those with involved nodes.

## PAGET'S DISEASE OF THE NIPPLE

Paget's disease of the nipple is a chronic eczematoid eruption of the nipple. An underlying mass is present in about half of the cases. Ninety percent of these masses are invasive carcinoma. In cases that are not associated with a mass, 30% later have an invasive cancer; the remainder will have in situ disease. In one third of patients axillary nodes are involved at time of diagnosis.

Patients should be evaluated with mammography to detect any underlying lesions. Next cytology by means of scraping or imprinting is necessary. If these means are nondiagnostic, a wedge skin biopsy is performed. Microscopically, intraepithelial tumor shows pathognomonic Paget's cells—large, pale, vacuolated cells—in the rete pegs of the epithelium. Intraductal lesions are often multifocal.

If the patients have a palpable mass, a mastectomy and axillary node dissection is necessary. If no mass is present, mastectomy or wide local excision with an axillary staging procedure is appropriate. Adjuvant therapy is the same as for other breast cancers.

## II. TYPICAL PRESENTATION

Women can present with a palpable lump diagnosed on self–breast examination or routine physical examination. Commonly now patients present with a nonpalpable mass diagnosed on routine mammography. Patients require a complete history with specific documentation of the preceding risk factors. In addition, a physical examination should document size, location, mobility, texture, and surface characteristics of any breast mass. Palpation of any axillary lymph nodes should be documented, along with any other skin or nipple changes.

## III. PREOPERATIVE WORKUP

### EVALUATION OF THE PALPABLE BREAST MASS

The first choice is usually mammography (sensitivity 85%-95%; specificity 60%-75%). Signs of malignancy include microcalcifications and density changes. Suspicious lesions should undergo histologic diagnosis. Ultrasonography is useful to differentiate solid from cystic lesions, especially in dense premenopausal breasts.

### Methods for Tissue Diagnosis

1. Fine-needle aspiration biopsy (FNAB); sensitivity ranging from 90% to 98%. Nondiagnostic aspirates mandate a surgical biopsy. The presence of hormone receptors (estrogen receptor–progesterone receptor [ER-PR]) can be ascertained on FNAB specimens by immunocytochemistry.
2. Core biopsy is of value when an unequivocal diagnosis cannot be obtained by cytologic studies.
3. Excisional biopsy is necessary when a definitive diagnosis cannot be established by needle biopsy techniques. Quantitative ER-PR assays require 1 cm$^3$ of fresh tumor.
4. Incisional biopsy is indicated for patients with large primary lesions (>4 cm) for whom preoperative chemotherapy, radiation therapy, or both are desirable.

### EVALUATION OF NONPALPABLE LESIONS

Mammographic findings most predictive of malignancy include speculated masses with associated architectural distortion and clustered microcalcifications in a linear or branching manner. All patients should have a tissue diagnosis before proceeding to definite surgery. This is increasingly made by cytologic examination rather than open biopsy. Several options exist for obtaining tissue for nonpalpable breast masses.

1. Needle localized biopsy: under mammographic guidance and with local anesthesia, a hookwire is placed within the suspicious area.
2. Stereotactic core needle biopsy is best reserved for patients with either a mass not seen by ultrasonography or for microcalcification.
3. Ultrasonographically or mammographically guided FNAB is less accurate and less commonly used.

### PREOPERATIVE ORDERS

Preoperative orders should include CBC, SMA 18, and CXR. Bone scanning is controversial. Scans are indicated in the presence of osseous symptoms, elevated

**32**

**BREAST CANCER**

serum calcium or alkaline phosphatase, in the presence of lymph node metastases (N1, N2, N3), and advanced local disease (T3, T4). Alterations in liver function are an indication for CT of the liver. The use of tumor markers such as CEA and CA 15-3 have a place in the follow-up of advanced cases.

## IV. SURGICAL ANATOMY

The breast is a modified sweat gland located within the superficial fascia. It receives its blood supply from the internal mammary, lateral thoracic, posterior intercostals, superior thoracic, and pectoral branch of thoracoacromial artery. Lymphatic drainage is by means of the axilla and the internal mammary nodes. The axillary lymph nodes are located below (level I), deep (level II) and medial to (level III) the pectoralis minor muscle. There are three major nerves within the axilla. The intercostobrachial nerve is a sensory nerve supplying the medial aspect of the arm. Transection of this nerve results in numbness. The long thoracic nerve supplies the serratus anterior muscle, and division of this nerve results in a winged scapula. The thoracodorsal nerve supplies the latissimus dorsi muscle, and transection results in shoulder weakness.

## V. CONDUCT OF OPERATION

### MODIFIED RADICAL MASTECTOMY

A transverse elliptical incision is made including the nipple and areola. Next, flaps are raised superiorly up to the clavicle and inferiorly to the inframammary fold. Medially the dissection is carried to the edge of the breast to the sternum. Perforators from the internal mammary and lateral thoracic arteries should be controlled. Care should be taken while developing the flaps to keep them both thin enough not to leave any breast tissue behind and yet not so thin that the skin is perforated or that the flaps will become ischemic. The average thickness should be approximately 5 mm. Finally, the breast is dissected off the pectoralis major muscle with the fascia included in the specimen. This completes a simple mastectomy. The axillary contents are included in a modified radical mastectomy. A closed-suction drain is placed.

### LUMPECTOMY

A lumpectomy (segmental mastectomy) is essentially an enlarged excisional biopsy. It is usually performed in cases of a previous excisional biopsy that revealed positive margins. The previous biopsy cavity should be removed intact without violating the cavity. A circumferential margin of 1 cm should be obtained.

### AXILLARY DISSECTION

Muscle relaxants should be avoided to allow adequate stimulation of the long thoracic and thoracodorsal nerves to aid in their identification. The incision is made between the pectoralis major and latissimus dorsi muscles within the hairline. The dissection is carried down to identify the borders of the axilla. Initially, the latisimus dorsi is identified, and the insertion of the thoracodorsal nerve into the medial aspect of this muscle is identified. Gentle compression of this nerve should be followed by contraction of the latissimus dorsi muscle. Next, the lateral boarder of the pectoralis major is dissected. The medial pectoral nerves are identified and preserved. Meticulous dissection along the lateral aspect of the chest wall should reveal the long thoracic nerve. Then attention is returned to the thoracodorsal nerve, and it is dissected proximally to reveal the axillary vein. Now that all the borders of the axillary compartment are identified, the nodal tissue is removed, taking care not to injure the surrounding nerves or vessels. Of note, the intercostal brachial nerve (T2) is encountered and should be preserved to prevent numbness along the medial aspect of the arm. A closed-suction drain is placed, and the wound is closed in two layers.

Axillary node status remains the single best prognostic factor. The aim of axillary dissection is to stage and treat the local disease. Clinical examination of the axilla correlates poorly with the true nodal status as assessed histologically. In one series of T1N0 patients, 17% had histologically positive nodes; and this figure rose to 27% for patients with T2N0 disease.

There are three levels of nodal involvement in the axilla. Level I nodes are lateral to the pectoralis minor, level II nodes are deep to the muscle, and level III nodes are medial to the muscle. In the absence of level I involvement, few patients (1.3%) have lymph nodes at level II or III (skip metastases). With one node positive at level I, there is a 12% chance of nodes at level II and III. With level II involvement, 50% have disease at level III.

### The Three Methods of Axillary Surgery

1. Sentinel node biopsy is used in cases of clinically node-negative patients with small tumors (less than 2 cm). The sentinel node is the first drainage lymph node from the tumor and will accurately predict the status of the remaining nodes in greater than 95% of cases. Injection of radiolabeled (technetium) sulfur colloid or a blue dye into the tumor or skin overlying the tumor allows identification of the sentinel node in 90% of cases. Axillary dissection is then limited to patients with involvement of the sentinel node. When frozen section is used to assess the status of the sentinel node, there is a 10% false-negative result, which requires reoperation.

2. Axillary node sampling: Much debate has surrounded the use of axillary node sampling and the extent of dissection. Some advise four-node sampling, others advise axillary dissection to a particular level (the intercostobrachial nerve), in which case a minimum of 10 nodes are needed.

3. Axillary node clearance: Complete clearance including level III for patients with palpable clinically involved nodes.

## BREAST CONSERVING SURGERY

This includes lumpectomy with microscopically uninvolved margins, axillary dissection, and breast irradiation. T1, T2 (<4 cm); N0, NI, M0, or T2 >4 cm in large breast are indications for breast-conserving surgery. Some contraindications include T3-T4, N2, MI tumors; large or central tumors in small breasts; multifocal/multicentric disease; collagen vascular disease; prior irradiation of the breast region; and pregnancy. Subareolar lesions no longer are considered a contraindication. Extensive intraductal component (EIC) is not considered a contraindication, provided that negative microscopic margins are obtained.

Factors that are not contraindications include tumor size (except relative to breast size), location, histologic type or grade, patient age, and a family history. No data are available on patients who have mutation of *BRCA1* or *BRCA2*. With appropriate selection and the use of adjuvant systemic therapy, local failure appears in 8% of patients at 10 years.

## POSTOPERATIVE ORDERS

**Admit to:**
**Diagnosis:** s/p mastectomy
**Condition:** stable
**Vital signs:** per routine
**Activity:** OOB and ambulate
**Allergies:**
**Nursing:** strict I&Os, check drain outputs every shift, change dressing in AM; postoperative day 1 evaluate flaps, Pneumoboots, PAS
**Diet:** clear liquids and advance as tolerated
**IV fluids:** $D_5$/0.45% NS with 20 mEq KCl at 85 ml/h; D/C when tolerating PO
**Medications:** cefazolin (Ancef) 1 g IV q8h
pain medications prn
**Laboratory tests:**

## VI. COMPLICATIONS

Complications of mastectomy include damage to the long thoracic nerve, which causes a winged scapula. The thoracodorsal nerve can be injured, resulting in shoulder weakness. If the intercostobrachial nerve is divided, there will be numbness along the inner aspect of the arm. Seroma, infection, and flap necrosis are known complications as well. Pneumothorax and injury to neurovascular structures are rare complications.

Lymphedema after axillary lymph node dissection carries a lifetime risk of 10% to 15%. The incidence increases with the extent of axillary surgery performed. The combination of axillary surgery and radiotherapy further increases the incidence.

## VII. DISCHARGE INSTRUCTIONS

### ADJUVANT SYSTEMIC THERAPY

**Node-positive Patients.** All node-positive patients should receive adjuvant hormonal or chemotherapy, depending on the menopausal status and the ER status of the tumor. Premenopausal women with positive nodes should undergo chemotherapy. Hormone receptor–positive patients should add tamoxifen to their regimen. Postmenopausal women with positive nodes with negative hormone receptors should undergo chemotherapy. For postmenopausal women with positive nodes who are hormone receptor positive, tamoxifen is the treatment of choice. Chemotherapy may be added, depending on the patient's status.

**Node-negative Patients.** The potential toxicity of chemotherapy must be balanced against the potential benefit. The tumor size, ER status of the tumor, and nuclear grade are the most important prognostic indicators for treatment. Other prognostic indicators include histologic types (eg, tubular, papillary and colloid are favorable variants), blood vessel and lymphatic invasion, percentage cells in S phase, ploidy, Her-2 neu expression, mutated p53 expression, cathepsin and Ki-67 expression.

The decision to treat node-negative patients is based on a stratification of certain risk factors. Patients with a low risk of recurrence either receive no adjuvant treatment or receive tamoxifen if hormone receptor positive. High-risk cases should receive adjuvant therapy.

Currently recommended adjuvant chemotherapy consists of six courses of CMF: cyclophosphamide (C), methotrexate (M), and 5-fluorouracil (F). In high-risk patients a doxorubicin (D)-based regimen may be chosen (CD or CDF). High-dose chemotherapy with bone marrow support or the use of peripheral blood progenitors is under investigation for high-risk patients such as those with greater than 10 positive nodes or locally advanced cancers.

### ADJUVANT RADIATION THERAPY

The aim is to reduce the chance of local recurrence in the chest wall or axilla. Patients eligible for radiation therapy are those with direct involvement of the fascia or muscle underlying the breast, pathologic tumor size >4 cm, grade 3 tumor, lymphatic or vascular permeation, ≥4 positive axillary nodes, N2 (fixed axillary nodes), extracapsular extension, inadequate dissection (<6 nodes in specimen), residual tumor along axillary vein, and measurement of any axillary lymph nodes 2.5 cm in diameter. It is a common practice to irradiate a supraclavicular field that includes the axillary apex when four or more nodes contain metastases.

Follow-up after mastectomy involves examination every 3 months for 3 years, every 6 months for the next 2 to 3 years, then yearly. Mammography of the opposite breast should continue yearly. SMA18 and CBC at each office visit and chest x-ray done yearly.

Follow-up after BCT includes a mammogram 6 months after completion of the radiation and then every 6 months for the first 2 years followed by annual mammography. Yearly mammography should be performed on the opposite breast as well.

# PART IX

## Vascular

# CAROTID ENDARTERECTOMY

*Babak Dadvand*

The first carotid endarterectomy was performed in 1954. By 1984, it had become the most common vascular surgical procedure performed in the United States. Enthusiasm declined in the 1980s after controversy over morbidity and mortality rates following the procedure. Recently, though, a number of prospective randomized studies have established the efficacy of carotid endarterectomy in the treatment of cerebrovascular disease.

## I. PATHOPHYSIOLOGY

**33**

Atherosclerosis is the most common cause of stroke in adults. The cause of atherosclerosis remains incompletely understood. However, it usually develops at areas of turbulence, such as vessel bifurcations. The carotid bifurcation is the most common site of atherosclerosis in the cerebral circulation. Carotid bifurcation plaques initially appear as a fatty streak of the intima. With increasing size, plaques may ulcerate and embolize or thrombose the artery. Mature plaques are covered by a fibrous cap. The disruption of this fibrous cap can lead to a plaque becoming symptomatic. Stroke secondary to cerebrovascular disease may occur by two distinct mechanisms: ischemia due to low flow states or embolism.

## II. TYPICAL PRESENTATION

Some of the indications for carotid endarterectomy include transient ischemic attack (TIA) with significant carotid artery stenosis. Another indication is patients with asymptomatic carotid artery stenosis >60% diameter reduction (ACAS study; note, this number may vary slightly from one institution to another). Patients who experience a cerebrovascular accident (CVA) with substantial neurologic recovery in the face of significant carotid artery stenosis are candidates for carotid endarterectomy. Also, patients with nonfocal neurologic symptoms and bilateral high-grade stenoses or unilateral occlusion and contralateral stenosis should undergo carotid endarterectomy.

Other indications include acute stroke. In patients with mild to moderate deficits, one should wait 4 to 6 weeks or wait for a plateau in recovery before proceeding with carotid endarterectomy. In patients with crescendo TIAs or stroke in evolution the risk of carotid endarterectomy is greatly increased, but surgical results are better than medical therapy alone. However, severe neurologic deficits indicate that the patient is not a candidate for carotid endarterectomy. Patients typically present with one or more of the following symptoms:

1. TIA: an acute, focal, neurologic deficit (usually contralateral motor, or sensory, or both) that resolves within 24 hours with no residual effects

2. Reversible ischemic neurologic deficit (RIND): same as TIA; however, RIND lasts more than 24 hours but clears completely within 1 week

3. CVA or stroke: an acute, focal neurologic deficit but with incomplete recovery

4. Crescendo TIAs: repeated TIAs with a pattern of complete recovery between ischemic events

5. Stroke in evolution: an acute neurologic deficit of modest degree that within hours or days progresses to a major neurologic deficit with progressive cerebral infarction

6. Amaurosis fugax: temporary monocular blindness, "curtain being pulled over one eye"

7. Speech disturbance

## III. PREOPERATIVE WORKUP

The diagnosis of cerebrovascular occlusive disease is made using both history and physical examination, as well as radiologic modalities.

A careful history to elucidate any of the preceding forms of presentation is necessary. It is of paramount importance to establish the distinction between focal and nonfocal neurologic deficits. Emphasis during the physical examination should be placed on the neurologic examination, evaluation for carotid bruits, pulse examination for dysrhythmias, and comparison of blood pressure between arms to rule out vertebral basilar insufficiency.

A number of noninvasive and invasive studies can be done to determine the cause and effect of stroke. With carotid duplex scanning, the extent of stenosis is based on velocity criteria. As the stenosis increases, so does the velocity of blood in that area so that the total volume of flow remains constant in the vessel. It is most accurate when stenosis results in a greater than 50% diameter reduction.

Carotid duplex scanning is the most common modality used to assess carotid stenosis, but angiography remains the "gold standard." The advantage of angiography is that it provides a complete and detailed visualization of intracranial and extracranial arterial circulation. However, angiography can be painful, cannot be used in patients with dye allergy, and can cause renal toxicity, as well as stroke (2%-4%).

The computed tomography (CT) scan is useful to differentiate between hemorrhage and infarction. Furthermore, a CT scan can rule out neoplasm, arteriovenous malformation, or subdural hematoma, which can cause similar symptoms.

Magnetic resonance imaging (MRI) is more sensitive than CT scan for detecting acute stroke, but cerebral hemorrhage is less well identified by MRI than CT scan. Magnetic resonance angiography (MRA) allows evaluation of intracranial and extracranial arterial circulation, but its precision is inferior to standard angiography.

**PREOPERATIVE ORDERS**

> **Admit to:** Dr. _____
>
> **Diagnosis:** carotid stenosis
>
> **Condition:** stable
>
> **Vital signs:** as per routine
>
> **Activity:** no restrictions
>
> **Allergies:**
>
> **Nursing:** strict I&Os
>
> **Diet:** regular, NPO after midnight
>
> **IV fluids:** heparin lock IV fluids, $D_5$/0.45% NS + 20 mEq KCl at 100 ml/h after midnight
>
> **Medications:** patient's home medications
> cefazolin (Ancef) 1 g IV on call to OR
>
> **Laboratory tests:** CBC, electrolytes, BUN, Cr, glucose, PT, PTT-INR, and T&C 2 U PRBCs

33

CAROTID ENDARTERECTOMY

## IV. SURGICAL ANATOMY

The carotid artery is located within the carotid jugular sheath. The internal jugular vein courses lateral to the common carotid artery. The vagus nerve lies posterior to and between the two vessels. The ansa cervicalis loops around the internal jugular vein at the level of the crycothyroid ligament and runs along the anterolateral aspect of the carotid artery. The carotid bifurcation occurs at the level of C4. The internal carotid artery lays posterolateral to the external carotid artery. The facial vein crosses the bifurcation. The internal carotid artery is identified by its lack of extracranial branches. The superior laryngeal nerve is adjacent and medial to the superior thyroid artery, the first branch of the external carotid artery. As the hypoglossal nerve courses medially, it crosses posterior to the occipital artery, then anterior to the external carotid artery, and then posterior to the stylohyoid and mylohyoid muscles. The hypoglossal nerve crosses 1 cm above the bifurcation running parallel to the mandible.

## V. CONDUCT OF OPERATION

The patient is placed in the supine position, and general endotracheal anesthesia is administered. The neck and ipsilateral upper thigh are prepped and draped in the usual manner. A linear incision is made overlying the anterior margin of the sternocleidomastoid muscle. Dissection is carried through the platysma. The carotid jugular sheath is identified and entered just above the omohyoid muscle. Dissection is then carried superiorly along the anterior surface of the carotid artery. The facial vein is identified and ligated. The hypoglossal nerve is also identified. The superior thyroid artery and external carotid artery are controlled with a vessel loop.

The patient is then given intravenous heparin. The internal, external, and common carotid arteries are clamped, and an arteriotomy is made across the bifurcation. A small Sundt-loop shunt is placed in the internal and common carotid arteries and held securely with Javid clamps. An endarterectomy is then carried out using the standard technique.

A segment of vein is exposed in the left upper thigh through an incision parallel to the groin crease. This segment of vein is excised and opened longitudinally. The vein is then sewn in place as a patch angioplasty using a running 6-0 Prolene suture. Just before the patch closure is completed, the shunt is removed. Vessel clamps are released to fill the required segment. The final sutures are placed and tied, and blood flow is established to the external and internal carotid arteries. Heparin is reversed partially with protamine sulfate. The wound is checked for hemostasis. A Jackson-Pratt drain is placed behind the sternocleidomastoid. The platysma is reapproximated with a running suture of 3-0 Vicryl. The skin is reapproximated with interrupted vertical mattress suture of 4-0 Dermalon. The groin incision is closed in two layers with a running suture of 2-0 Vicryl in the subcutaneous tissue and a running subcuticular suture of 3-0 Monocryl. Benzoin and Steri-Strips are applied. The patient is awakened and extubated, and neurologic function is tested. The patient is then transported to the recovery room.

## VARIATIONS OF OPERATION

There are slight variations to the carotid endarterectomy. If the patient has had prior carotid endarterectomy or vein harvested for other reasons (eg, coronary artery bypass graft), the surgeon may choose to use Dacron, a synthetic material, for the patch angioplasty. There are occasions where a patch angioplasty is not used; rather, the endarterectomized vessel is closed primarily. The disadvantage of this procedure is narrowing of the vessel lumen.

## POSTOPERATIVE ORDERS

**Admit to:** Dr. _____
**Diagnosis:** s/p carotid endarterectomy
**Condition:** stable
**Vital signs:** q15min until stable, then q1h; notify house officer if SBP <90 or >170
**Activity:** bed rest, OOB in AM
**Allergies:** NKDA
**Nursing:** strict I&Os, Jackson-Pratt drain to bulb suction, Foley to gravity, PAS, IS × 10/h, neurologic check (motor and cranial nerves) q2h × 4, then every shift, check for signs of hematoma
**Diet:** sips of clear fluids, advance as tolerated in the AM
**IV fluids:** D$_5$/LR at 125 ml/h, heparin lock IV fluids when tolerating PO well

**Medications:** patient's preoperative medications
analgesia
aspirin 325 mg PO qd
no hypnotic medication unless specifically ordered
**Laboratory tests:** stat in recovery room: CBC, electrolytes, CXR

## VI. COMPLICATIONS

1. Myocardial infarction (most common): May occur in immediate post-operative period or later. Workup includes ECG, CBC, CK, CKMB/MB% q8h $\times$ 3, troponin, $O_2$ nasal cannula, NTG, $MSO_4$, transfer to SICU/telemetry
2. Stroke: May occur during or after carotid endarterectomy. Neurologic examination (ie, focal deficits) and radiologic modalities (eg, CT brain/MRI)
3. Bleeding (1%-5% of patients): Check coagulation markers; may need to go to OR
4. Wound infection
5. Cranial nerve injury: Hypoglossal nerve: tongue deviates to ipsilateral side
   Vagus nerve: hoarseness
   Marginal mandibular nerve: inability to pull down lower lip
   Superior laryngeal nerve: loss of high notes, voice fatigue
6. Recurrent carotid stenosis: up to 30%, but <3% are symptomatic.
   Two forms: (1) within 6 months of carotid endarterectomy (intimal hyperplasia)
   (2) >2 years after carotid endarterectomy (recurrent atherosclerosis)
   Follow with carotid duplex scan; may need to reoperate if meets any of the preceding indications

If a neurologic deficit develops in the immediate postoperative period, return patient to the OR:
a. If internal carotid artery is filled with thrombus, clamp the common carotid artery proximally, open an endarterectomy site, and perform a thrombectomy.
b. If no thrombus, perform an intraoperative arteriogram or carotid duplex scan.

33

CAROTID ENDARTERECTOMY

## VII. DISCHARGE ORDERS

Patients are discharged home usually on the first postoperative day. The patient must be afebrile and tolerating a regular diet. In addition, hypertension must be controlled. The Jackson-Pratt drain is removed on POD 1. Some surgeons remove the skin sutures on POD 2, whereas others have the patient return to clinic 5 to 7 days later for suture removal. There are no dietary restrictions. Patients should not drive while taking narcotic medication. The patient may shower. A follow-up visit is scheduled 1 to 2 weeks after discharge.

# MESENTERIC ISCHEMIA

*Jeffrey Hazey*

Arterial perfusion to the abdomen is supplied by three branches of the intraabdominal aorta, the celiac axis (CA), the superior mesenteric artery (SMA), and the inferior mesenteric artery (IMA). Ischemia as a result of occlusion or decreased flow in any of these vessels may be divided into acute and chronic processes and will be addressed individually. The key to treatment is prevention and timely/early recognition of gut ischemia before development of intestinal gangrene or necrosis. Once infarction has occurred, the respective segment must be resected, and mortality increases to more than 50%. Initial long segment resection or repeated resection may lead to short bowel syndrome and lifelong dependance on hyperalimentation, exposing the patient to all risks inherent to total parenteral nutrition.

**34**

## I. PATHOPHYSIOLOGY

### ACUTE MESENTERIC ISCHEMIA

Sudden loss of flow in any of these vessels may result from arterial embolism, thrombosis, or venous thrombosis. Another entity, referred to as nonocclusive mesenteric ischemia, describes a condition of inadequate perfusion, resulting in symptoms and ischemia in the absence of complete occlusion of the named vessels.

The abrupt onset of abdominal pain in the absence of physical findings is the hallmark of mesenteric arterial embolism. The typical presentation is pain out of proportion to physical findings with vomiting or diarrhea. The diarrhea may be bloody in response to mucosal ischemia and intestinal "spasm" causing a cathartic effect in the ischemic gut. This pain may progress to peritonitis, because mucosal ischemia progresses to transmural ischemia and full-thickness necrosis of the bowel wall. Once necrosis and peritonitis ensue, surgical exploration is mandatory, and mortality increases significantly. Patients exhibit a leukocytosis and metabolic acidosis on routine laboratory values, but these should not delay definitive diagnosis by means of mesenteric arteriography or surgical exploration if the index of suspicion is high. The embolic source is almost universally cardiac, with patients having a history of atrial arrhythmia or recent myocardial infarction with ventricular aneurysm or wall motion abnormality. This pattern of ischemia tends to spare the proximal jejunum and distal colon, because the embolism lodges in the proximal SMA distal to the proximal jejunal branches. The distal colon is then spared by means of the IMA.

Arterial thrombosis is often the result of longstanding atherosclerotic disease of the CA, SMA, and IMA. This occurs in elderly patients with a history of abdominal angina, coronary artery disease, and frequently aortoiliac occlusive disease or peripheral vascular disease. In patients who have had a aortoiliac reconstruction, suspicions should be raised regarding this diagnosis when they complain of abdominal pain in the absence of physical signs. These lesions often involve the ostia of the mesenteric vessels, and typically all three vessels are occluded before symptoms appear. The IMA usually is occluded as the result of longstanding aortoiliac disease, and patients usually have developed a rich collateral circulation compensating for the chronic relative ischemia. These patients may present during concurrent illness that produces relative hypotension or hypoperfusion. Dehydration with vomiting or diarrhea or sepsis may precipitate occlusion of a previously stenotic vessel. Abdominal distention, increasing fluid requirements, oliguria, and metabolic acidosis ensue as the patients progress from relative ischemia to necrosis and peritonitis.

Patients without longstanding atherosclerotic disease of the mesenteric vessels but severe cardiopulmonary dysfunction with cardiogenic or septic shock may present with signs and symptoms of intestinal ischemia. Nonocclusive mesenteric ischemia is the end result of splanchnic vasospasm. This may result from vasopressors in critically ill patients or postcocaine intoxication, and historically it is thought to have some link to digitalis therapy. The absence of a stenotic lesion on angiogram with arterial spasm is the hallmark. Treatment with surgical exploration for signs of peritonitis and intraarterial infusion of papaverine have shown benefit. The most important intervention a clinician can perform to reverse mesenteric ischemia is stabilization and improvement of the underlying hemodynamic instability.

Venous thrombosis can occur in hypercoagulable patients (antithrombin III, protein C or S deficiencies), portal hypertension, congestive heart failure, patients with intraabdominal sepsis, malignancy, or a history of deep venous thrombosis. These patients lack the classic history seen in chronic ischemia and typically are young. This may progress to gut necrosis and peritonitis, with equivalent mortality rates to that seen in acute arterial embolism or thrombosis. In distinction, this may be diagnosed by computed tomography (CT) scan with visualization of clot within the portal vein or SMV. Treatment is heparinization in those patients who are stable and without peritoneal signs. Surgical exploration is mandatory should a patient show signs of peritonitis.

## CHRONIC MESENTERIC ISCHEMIA

Longstanding atherosclerotic occlusive disease of the aorta and mesenteric vessels can produce a classic pattern of abdominal angina. This postprandial abdominal pain due to relative ischemia when the normal postmeal hyperemic response cannot occur because of atherosclerotic disease results in food avoidance and weight loss. Women are affected 3:1 relative to men, with a mean age of 60. Coronary artery disease, peripheral vascular disease, and aortoiliac occlusive disease with occlusion of the IMA compromise collateral flow. Occlusion of two or more mesenteric vessels typically precedes these symptoms. Treatment revolves around early recognition, angiogram, and comprehensive revascularization of affected vessels.

The celiac artery compression syndrome with compression of the celiac axis by the median arcuate ligament of the diaphragmatic crura may present as intermittent, reversible ischemic abdominal pain in the absence of intrinsic arterial or venous disease. This entity is difficult to diagnose, and careful selection of patients for surgery and division of the median arcuate ligament is mandatory.

Other causes of mesenteric ischemia include autoimmune disorders resulting in vasculitis and allergic or radiation arteritis. Fibromuscular dysplasia and intimal hyperplasia may involve the trunk of the CA or SMA in young women taking birth control pills and who smoke heavily.

## II. TYPICAL PRESENTATION

**34**

**MESENTERIC ISCHEMIA**

Acutely, the typical presentation is one of abdominal pain out of proportion to physical findings. Intestinal spasm may result in diarrhea, with bloody muscosal sloughing. Progression to transmural ischemia and necrosis will produce symptoms of peritonitis. Patients may become oliguric with increasing fluid requirements, and a metabolic acidosis may develop that will progress to hypotension and septic shock unless the inciting event is reversed and the ischemic bowel resected.

Chronic mesenteric ischemia on the other hand presents with chronic postprandial abdominal pain (intestinal angina), with food avoidance and weight loss. The classic scenario is cachectic-appearing elderly women with a history of aortoiliac occlusive disease or peripheral vascular disease.

Surgery is contemplated acutely in patients who present with signs of intestinal ischemia and necrosis or electively in patients with evidence of chronic ischemia. Patients presenting with signs and symptoms of peritoneal irritation or peritonitis should undergo abdominal exploration to assess bowel viability and the need for resection. A high index of suspicion with early intervention is the best chance these patients have for recovery. Delay with progression to bowel necrosis increases mortality to more than 50%.

Angiographic visualization of embolism, thrombosis, or stenosis in the acute or chronic presentation directs the surgeon to the cause. Elective revascularization of all involved vessels in patients with chronic ischemia is clearly preferable to acute revascularization in the setting of bowel ischemia.

## III. PREOPERATIVE WORKUP

A high index of suspicion in a patient with a classic clinical history is paramount for the prompt recognition and diagnosis of acute and chronic mesenteric ischemia. Complaints of severe, poorly localized abdominal pain in the setting of an unremarkable physical examination should raise suspicion. Laboratory values may show leukocytosis in the setting of metabolic acidosis. Fluid requirements will increase as the patient progresses to necrosis, and oliguria ensues. Sepsis and hemodynamic instability will ultimately occur in the absence of timely diagnosis and treatment of intestinal ischemia.

Duplex scanning of the mesenteric vessels can be used as a screening technique but has its limitations, especially in the setting of abdominal distention and gas. Decisions to operate rarely can be made on the basis of this study and should not delay definitive evaluation by angiography or surgical exploration.

Angiography remains the "gold standard" for diagnosis and potential treatment of mesenteric ischemia. A lateral angiogram is necessary to visualize the anterior takeoff of the CA and SMA. Ostial and proximal lesions are easily missed without a lateral view.

Thrombolytics may be used in the event an embolic source is localized on angiogram, and the catheter may be placed to infuse thrombolytics directly into the clot. This may result in clot lysis quickly, with corresponding clinical improvement. This can only be attempted in the absence of peritonitis and in patients who are clinically stable. Surgical exploration should not be delayed if a diagnosis of intestinal necrosis is entertained or there is any question of bowel viability.

## PREOPERATIVE ORDERS

In the acute setting of hemodynamic instability and active ongoing ischemia, aggressive resuscitation and stabilization is imperative before prompt surgical exploration. Attention must be paid to maintenance of hemostasis with monitoring of urine output, evaluation of electrolytes, hematocrit, and coagulation studies. Broad-spectrum antibiotics with aerobic and anaerobic coverage in the setting of intestinal necrosis and peritoneal contamination are important.

Patients undergoing elective revascularization for chronic mesenteric ischemia should have comprehensive preoperative evaluation of cardiopulmonary status. Any significant cardiac disease should be addressed and treated preoperatively, as it is in elective peripheral revascularization.

## IV. SURGICAL ANATOMY

The CA and SMA exit the anterior abdominal aorta proximal to the renal vessels high in the abdomen. The IMA has its takeoff below the renal vessels and proximal to the aortic bifurcation just off to the left of the anterior abdominal aorta. The celiac artery immediately branches into the splenic artery, left gastric artery, and common hepatic artery. This supplies blood to the foregut, liver, biliary tree, and spleen. The SMA provides blood flow to the midgut (small bowel, proximal colon) by way of the main branch of the SMA and the ileocolic, the right colic, and middle colic arteries. The IMA supplies the hindgut, including the distal colon and rectum by way of the left colic, sigmoid branches, and superior rectal and hemorrhoidal arteries.

Important collaterals interconnect these vessels, protecting the respective areas each vessel supplies should one or two vessels occlude. These collaterals develop and are most important during periods of chronic ischemia.

They offer some protection in the acute scenario but frequently have not had the time and stimulus to develop to the point where they can provide adequate flow in the event of an acute occlusion. The CA and SMA are connected by means of the superior and inferior pancreaticoduodenal arteries. The SMA and IMA collateralize by way of the marginal artery of Drummond and the arc of Riolan. In addition, there may be meandering retroperitoneal vessels that develop, and over time they may supply a significant amount of flow to other areas. The distal hemorrhoidal arterial and venous systems possess several collaterals with the systemic pelvic circulation.

## V. CONDUCT OF OPERATION

Surgical exploration should occur through a midline abdominal incision with complete abdominal exploration. Exposure of the celiac axis is notoriously difficult and is best addressed in a vascular surgery text. Retroperitoneal exposure of the SMA is accomplished by incising the retroperitoneal space lateral to the fourth portion of the duodenum and reflecting this to the right. The dissection is carried to the patient's right over the left renal vein, and the SMA is isolated as it exits from beneath the pancreas. The IMA is easily identified as it exits the aorta to the left below the renal vessels and proximal to the aortic bifurcation.

### ACUTE MESENTERIC ISCHEMIA

Patients presenting with signs and symptoms of peritonitis and bowel necrosis must undergo exploration by means of midline laparotomy. The cause should be determined on the basis of history, clinical presentation, and pattern of bowel necrosis on surgical exploration. If an embolic phenomenon is thought to be the cause, exposure of affected vessels with embolectomy may avoid resection of a large portion of bowel. Assessment of bowel viability should occur after any revascularization procedure. Frankly necrotic bowel must be resected. Often, bowel with marginal or uncertain viability is discovered. A number of procedures can be used to assess viability. Doppler ultrasonography detection of pulsatile flow on the antimesenteric border can be used to indicate adequate perfusion. Injection of intravenous fluorescein and photoplethysmography can be used as well. Despite having these diagnostic tools, viability may remain uncertain. In this event, two techniques may avoid leaving soon-to-be necrotic bowel behind. Exteriorization of questionable bowel segments rather than anastomosis allows direct visualization of mucosa. Also, a planned second-look laparotomy 24 to 36 hours later to assess viability and perform a delayed anastomosis is acceptable.

### CHRONIC MESENTERIC ISCHEMIA

Patients presenting with chronic mesenteric ischemia and elective revascularization of the CA, SMA, or IMA are approached similarly to other revascularization techniques. The CA, SMA, or IMA can have its flow restored by means of mesenteric endarterectomy or the more widely accepted aortomesenteric vein bypass to revascularize the CA or SMA. Angioplasty has been used in a limited number of cases with variable results.

Aortomesenteric vein bypass of the CA or SMA can be used in the acute presentation of arterial thrombosis secondary to longstanding atherosclerotic disease or in the elective setting during revascularization for chronic mesenteric ischemia. Saphenous vein bypass of affected segments should be done expeditiously if performed in the face of acute ischemia and before the decision to resect affected segments of bowel.

## VARIATIONS OF OPERATION

A number of surgeons are performing a minilaparotomy at the bedside of a critically ill patient. This is done under local anesthesia and used only for diagnostic purposes. If bowel is viable, the incision is closed at the bedside. Should necrotic, ischemic or nonviable bowel be found, the patient is immediately taken to the operating room for definitive procedure. This is useful to rule out those in the intensive care unit who do not need formal operative exploration but has its limitations as to what can be done at the bedside.

Increasingly, surgeons are performing laparoscopy to assess bowel viablity. This has its limitations in patients with adhesive disease. Techniques to assess bowel viability laparoscopically have not been perfected, and the cause of the ischemic disease is not so easily determined using this technique as it is with open surgery.

## POSTOPERATIVE ORDERS

Careful attention should be paid to urine output and hemodynamic stability. Fluid requirements should improve and pressor support decrease. Metabolic acidosis should improve if all involved bowel was resected. Nasogastric decompression with bowel rest to protect anastomoses and treat distention is imperative. Hemodynamic monitoring in the form of an arterial line and Swan-Ganz catheter is necessary to optimize cardiovascular performance. Broad-spectrum antibiotics should be continued until assurances of appropriate resection and treatment of all affected bowel can be made.

**Admit to:** ICU
**Diagnosis:** s/p mesenteric ischemia bowel resection
**Condition:** guarded
**Vital signs:** q1h
**Activity:** bed rest
**Allergies:**
**Nursing:** NGT to LCWS, Foley to gravity, drains to bulb suction, routine central and arterial line care, PAS, respiratory vent settings if necessary
**Diet:** NPO

**IV fluids:** lactated Ringer's at 150 to 250 ml/h to maintain urine output
**Medications:** ampicillin, gentamicin, and metronidazole (Flagyl)
               IV pressor support if necessary
**Laboratory tests:** CBC, BMP, LFTs, PT, PTT, ABGs

## VI. COMPLICATIONS

No complications are unique to surgical exploration with or without bowel resection for mesenteric ischemia. Infectious complications as a result of peritoneal contamination from perforation or necrosis include wound infection, dehiscence, intraabdominal abscess, and sepsis.

34

MESENTERIC ISCHEMIA

# DIALYSIS ACCESS: CHRONIC AMBULATORY PERITONEAL DIALYSIS

*Jeffrey Hazey*

The ability of the body to clear serum of potentially toxic metabolites, acids, and products of protein breakdown (nitrogens) is significantly impaired in patients with chronic renal insufficiency and absent in end-stage renal failure. In the absence of kidney transplantation the method of choice to clear the blood in patients with acute and chronic renal failure include hemodialysis and peritoneal dialysis. Hemodialysis includes many different methods of filtration, including traditional dialysis by means of an arteriovenous (AV) fistula, AV graft, Scribner shunt, or hemodialysis catheter. Newer critical care techniques include continuous AV hemofiltration with or without dialysis (CAVH ± D). This is driven by the patient's mean arterial pressure. Continuous venovenous hemofiltration with or without dialysis (CVVH ± D) is driven by a pump.

35

Peritoneal dialysis uses the peritoneal surface to facilitate fluid and solute exchange. This technique requires placement of a chronic indwelling catheter in the peritoneal space with access provided to the patient for continuous infusion or withdrawal of fluid and electrolytes. Placement and management of these catheters will be the focus of this chapter.

## I. PATHOPHYSIOLOGY

The peritoneal surface approaches that of total body surface area. The rich vascular supply and capillary network is thought to be the membrane responsible for the movement of solutes and fluid from the serum into the peritoneal cavity and vice versa. This is supported by the fact that vasoconstrictors have been shown to decrease clearance rates and vasodilators to facilitate clearance of solutes. In addition, vascular limitations; fistula, graft, or catheter dysfunction; and complications such as hypotension as seen with hemodialysis are eliminated. Circumstances that limit available peritoneal surface area also decrease the effective solute clearance. The movement of fluid and electrolytes is manipulated by differential concentration gradients of select solutes. Continuous ambulatory peritoneal dialysis (CAPD) uses osmotic shifts to withdraw excess fluid from the serum.

## II. TYPICAL PRESENTATION

Patients being considered for chronic ambulatory peritoneal dialysis typically come to the surgeon in one of two scenarios. They may present with acute renal failure or an acute need for dialysis as outlined later. These patients may require a short-term bridge of hemodialysis by means of a temporary

249

dialysis catheter until the CAPD catheter "matures" and is ready for use. Another subset of patients are those with chronic renal failure or a condition in which CAPD is anticipated in the near future. These patients are not undergoing any form of dialysis at presentation, and placement is elective.

Patients presenting for CAPD catheter placement carry a diagnosis of end-stage renal disease, necessitating dialysis to maintain their fluid, electrolyte, and nitrogen status. Others with intraabdominal (mucinous or pseudomyxomatous malignancy) or hepatic malignancy will typically be referred by their oncologist. The rare patient with intractable ascites and end-stage liver disease should have had aggressive medical management by the hepatologist fail before referral to a surgeon for placement of a CAPD catheter.

Placement of an indwelling CAPD catheter is considered a surgical procedure with specific indications and complications that surgeons need to be familiar with. Indications for placement of a CAPD catheter are not limited to chronic dialysis and include the following:

1. Acute renal failure: Patients may opt for this short-term approach while awaiting return of renal function.
2. Chronic renal failure.
3. As a bridge to hemodialysis.
4. Infusion of intraperitoneal chemotherapeutic agents for metastatic abdominal or hepatic malignancy.
5. In select patients with intractable ascites and manifestations of problems secondary to intraperitoneal fluid volume, a CAPD catheter may be placed to withdraw fluid as necessary.
6. Patients desiring home dialysis and the ability to freely move about.
7. Inability to tolerate hemodialysis because of cardiac disease or hypotension during hemodialysis.
8. Contraindications to hemodialysis. These include lack of vascular access, repeated infections, or inability to tolerate anticoagulation (ulcer disease, history of bleeding complications).
9. Diabetics may benefit from insulin infusion into the peritoneal cavity.
10. Patients infected with HIV (human immunodeficiency virus).
11. Some small children.

## III. CONTRAINDICATIONS TO CAPD

The surgeon needs to be aware of a number of contraindications to CAPD. These include the following:

1. Lack of effective peritoneal surface area to support dialysis.
2. Loss of abdominal domain with movement of fluid out of the peritoneum and into the chest or other inaccessible body cavities.

This may include hernias or other spaces where the dialysate would not readily exchange.

3. Respiratory compromise when the abdominal space is filled, with fluid limiting diaphragmatic motion.

4. Intraabdominal malignancy except for the indication of infusion of chemotherapeutic agents.

5. Previous abdominal surgery preventing safe placement of a CAPD catheter or that would increase the likelihood of catheter dysfunction.

## IV. PREOPERATIVE WORKUP

Preoperative evaluation should include basic laboratory values, blood count with attention to the hematocrit. Renal failure patients typically are anemic. Electrolytes including potassium and blood urea nitrogen and creatinine should be obtained especially if the patient is currently undergoing dialysis. Coagulation studies need to be addressed, especially if the patient undergoes the procedure shortly after a dialysis session. Patients with renal failure should be optimized medically before undergoing CAPD catheter placement. The operative time is usually chosen during a nondialysis day so that the patient may be dialyzed the day before the procedure to correct any electrolyte abnormalities and then dialyzed the day after the procedure to remove any excess fluid they may have received during the procedure. Patients are kept nothing by mouth the evening before the procedure and receive perioperative antibiotics to prevent infectious complications of an intraabdominal foreign body.

### PREOPERATIVE ORDERS
**Diet:** NPO
**Medications:** preoperative antibiotics
**Laboratory tests:** CBC, PT, PTT, BMP, LFTs

## V. SURGICAL ANATOMY

Knowledge of the abdominal wall muscle and fascial layers is imperative for accurate and safe placement of a CAPD catheter. This is essential for proper placement of the Dacron cuff within the subcutaneous tissue or rectus abdominis muscle. These cuffs will incorporate into the tissue, preventing tract site infection or drainage of dialysate from the peritoneum.

Placement of the catheter is in the infraumbilical location. Both the percutaneous and surgical CAPD catheter are placed below the umbilicus and into the intraperitoneal pelvis. The catheter tip or "coil" should reside in the pelvis with confirmation by means of fluoroscopy or plain abdominal film.

## VI. CONDUCT OF OPERATION

The percutaneous placement of CAPD catheters can be performed at the bedside. The skin and subcutaneous tract are anesthetized with local anesthesia, and a small skin incision is made. The catheter is inserted into the peritoneum pointing toward the pelvis and threaded over the trocar introducer until the Dacron cuff resides in the subcutaneous pocket. A suture may be used to close the entrance site, and placement is confirmed by plain abdominal films. Functioning of the catheter should also be confirmed at the time of placement. This is accomplished with the aid of a peritoneal dialysis nurse clinician with infusion of saline and return of appropriate amounts of fluid.

### VARIATIONS OF OPERATION

Surgical placement requires a transverse 3- to 4-cm infraumbilical incision to expose the anterior rectus sheath, rectus abdominis muscle, posterior rectus sheath, and peritoneum. The catheter is placed under direct vision through a purse-string stitch in the peritoneum and tunneled into the pelvis. The distal cuff is secured just above the peritoneum or posterior fascia within the belly of the rectus abdominis muscle. The anterior rectus sheath is closed, and the proximal catheter is then tunneled to a counter incision 4 to 5 cm away. It is brought through the skin with the proximal cuff residing in the subcutaneous space. The transverse incision is closed with a subcuticular stitch, and the exit site for the CAPD catheter is secured with a Prolene suture. Again, the catheter is tested to ensure easy flow of dialysate into the abdomen and unrestricted return of dialysate. Should flow into the abdomen or return of fluid be inadequate or slow, repositioning of the catheter is paramount to longevity of the catheter and successful peritoneal dialysis.

Laparoscopy can be used to place the catheter as the primary procedure or as an adjunct to reposition a nonfunctioning or poorly functioning catheter. It may be used to lyse adhesive disease that may be interfering with catheter function.

### POSTOPERATIVE ORDERS

Postoperatively, patient compliance is a necessity. Patient education and teaching are an essential part of their management and successful outcome with this method of dialysis. Sterile technique while handling and infusing fluid is paramount to avoid infection.

Patients may resume their normal activity almost immediately postoperatively. They should continue their normal renal diet.

## VII. COMPLICATIONS

Complications can be divided into those occurring as a result of catheter placement and those resulting from longstanding residence and daily manipulation.

Surgical complications include leaking of dialysate, bowel injury, bladder injury, bleeding (intraperitoneal or within the layers of the abdominal wall), and ileus. These can be avoided with good surgical technique and should be recognized at the time of placement.

Nonsurgical complications are most commonly infectious in nature. A variety of potential sources may seed the catheter or involve the peritoneum. Organisms can gain access to the peritoneum through the catheter tract as a catheter infection or through the gastrointestinal tract as with diverticulitis. Up to three quarters of the infections are due to gram-positive organisms, with approximately 20% being gram negative. These infections can be treated with intravenous and intraperitoneal antibiotics as long as the catheter and Dacron cuff are not directly involved. Once the cuff is infected, thus acting as a foreign body, it must be removed.

The catheter will likely malfunction over the course of a patient's dialysis. Approximately 85% of catheters are functional after 1 year. Catheter malfunction as a result of adhesions or omental wrapping of the catheter can be avoided with proper placement or corrected with laparoscopic repositioning of the catheter.

Adhesions or loops of bowel may contribute to areas of fluid loculation, making this inaccessible for an effective dialysis membrane. Again, laparoscopic adhesiolysis may improve and correct this complication.

The increase in intraabdominal pressure may facilitate hernia formation through a preexisting weakness in the abdominal wall or recanalization of a processus vaginalis.

## VIII. DISCHARGE INSTRUCTIONS

Dialysate concentrations and formulations will be addressed by the nephrologist. A typical dialysate exchange is 2 L four times a day. In general, dextrose is used to facilitate removal of fluid with a higher dextrose concentration in the dialysate to generate a net loss of fluid.

**35**

**DIALYSIS ACCESS**

# PART X

## Skin and Soft Tissue

# WOUND HEALING AND MANAGEMENT

*Edward E. Cherullo*

A wound is an intentional or accidental disruption in tissue continuity. The creation of this disruption initiates a series of events that culminate in healing and restoration of the tissue's integrity. An understanding of the multiple factors that contribute to the healing process will form the basis for the management of surgical and traumatic wounds and their complications.

## I. PATHOPHYSIOLOGY

Classically, wound healing is described as a continuum of three overlapping processes: inflammation, proliferation, and maturation. These processes are divided into three phases of wound healing: the lag phase, the proliferative phase, and the maturation phase. These phases of wound healing ultimately result in the return of both tissue strength and the protective epithelial barrier to infection.

The lag phase typically lasts for 2 to 3 days and has several distinct characteristics. An acute inflammatory response occurs immediately after injury and is dominated by vasoconstriction and dilation, platelet aggregation, and the release of the chemical mediators—prostaglandins and cytokines. These cytokines stimulate the migration of neutrophils into the wound. Polymorphonuclear neutrophil leukocytes predominate within the wound area for the first several hours of healing and engage in bacterial phagocytosis. Circulating monocytes are the second cellular type to move into the wound and become the tissue macrophages that aid in bacterial control and continue to release the chemokines that mediate repair. Epithelialization is complete by 48 hours in uncomplicated wound healing, and the approximated wound edges are then completely sealed.

The proliferative phase is marked by the migration of fibroblasts into the wound around postoperative day 4. These fibroblasts produce the collagen-rich extracellular matrix on which capillary buds grow from existing venules across the wound to supply nutrients to the healing tissue. Wound strength slowly increases during this phase of healing, and after the first month, an uncomplicated wound has reached approximately 50% of its final strength.

The maturation phase of wound healing begins in the third to fourth postoperative week and continues indefinitely as long as the tissue is alive. During this phase the cellular activity in the wound decreases substantially. The strength of the wound continues to increase because of the formation of collagen cross-linking, remodeling, and contraction. Remodeling of collagen takes place along lines of tension, and wound strength can eventually reach a maximum of 70% to 80% of that of intact skin. Contraction of the wound is mediated by myofibroblasts and results in the edges of the wound moving closer together until closed. Contraction plays a minimal role in wounds that are closed primarily.

Cytokines and growth factors are released at the site of injury and are directly responsible for the initiation of wound healing and mediating its progression. Platelet-derived growth factor (PDGF) is a potent attractant for inflammatory cells and fibroblasts. In addition, transforming growth factors alpha and beta, epidermal growth factor, fibroblast growth factors, monocyte-derived growth factor, and interleukin 1 and 2 act in concert with myriad other chemical signals to mediate the wound healing process.

## TYPES OF WOUND HEALING

Wound healing is typically divided into two broad processes that differ in presentation, healing and management. Healing by *first (primary) intention* occurs when surgical wounds and lacerations that are cleanly created are directly reapproximated and in which tissue repair takes place in an uncomplicated manner. Tissue edges healing by *secondary intention* are left unopposed and open and require the formation of healthy granulation tissue and epithelialization for coverage of the defect and underlying exposed tissues. *Granulation tissue* is beefy red, moist tissue overlying a wound surface. This tissue is rich in inflammatory cells, chemical mediators, and capillaries and supports the ingrowth of epithelial cells from the lateral edges of the wound. This tissue is not sterile, yet a large number of immune cells act as a barrier to infection. Chronic granulation tissue refers to unhealthy granulation tissue often with a superficial fibrin exudate. This tissue will not support epithelialization and must be debrided to allow new healthy tissue to grow in its place. Primary and secondary healing can be combined in a *delayed primary closure (third intention healing)* in which an open wound is closed under sterile conditions primarily after 4 to 5 days when bacterial counts are greatly reduced, thus decreasing the risk of infection. The success of delayed primary closure is directly related to the surgeon's ability to identify minor signs of infection in the wound before closure. Wounds closed in this manner heal with few complications and similarly to those treated by primary closure. Wounds initially closed primarily may become infected and thus require open drainage and conversion to secondary healing.

Skin grafts may be used to cover open wounds that are healing by secondary intention and have healthy granulation tissue. The grafted tissue receives its blood supply from the capillary-rich granulation tissue on which it is laid. To promote adequate healing in this instance minimal movement of the graft should occur so as to avoid disruptive shearing forces.

## FACTORS AFFECTING WOUND HEALING

**Extremities of age:** Children 2 to 7 years of age exhibit the most effective wound healing. In older adults, comorbid factors are present that interfere with optimal wound healing.

**Severe malnutrition:** Healing wounds require carbohydrates and fats in addition to multiple enzymatic cofactors for adequate closure. In general, wounds receive priority over other tissues for limited nutrients. In vitamin C deficiency (scurvy), wound healing is impaired because of altered collagen synthesis and cross-linking.

**Vascularity:** Areas of high vascularity such as the face heal quicker and with fewer complications than areas of lower vascularity such as the pretibial area. Systemic (diabetes mellitus) or local (peripheral vascular disease) processes that decrease the blood flow to a wound significantly compromise the healing process.

**Antiinflammatory drugs and immunosuppression:** Steroids given in the immediate postoperative period have an adverse effect on wound healing because of the importance of immunologic function and inflammation in the early phases of wound healing. Subsequently, these agents given after the first stages of wound healing have little effect on overall outcome.

**Foreign body:** A foreign body may act as a nidus of infection and decreases the bacterial count necessary to result in a clinical infection.

**Renal failure:** Uremia may contribute to poor wound healing.

**Obesity:** Adipose tissue is poorly vascularized. Obese patients also frequently have other conditions that impede wound healing such as diabetes and peripheral vascular disease.

**Radiation:** Irradiated tissue often has significantly decreased blood flow.

**Cigarette smoking:** Classically, nicotine and other agents present in cigarette smoke constrict small blood vessels and thus decrease oxygen delivery to the healing wound. The factors contribute to inefficient healing and potential infection.

## II. TYPICAL PRESENTATION

### SURGICAL WOUNDS

Surgical wounds are classified by the degree of suspected bacterial contamination and therefore stratified by the likelihood of infection. A clean wound is formed under sterile conditions. By definition the genitourinary, gastrointestinal, and tracheobronchial systems are not entered. A clean-contaminated wound is defined as one in which one of these systems is entered but minimal spillage has occurred. Clean and clean-contaminated wounds may be primarily reapproximated and healing occurs by first intention. A wound is classified as contaminated when gross contamination with enteric contents or purulent material has occurred. These wounds are likely to become infected and are often left open to heal by secondary intention. Dirty or infected wounds are routinely treated as open wounds and left to heal by secondary intention because of the high likelihood for the development of infection if the wound is closed.

| Clean (skin, vascular) | 1.5%-5% |
| Clean-contaminated (gastrointestinal, genitourinary, reproductive, respiratory tract) | 7%-11% |
| Contaminated (penetrating trauma, bowel spillage) | 10%-15% |
| Dirty/infected (gross pus, gangrene, bowel perforation) | 15%-40% |

## TRAUMATIC WOUNDS

Traumatic wounds present in a variable manner and may be associated with other significant injuries.

## III. PREOPERATIVE WORKUP

### SURGICAL WOUNDS

Prophylactic, preoperative antibiotics have not been proven to decrease wound infection rates for clean surgical wounds. Prophylactic antibiotic use has proven to be most effective in decreasing wound infection rates associated with clean-contaminated wounds. In general the choice of antibiotic should reflect the likely pathogens to be encountered. For example, in colon surgery the patient should receive antibiotic agents that are effective against aerobic and anaerobic colonic flora. The antibiotics need to be given at least 1 hour before the surgical incision is made to ensure adequate tissue levels are reached. Antibiotics should be discontinued within 48 hours of uncomplicated procedures, because they are of little benefit after this time and predispose to the development of antibiotic resistance and superinfection. For gastrointestinal procedures the patient may also receive a mechanical or antibiotic bowel preparation to further decrease the number of bacteria that could cause infection. Mechanical bowel preparations work by initiating a cleansing of the intestinal tract with unabsorbable inert agents. Commonly prescribed agents include GoLYTELY and Fleets Phospho-Soda.

### TRAUMATIC WOUNDS

No advantage has been demonstrated for the administration of antibiotics for minor uncomplicated soft-tissue wounds. Antibiotics are indicated for high-risk wounds or patients including those with prosthetic cardiac valves, orthopedic prostheses, diabetes, and deep, old wounds.

## IV. CONDUCT OF OPERATION

Surgical wounds are closed systematically in layers. Small wounds are ideally closed with interrupted sutures placed loosely, approximating the wound edges. In abdominal cases the peritoneum does not need to be reapproximated. The abdominal fascia is sutured with minimal tension with slowly absorbable (polydioxanone suture) or nonabsorbable (Ethibond) suture. It is important that when closing the fascia the stitches approximate the tissue but are not strangulating, because this can contribute to wound dehiscence or infection. The subcutaneous tissues should not routinely be reapproximated, because this adds nothing to the strength of the closure, but instead introduces a foreign body into the healing tissue and additionally acts to decrease blood flow to the wound. This subcutaneous suture thus contributes to the formation of potential postoperative wound infections. In some instances the subcutaneous tissues are reapproximated, such as Scarpa's fascia in pediatric inguinal surgery. Skin is closed with material suitable to the wound.

Patients with traumatic wounds require thorough investigation to reveal any associated injuries that are not readily apparent. The status of the vascular and neurologic structures should be assessed distal to the site of injury. The neurologic examination should be performed before the administration of local anesthetics or narcotic analgesia. The surrounding skin should be cleaned thoroughly using standard aseptic technique. The wound should be irrigated copiously with normal saline. Use of antimicrobial solutions should be avoided, because they interfere with wound healing. A bulb syringe or 16-gauge angiocatheter are effective delivery systems. Gross debris may be removed with gentle scrubbing. Hemostasis is achieved by elevation and direct pressure. Suture ligation or electrocautery can be used to control larger bleeding vessels. The wound must be completely explored to assess the complete degree of injury and identify the presence of any foreign bodies. Débridement is the surgical removal of any nonviable tissue not cleared by irrigation. This process can also allow for the more direct reapproximation of jagged wound edges. The decision to close a traumatic wound primarily is clinical, and many factors should be considered. Wounds open for greater than 4 hours have a high likelihood for significant bacterial colonization and may best be treated as open wounds.

## VARIATIONS OF OPERATION

Multiple techniques exist for effective wound closure. Adherence to good surgical technique will optimize wound healing. The wound edges should be protected from desiccation during long procedures, electrocautery and suture ligation should be used judiciously, and tissues should be handled gently. Closing sutures should reapproximate not strangulate tissues, and there are few indications to close "dead space" in obese patients. In patients with a large amount of subcutaneous adipose tissue, gauze packing is sometimes closed within the wound to wick exudates from the wound. This prevents the development of a subcutaneous seroma that can predispose to infection. These wicks are then removed on postoperative day 1 or 2.

## POSTOPERATIVE ORDERS

Wounds heal most effectively in the presence of adequate nutrients and oxygen. Ensuring adequate tissue perfusion is critical to postoperative wound management. This can be accomplished by ensuring nutritional needs are met and proper fluid balance is maintained. Protection from trauma and cleanliness is also critical to efficient wound healing. A small amount of stress to the wound edges stimulates effective repair. Therefore early patient movement and ambulation are helpful for wound healing. Postoperative prophylactic antibiotics should be discontinued within 48 hours, because prolonged use has no additional benefit.

## V. COMPLICATIONS

### INFECTION

*Superficial wound infections* constitute 75% of all wound infections and involve the skin and subcutaneous tissues superficial to the muscle and fascia. The usual source of bacterial contamination is the patient's own flora. Environmental causes account for only about 5% of wound infections. *A wound infection typically presents around the fifth to the eighth postoperative day.* Wounds should be inspected daily and the dressing changed as necessary. Patients manifesting a superficial wound infection may have spiking fever, wound erythema, tenderness, wound site warmth, swelling, fluctuance, drainage, and nonhealing. (The four cardinal signs of infection are rubor, calor, tumor, and dolor.) *Postoperative fever mandates examination and documentation of wound status.* The management of a superficial wound infection begins with opening the wound and obtaining aerobic and anaerobic cultures. The wound is then probed to ensure the fascial layer is intact. Broad-spectrum systemic antibiotics are indicated initially in patients with prosthetic devices (cardiac valves), systemic toxicity, compromised immune systems, or if significant cellulitis is also present. These antibiotics are changed to organism-specific agents when the culture results are available. Routine antibiotics are not necessary. The open wound is then packed (wet to dry) with damp gauze and a dry dressing placed over the packing. This is changed two to three times daily. The wound is then managed as an open wound and allowed to heal by secondary intention. Wound packing with wet-to-dry dressings aids healing by manually debriding fibrinous exudates from wounds with each dressing change. Dakin's solution, 2% boric acid, 0.25% acetic acid, and provodine-iodine solutions inhibit the successful growth of granulation tissue, but their antiseptic properties occasionally justify their use in heavily contaminated or infected wounds.

### DEHISCENCE

Wound dehiscence is the unplanned, undesired, complete separation of the wound edges. This process can occur in any patient with risk factors for poor wound healing. The most common technical causes of dehiscence are infection and excessively tight sutures. These tight sutures constrict the approximated tissues and cause local ischemia and ultimately tissue necrosis. Wound dehiscence generally occurs 7 to 10 days postoperatively when wound strength is low and wound stress is high because of movement, abdominal distention, or ileus. Patients may provide a history of a "tearing" sensation with coughing or notice a sudden gush of fluid. Wound dehiscence usually mandates immediate surgical exploration and repair to prevent evisceration.

## VI. DISCHARGE ORDERS

Patients should avoid stress to the wound, because it will not reach an acceptable strength level until about 6 weeks postoperatively. Patients undergoing abdominal procedures should avoid lifting greater than 15 pounds. In addition, patients should avoid straining and will benefit from a stool softener (narcotic analgesics can be constipating). Walking and limited activity should be encouraged. If the skin was closed with absorbable suture, the patient may remove the dressing and shower on postoperative day 2. Adhesive strips or an occlusive polymer (Calodion) may be present on the wound, and patients and families should be instructed these agents fall off in about 5 to 7 days. Patients should also be informed the wound will undergo significant remodeling for up to 1 year, and its appearance is likely to change (for the better) significantly with time. Patients with wounds closed with skin staples (clips) should have these removed around postoperative day 8. This will minimize the tissue reaction to the clip that results when they are left in place too long and the resultant poor cosmetic result. Finally, drainage from a previously closed wound, erythema, new pain, or swelling is not normal in the postoperative period, and the patient should be instructed to seek evaluation should these signs of possible infection develop.

36

WOUND HEALING AND MANAGEMENT

# SKIN AND SOFT TISSUE TUMORS

*Brett Butler*

Soft tissue tumors encompass a large group of cancers that arise from mesodermal elements, including bone, nerve, cartilage, connective tissue, fat, and muscle. Soft tissue tumors are classified by the tissues in which they originate. Sarcoma is added when the tumor exhibits malignant characteristics (ie, benign fatty tumor = lipoma and malignant tumor = liposarcoma). Sarcomas are rare, with only 6400 cases occurring each year in the United States.

## 37

## I. PATHOPHYSIOLOGY

These tumors occur equally in males and females. They occur in all age groups with no ethnic or racial predisposition. Sarcomas can be linked to radiation exposure, chemicals, herbicides, viruses, long-standing lymph-edema, neurofibromatosis-1, and Li-Fraumeni disease.

The sarcomas usually are contained in a pseudocapsule and typically grow by direct extension and generally along tissue plains. These lesions can occur in a variety of locations from the extremities to the retroperi-toneum, head, and neck. Treatment depends on the location of the lesion. Surgical resection is the mainstay of treatment, but some lesions respond to chemotherapy and radiation.

Sarcomas are classified by tumor histology and grade. Tumor grade is determined by the number of mitotic figures per high power field, the amount of stromal cellularity, and the amount of cellular atypia and is divided into low, intermediate, and high grade. Of note, tumor grade is the most significant prognostic factor in staging sarcomas.

Epidermal cysts, often referred to as sebaceous cysts, consist of a layer of epidermis superficially and more mature layers deeper. Keratin collec-tions in the center give a white creamy appearance. Lipomas are lobulated tumors containing normal fat cells. The malignant variant, liposarcoma, usually occurs in deeper plains and mostly in the thigh.

## II. TYPICAL PRESENTATION

Soft tissue tumors often present with minimal symptoms, and consequently patients will present with locally advanced tumors. Often some unrelated trauma brings the lesion to the patient's attention. These lesions are usually benign, but patients may wait months before presentation. Usually they have a painless mass that they have noticed for several months.

Cysts can range from soft to firm, typically arising on the scalp, face, ears, neck, and back. The patient usually ignores them until they rupture, cause local inflammation, or become infected. Once infected, they become warm and erythematous and often progress to an abscess.

Lipomas are soft, subcutaneous masses usually not fixed; they can be easily palpated in the fat and are typically visible. Often they are multiple and found on the trunk, but they can be anywhere on the body. Persons typically present for excision for cosmetic reasons.

Because of their location, retroperitoneal tumors usually present late in the course of the disease. These tumors can present with an abdominal mass, fullness, early satiety, and vague pain; it is rare to have any nodal metastasis on presentation. The lungs account for 75% of distant metastasis, but roughly only 10% of patients will have metastatic disease at original presentation.

## III. PREOPERATIVE WORKUP

### EXAMINATION

A complete history and physical should define the area of involvement, evaluate nodal involvement, include neurologic and motor examinations, and check for edema. If a mass has persisted longer than 6 weeks, one should proceed with a biopsy. In addition, any mass greater than 5 cm or an enlarging symptomatic lesion should be biopsied. This can include fine-needle aspiration (FNA), core needle, incisional, or excisional (if less than 3 cm).

### DIAGNOSTIC STUDIES

Further diagnostic studies include computed tomography (CT) or magnetic resonance imaging (MRI). CT is favored for evaluating the lungs and cortical bone involvement, whereas MRI is helpful in evaluating different tissue plains. Chest x-ray is useful in determining the baseline of lung involvement. Angiograms are occasionally necessary for large retroperitoneal tumors. Positron emission tomography scan can detect local extension and determine tumor grade. Abdominal CT scans are used to evaluate liver involvement with retroperitoneal sarcomas or liposarcomas.

### NEOADJUVANT THERAPY

With some intermediate- to high-grade sarcomas of the extremities, neoadjuvant chemotherapy (doxorubicin) and radiation are given preoperatively in an attempt to make limb-sparing surgery possible.

The preoperative workup for cysts depends on the patient's presentation. If the cyst is infected, start with a local incision and drainage in the clinic and packing three times a day. The patient should be started on an oral antibiotic such as cephalexin (Keflex) to cover gram-positive organisms. The patient should be instructed to clean the wound daily with a cotton-tipped applicator and hydrogen peroxide, and if the infection is cleared in 2 weeks, the patient should be scheduled for elective excision.

## PREOPERATIVE ORDERS

Antibiotics

Appropriate counseling on possible need to resect muscle and nerves impairing subsequent limb functioning

In retroperitoneal tumors, complete bowel preparation and possibility of stoma discussed with patient

## IV. SURGICAL ANATOMY

Soft tissue tumors can be extensive and can occur throughout the body. Tumors in the thigh, buttocks, and groin account for about half of these tumors, the torso accounts for around 18%, and 13% of tumors occur in the retroperitoneum.

## V. CONDUCT OF OPERATION

Operations can be quite varied and extensive, depending on the size and location of the tumor. However, the unifying principle involves complete resection with negative margins. A small mass less than 3.5 cm has a low probability of malignancy and should be treated with an excisional biopsy. For larger lesions or if insufficient cores were obtained by FNA, an incisional biopsy should be done. The incision needs to be properly placed in the extremity along the long axis. On the trunk or retroperitoneum an incision should be placed over the tumor. The placement is critical, because if a sarcoma is found, the scar will need to be excised during the definitive treatment. Care should be taken not to raise flaps or disturb planes superficial to the tumor. The specimen should be sent for frozen section to document negative margins. Finally, proper hemostasis is important to avoid difficulty with radiation or a re-resection. The placement of drains should be limited, but if a drain is necessary, it should be brought out the incision site to avoid tracking tumor cells.

The standard treatment of sarcomas of the extremity involves wide local excision. Margins of 3 to 5 cm of normal tissue proximally and distally are acceptable. Lateral and deep margins should extend to an area of grossly intact fascia. Nerves and vessels should be resected as needed, especially for high-grade tumors. Violating the tumor capsule should be avoided at all times. Radical amputation, which involves amputating one joint space above the tumor, is reserved for poor candidates with bony invasion, large tumor size, or recurrent tumors.

Retroperitoneal sarcomas are more difficult to treat because of their advanced presentation. Complete excision is only successful about half the time. Often it is necessary to resect adjacent organs to achieve negative margins. A transperitoneal approach is preferred to the flank approach, because it allows early control of the vascular supply and provides a better chance of complete resection.

Cysts are removed either before they rupture or after an abscess has been adequately drained. The most important point is to excise the entire cyst wall. With incomplete excision, there is a high recurrence rate.

## POSTOPERATIVE ORDERS

Sutures should be removed after 10 to 14 days, or longer if there is excessive tension on the extremity.

## VI. POSSIBLE COMPLICATIONS

Seromas can occur with large amounts of tissue undermining. Occasionally, they require percutaneous drainage.

Wound complications are not uncommon, especially when surgery was in a radiated field.

There can be local recurrence if negative margins are not achieved.

## VII. DISCHARGE ORDERS

With intermediate- to high-grade sarcomas, most patients will receive radiation therapy postoperatively. In low-grade sarcomas, radiation is advised only if there are positive margins. Depending on the nature of the sarcoma, such as bone, chemotherapy may be recommended. Chemotherapy has shown no benefit in retroperitoneal sarcomas. Many of these patients, especially those with extremity sarcomas, may need extensive rehabilitation after recovery. If the patient has a sarcoma, he or she will need a postoperative chest CT scan (if not previously done) followed by yearly imaging (alternating chest radiograph and chest CT).

# MELANOMA

*Lee Akst*

Melanoma occurs in the United States with an incidence of approximately 30,000 new cases per year. Although accounting for only 3% of all newly diagnosed cutaneous cancers, melanomas cause 65% of skin cancer deaths. Melanoma is treated surgically, with attention to both the primary site and the regional lymph nodes. Treatment recommendations in both these areas have been changing as knowledge of melanoma biology and melanoma behavior evolves.

## I. PATHOPHYSIOLOGY

## 38

Malignant melanoma is a neoplasm originating from melanocytes, which are the cells responsible for skin pigmentation normally found in the basal layer of the epidermis. Melanoma is typically found in patients with a fair complexion who sunburn rather than tan, and its incidence rises in populations living closer to the equator. Ultraviolet radiation is thought to be the agent driving both initiation and promotion of melanoma, as well as other cutaneous cancers.

Nonenvironmental factors associated with an increased risk for melanoma include a previous melanoma, the presence of dysplastic or congenital nevi, and a family history of melanoma. Although the lifetime risk of melanoma in the general population is approximately 0.5%, patients who have already had one melanoma have a 3% to 5% risk that a new primary melanoma will develop. Patients with dysplastic nevi have a 10% lifetime risk that a melanoma will develop, either de novo or within an existing dysplastic nevus. Although melanoma is not generally associated with small congenital nevi, the rare patient with a large (diameter >20 cm) congenital nevus has a lifetime risk of melanoma between 5% and 20%. Between 8% and 12% of malignant melanomas occur in patients with a family history of melanoma. These patients usually have a family history of dysplastic nevi as well. Evidence seems to indicate an autosomal dominant transmission, and chromosomes 1, 6, 7, 9, and 10 have been implicated.

## II. TYPICAL PRESENTATION

Malignant melanomas typically present as pigmented lesions noticed by visual inspection. Because other skin lesions may present with a similar appearance, biopsy is necessary to establish the diagnosis. Several characteristics differentiate melanomas from benign skin lesions. The color of a melanoma lesion classically varies, with brown or black lesions often containing areas of blue, white, or red. The perimeter of a melanoma is frequently "notched." The surface of a melanoma lesion typically is irregularly raised. Rapid growth, ulceration, bleeding, or darkening of a pigmented lesion increases concern for melanoma.

There are four types of cutaneous melanomas, based on different growth patterns and clinical characteristics:

1. **Lentigo maligna melanoma:** This least aggressive form represents 15% to 20% of all cutaneous melanomas. Typically they are large (>3 cm), flat lesions with brown or black pigmentation. Histologically, radial growth precedes vertical growth, and this type of melanoma may not invade the papillary dermis for several years.

2. **Superficial spreading melanoma:** Comprising about 70% of all melanomas, the superficial spreading variant is of intermediate malignancy. This form generally originiates in a preexisting nevus and grows both radially and vertically. These lesions typically have variation in color, irregular borders, and an irregular surface.

3. **Nodular melanoma:** This variant represents 15% to 30% of all melanomas and is the most aggressive. Nodular melanomas typically occur in uninvolved skin rather than in a preexisting nevus, and they grow predominantly vertically rather than radially. This growth makes early diagnosis difficult. Nodular melanomas typically are bluish black and more uniform in their coloration than other types and have smooth borders.

4. **Acral lentiginous melanoma:** This form of melanoma is rare within light-pigmented populations (2% to 8%) but represents between 35% and 60% of melanomas found in dark-pigmented populations. It occurs on the palms, soles, and in the nailbeds. They have a long radial growth phase, which presents as a flat lesion with color variation, followed by a vertical growth phase and increased metastatic potential. In the nails, this melanoma appears as an irregular tan/brown streak originating from the nailbed, which can be confused with a subungual hematoma.

The presence of any suspicious pigmented lesion is an indication for excisional biopsy with 1 to 2 mm margins. Because tumor thickness is the single characteristic that best determines prognosis and treatment, a full-thickness biopsy is necessary. If a suspicious lesion is transected with a partial-thickness shave excision and later proves to be melanoma, the ability to perform microstaging is lost. Lesions too large for complete excisional biopsy should undergo a full-thickness incisional biopsy or punch biopsy through the most raised or most pigmented area of the lesion. Once the diagnosis of malignant melanoma is confirmed, surgical re-excision of the primary site and surgical treatment of the regional lymph nodes are indicated.

### III. PREOPERATIVE WORKUP

Once the diagnosis of melanoma has been confirmed by biopsy, the patient is scheduled for surgery. This surgery should address both the primary site and the regional lymph nodes. Rarely, surgery might be used to palliate distant metastatic disease as well. The depth of tumor invasion determined at initial biopsy is critical in planning the surgical approach. Full-thickness excisional/incisional biopsies of suspicious pigmented lesions are always favored over partial shave excisions, because the latter cannot accurately determine the depth of invasion.

The most common sites of distant metastasis for melanoma are the lungs, liver, brain, bone, and gastrointestinal tract. Therefore, preoperative workup for patients with melanoma should also include a chest x-ray and liver function tests. In addition, any gastrointestinal or central nervous system complaints should be evaluated appropriately as directed by history and physical examination.

### PREOPERATIVE ORDERS

**Diet:** NPO after midnight
**Medications:** antibiotic on call to OR
                    PAS on call to OR
**Laboratory tests:** CMP, CBC, LFTs, CXR

## IV. SURGICAL ANATOMY

The most important anatomy with regard to melanoma is the histologic layers of the skin. The depth of invasion of the primary melanoma has been found to be the single best predictor of both local and regional spread of disease. Therefore the depth of invasion dictates the surgical approach used for both the primary site and the regional lymph nodes. The most superficial skin layer is the epidermis, which itself has five morphologic layers. Melanocytes occupy the *stratum basale,* which is the deepest epidermal layer, closest to the basement membrane. Deep to the basement membrane is the dermis, which has a more superficial papillary layer and a deeper reticular layer. The papillary dermis is a loose and highly vascular structure with fine collagen fibers, whereas the much thicker reticular dermis has thick, interlacing bundles of coarse collagen fibers. Underlying the dermis are the hypodermis and subcutaneous tissues.

There are two methods of microstaging based on the depth of invasion of the primary tumor (Table 38-1). The Clark system is based on the layers of the skin, whereas the Breslow system uses depth from the top of the granular layer of the tumor to the base of the tumor as measured by an ocular micrometer.

Overall, tumor thickness as measured directly has superseded the Clark level of invasion as the microstaging method of choice. It is more reproducible and less subjective than determination of the Clark level. Also, even within a single Clark level, tumor thickness has been shown to have an independent prognostic significance. Several studies have confirmed the usefulness of the Breslow system in predicting local recurrence, regional spread, and survival rates. For example, 10-year survival rates are greater

**TABLE 38-1**

METHODS OF MICROSTAGING

| Depth of Invasion | Clark Level | Approximate Breslow Equivalent |
|---|---|---|
| Contained within epidermis, no invasion of basement membrane | Level I | |
| Penetrates basement membrane, extends into papillary dermis | Level II | ≤0.75 mm |
| Tumor throughout papillary dermis, abuts but does not invade reticular dermis | Level III | 0.76-1.5 mm |
| Extends into reticular dermis | Level IV | 1.51-4 mm |
| Extends into subcutaneous tissues | Level V | >4 mm |

than 95% for lesions less than 0.76 mm thick and decrease to less than 50% for lesions thicker than 4 mm. Therefore current recommendations about treatment of the primary site and approach to the regional lymph nodes are based on tumor thickness.

## V. CONDUCT OF OPERATION

Surgery for melanoma involves both excision of the primary melanoma and treatment of the regional lymph nodes. With regard to the primary site, surgery can be seen as a staged procedure. Initial excisional biopsy should be performed with 1- to 2-mm margins. This biopsy confirms the diagnosis and establishes the depth of invasion of the tumor. This depth of invasion is the greatest predictor of tumor recurrence at the primary site, and deeper layers of invasion call for wider margins at the time of definitive resection. On the basis of several studies examining the relationship between tumor depth, the size of the margin, and tumor recurrence, the following guidelines have been established for control of the primary site:

> Melanoma in situ (no invasion through the basement membrane): 0.5-cm margin
> Thickness <1 mm: 1-cm margin
> Thickness 1-4 mm: 2-cm margin
> Thickness >4 mm: 3-cm margin

These guidelines should be modified on the basis of the site of the melanoma. For instance, lesions of the face may not allow for margins greater than 1 cm, because other vital structures might be nearby. In addition, subungual lesions should be treated with amputation at the appropriate metatarsophalangeal or metacarpophalangeal joint to allow for complete skin closure.

With regard to regional lymph nodes, surgical excision is the only potentially curative procedure that can be offered for regional metastases. Therefore, if there is palpable regional spread, a therapeutic lymph node dissection is clearly indicated. Even if such a resection is not curative, it can prevent future pain associated with tumor enlargement, skin breakdown, and tumor necrosis. The nodal drainage areas amenable to dissection include the ilioinguinal, axillary, cervical, and parotid regions. In the ilioinguinal region draining the lower extremities and lower trunk, a superficial groin dissection removes the superficial femoral nodes within the femoral triangle, whereas a deep groin dissection removes the iliac and obturator nodes as well. These deep nodes can be removed extraperitoneally through the same incision used to access the superficial nodes or intraperitoneally through a separate midline abdominal incision. This second approach allows evaluation of the paraaortic nodes as well. The approach to axillary dissection is the same for melanoma as for breast cancer, with care taken to remove levels I to III (the lymph nodes lateral, beneath, and medial to the pectoralis minor muscle). With extensive axillary involvement, supraclavicular disease might be present as well. If there is supraclavicular involvement, axillary dissection must be considered palliative rather than curative. In the head and neck, melanomas anterior to the ear and superior to the commisure of the lip spread first to the superficial parotid nodes and then to the cervical nodes. Melanomas posterior to the ear spread to the occipital and posterior cervical nodes, whereas those anterior lesions inferior to the commisure of the lip spread to the anterior cervical nodes.

Although there is universal agreement that management of palpable lymphadenopathy requires a therapeutic lymph node dissection, there is great controversy surrounding the use of elective lymph node dissection (ELND) for regional lymph nodes without clinical evidence of disease. Proponents of ELND argue that resection of occult micrometastases can reduce the risk of disseminated disease, whereas those who prefer to delay lymph node dissection until regional disease is palpable hope to save many patients the morbidity of possibly unnecessary surgery. Microstaging can help to select patients who might benefit from ELND. Patients with thin (<0.76 mm) tumors are at low risk for regional spread, and therefore do not benefit from elective lymphadenectomy. Patients with thick (>4 mm) tumors are at risk for distant spread at the time of presentation. Because of the likelihood of distant metastases, these patients also do not benefit from elective lymphadenectomy. Meanwhile, patients with intermediate (0.76–4 mm) tumors are at greatest risk for regional spread without distant metastases and therefore would benefit from ELND. Retrospective studies comparing wide local excision to wide local excision plus ELND support the survival benefit of elective dissection in the intermediate-thickness group. However, prospective studies have found no benefit to elective lymph node dissection compared with delayed dissection. Some of these studies were limited by a patient population with a preponderance of thin lesions, in whom no benefit was expected. Additional prospective, randomized trials are underway to further evaluate the benefit of ELND, but for now it remains one of the most controversial areas of surgical oncology.

Surgery for metastatic disease should generally be considered palliative. Occasionally there are patients with an isolated locoregional cutaneous or subcutaneous recurrence or an isolated pulmonary metastasis in whom surgical resection can be curative. However, these patients are the exception rather than the rule, and most patients with localized distant metastases cannot be cured by resection. Unfortunately, conventional chemotherapy and radiation therapy offer no benefit in an adjuvant role and are of limited use for the treatment of metastatic disease as well.

## VARIATIONS OF OPERATION

Sentinel node biopsy might help determine which patients would benefit from an ELND. In this technique, blue dye or a radionuclide is injected around the biopsy site at the time of definitive surgery. This blue dye or radioactivity marks the lymph drainage for the area of the lesion, and it is concentrated in the "sentinel" node. It is thought that melanoma involves a nodal basin in an orderly fashion and that involvement of the sentinel node is the first step. Studies have confirmed that in patients with a negative sentinel node biopsy, the remainder of the nodal basin was also uninvolved. In theory, then, sentinel node biopsy could be a factor in determining which patients with no clinical lymphadenopathy should undergo ELND. If the sentinel node contains micrometastases, elective dissection should be pursued, and if the sentinel node contains no metastases, an unnecessary procedure can be avoided. At present, sentinel node biopsy is still investigational, and a large multiinstitutional randomized trial is necessary before it becomes part of routine practice.

Another investigational therapy that might prolong survival in selected melanoma patients is adoptive immunotherapy. Adoptive immunotherapy involves the use of a patient's own lymphocytes to eliminate micrometastatic disease. There is evidence to suggest that interleukin-2 generates lymphokine-activated killer cells, which kill tumor cells nonspecifically. It is also possible that by harvesting and amplifying T lymphocytes that are manufactured by the patient in response to his or her own tumor, a more specific antitumor effect can be realized. As with sentinel node biopsy, adoptive immunotherapy remains investigational, and large randomized trials are necessary before it becomes a common part of clinical practice.

## POSTOPERATIVE ORDERS

Postoperative orders after surgery for melanoma will vary according to the site and degree of surgery performed. Some general postoperative orders include the following:

**Admit to:** surgey
**Diagnosis:** s/p

**Condition:** stable
**Vital signs:** per routine
**Activity:** (depends on site and extent of operation)
**Allergies:**
**Nursing:** routine I&Os, PAS, drains to bulb suction
**Diet:** as tolerated
**IV fluids:** lactated Ringer's at 100 ml/h; heparin lock IV fluids with
    good oral intake
**Medications:** analgesic, antiemetic, antibiotic
**Laboratory tests:**

## VI. COMPLICATIONS

The possible surgical complications also depend on the site and extent of the operation performed. Infection and hematoma are possible short-term complications of any operation. A long-term complication specific to lymph node dissection is lymphedema of the affected extremity. For example, in up to 25% of patients undergoing a deep groin dissection, edema will develop. Treatment is largely symptomatic.

## VII. DISCHARGE ORDERS

Patients with extremity resections and lymph node dissections should walk with assistance and keep the extremity elevated. Adequate pain medication should enable patients to be comfortable during ambulation. Patients require close follow-up with serial examinations for early detection of suspicious lesions.

# PART XI

Hematology

# SPLENECTOMY

*Bipand Chand*

Laparoscopic splenectomy has rapidly become the standard of care for most nontraumatic splenic disease. Laparoscopic splenectomy offers similar advantages as other laparoscopic procedures with significantly smaller incisions, decreased postoperative pain, less disruption of pulmonary function, and earlier recovery of normal activity levels. Indications for splenectomy include hematologic disorders, certain malignancies, and trauma.

## I. PATHOPHYSIOLOGY

39

The spleen functions to regulate cellular elements and has imunologic functions. The process known as pitting refers to the removal of nondeformable, intracellular substances such as Heinz bodies, Howell-Jolly bodies, and hemosiderin granules from red cells. The spleen can also remove aged red cells, abnormal neutrophils, and abnormal platelets. The removal of cellular elements involves either sequestration or the production of antibodies that result in the destruction of these cellular elements. In the normal condition, approximately one third of the platelet pool may be sequestered in the spleen, but this may increase to greater than 80% in splenomegaly. The opposite may occur in hypersplenism, which refers to the accelerated removal of any blood element leading to an anemia, leukopenia, or thrombocytopenia. The immunologic function includes the production of complement, tuftsin, opsonins, properidin, interferon, and IgM antibodies. The spleen also participates in phagocytosis of antibody-coated cells.

## II. TYPICAL PRESENTATION

### HEMATOLOGIC DISORDERS (ANEMIAS, THROMBOCYTOPENIAS, MYELOPROLIFERATIVE DISORDERS, MALIGNANCY)

**Anemias.** Hereditary spherocytosis (HS) is an autosomal dominant trait that results in a defective erythrocyte membrane. It presents with anemia, reticulocytosis, jaundice, and splenomegaly. Cholelithiasis is present in up to 30% of these patients. Splenectomy is the treatment of choice. After splenectomy the inherent abnormality persists, but the site of destruction is no longer present. Hereditary elliptocytosis is a variant of this disease process.

Thalassemia is transmitted as a dominant trait and results in a defect of hemoglobin synthesis. The disease is classified into alpha, beta, and gamma subtypes and has two degrees of severity: homozygous (major) and heterozygous (minor). The clinical manifestations of thalassemia major include pallor and poor growth and development in early age. Nucleated red cells, known as target cells, reticulocytosis, leukocytosis, and the presence of circulating fetal hemoglobin are present in this condition. Splenectomy may reduce the hemolytic process and therefore decrease the need for blood transfusions.

Hereditary hemolytic anemia may include enzyme deficiencies such as pyruvate kinase and glucose-6-phosphate deficiency or may be idiopathic. Most patients maintain hemoglobins, but some benefit may be offered with splenectomy. Most idiopathic hemolytic anemia results from the production of circulating antibodies against red cells. Anemia occurs when the spleen sequesters these red cells, thereby removing them from the circulating blood volume. Treatment options include blood transfusions, steroids, and splenectomy.

**Thrombocytopenias.** Idiopathic thrombocytopenic purpura (ITP) is an acquired autoimmune disease resulting in the destruction of platelets. The diagnosis is confirmed by demonstrating a normal or increased number of megakaryocytes and the presence of thrombocytopenia in the absence of any systemic disease or drug toxicity. ITP accompanied with autoimmune hemolytic anemia is known as Evan's syndrome. Acute ITP has an excellent prognosis in children and rarely requires surgical intervention. In adults, however, a long-term response to steroids, plasmapheresis, immune globulin, and other medications is uncommon. Splenectomy offers a 75% to 85% permanent success rate in patients with ITP.

Thrombotic thrombocytopenic purpura (TTP) is another immunologic disease process that affects the vasculature of the spleen without a direct known cause. The pentad of fever, purpura, hemolytic anemia, neurologic manifestations, and renal disease is present in most patients with TTP. Laboratory studies reveal thrombocytopenia, reticulocytosis, and leukocytosis and occasionally renal manifested dysfunction as azotemia, hematuria, proteinuria, and casts. The clinical course has a rapid onset, fulminant course, and is usually fatal. Repeated plasmapheresis may reverse the course, but occasionally the use of high-dose systemic steroids and splenectomy is performed with some success.

**Myeloproliferative Disorders.** Myeloproliferative disorders result in an anemia and in splenomegaly. A peripheral blood smear shows fragmented red blood cells and immature red cells. Symptoms usually relate to the anemia and may manifest as spontaneous bleeding, secondary infection, or relate to the size of the spleen, causing pain or early satiety. Treatment consists of transfusions, hormones, chemotherapy, and splenectomy. Splenectomy has been performed, in conjunction with the use of chemotherapy and radiation, for the treatment of Hodgkin's disease, non-Hodgkin's lymphoma, and chronic lymphocytic leukemia. Palliative splenectomy is performed before the platelet count becomes excessively low. Splenectomy being performed for staging patients with Hodgkin's disease has decreased because of the greater reliance on abdominal computed tomography and liberal use of chemotherapy.

## TRAUMA

The spleen is the most common solid organ injured after blunt abdominal trauma. Signs and symptoms include tachycardia, hypotension, and left upper quadrant pain. Injury scales evaluate for subcapsular hematomas, parenchymal lacerations, and the proximity of these injuries with the splenic hilum. Management depends on the hemodynamic stability of the patient, with ongoing bleeding mandating exploration. Hemodynamically stable patients are managed nonoperatively. A large percentage of blunt abdominal trauma patients are evaluated by spiral computed tomography scans. This allows assessment of the extent of splenic injury and determination of whether there is other concomitant solid organ injury. Patients taken for operation should undergo splenic salvage, except in cases of splenic rupture or severe hilar injury, in which case splenectomy is indicated. A more conservative approach in the pediatric population avoids surgical management in 85% of patients with splenic injury. In adults, approximately one third are managed by observation and one third by splenic salvage, and one third require splenectomy.

## III. PREOPERATIVE ORDERS

Patients undergoing elective splenectomy receive a polyvalent pneumococcal, meningiococcal, and *Haemophilus influenzae* vaccine ideally 1 week before operation. They are admitted the day of operation and given prophylactic antibiotics immediately before surgery. Routine bowel preparations are not given.

## IV. SURGICAL ANATOMY

The spleen lies in the left upper quadrant of the abdomen, deep to the ninth, tenth, and eleventh ribs. It contacts the diaphragm, stomach, pancreas, left kidney, and splenic flexure of the colon through the splenorenal, phrenosplenic, splenocolic, and the gastrosplenic ligaments. All are avascular with the exception of the gastrosplenic ligament containing the short gastric vessels, the splenic artery, and vein. Accessory spleens are most common at the splenic hilum, gastrosplenic ligament, splenocolic ligament, splenorenal ligament, and the greater omentum. They have also been reported in the pelvis and in the scrotum.

The adult weight of the spleen ranges from 75 to 100 g. The spleen is covered by a fibrous capsule and contains pulp in the inner trabeculae. The pulp is divided into three zones: white, marginal, and red. The red zone contains the cellular elements.

## V. CONDUCT OF OPERATION

### LAPAROSCOPIC TECHNIQUE

The patient is placed on the operating table in the supine position, administered general endotracheal intubation, and has a urinary catheter placed. The patient is then placed in the right-lateral decubitus position with an

39

SPLENECTOMY

axillary roll and the arms secured on a double armboard. The right knee is bent and the left leg is straight with both padded and with pneumatic stockings. The operating table is then broken at the level of the umbilicus to lengthen the distance between the iliac crest and the costal margin. The surgeon and assistant then stand on the right side of the table facing the patient's abdomen and viewing a single video monitor over the patient's left shoulder. Typically, three 10-mm trocars and a 10-mm, 30- or 45-degree scope are used. Initial trocar placement is done close to the midline using the open technique. Once pneumoperitoneum is established, two additional 10-mm trocars are placed under direct visualization. The typical position of the lateral port is at the level of the eleventh rib tip, and the middle port is halfway between the midline and lateral port. Proceeding from an inferior to superior direction, the peritoneal attachments are sharply divided. The dissection continues lateral to medial, with minimal retraction on the spleen to prevent capsular tear, until the hilar vessels are identified. The inferior pole is mobilized by use of the harmonic scalpel to divide the branches of the epiploic vessels. The superior pole is then mobilized by dividing the short gastric vessels with the harmonic scalpel along the greater curvature of the stomach. The remaining hilar pedicle is divided by use of a vascular gastrointestinal anastomosis stapler. The spleen is then placed into an impermeable retrieval bag and then morcellated into pieces with ring forceps for removal. The abdomen is then reinsufflated, and the operative site is irrigated with hemostasis ensured. Drains are placed only if pancreatic injury is suspected.

## OPEN TECHNIQUE

The incision may be midline or subcostal. A self-retaining Thompson retractor is then placed for exposure. With the surgeon positioned on the right side of the table, exploration of the convex surface of the spleen will define the avascular ligaments. Transection of the avascular ligamentous attachments using electrocautery allows for medial rotation of the spleen. The short gastric vessels coursing between the greater curvature and the spleen are then ligated with 2-0 silk ties, allowing the surgeon to deliver the spleen into the wound. Blunt dissection of any remaining posterior attachments allows further mobilization. Dissection at the splenic hilum must be meticulous to avoid pancreatic injury and to clearly identify the splenic artery and vein. Each of these is doubly ligated with a 2-0 silk tie. The spleen is then removed. It is important to locate and remove any accessory spleens in patients with hematologic disorders. Investigation should include the hilum, gastrosplenic ligament, gastrocolic ligament, and greater omentum.

## VARIATIONS OF OPERATION

Techniques to preserve splenic tissue are dictated by the extent of damage. Compression or the application of topical hemostatic agents, such as oxidized cellulose, collagen, or fibrin glue, can manage small lacerations.

SPLENECTOMY

More extensive disruption may require suturing techniques, wrapping with the omentum, or placement of an absorbable mesh. Suturing should incorporate the parencyhma and is most commonly done in horizontal mattress fashion, preventing further trauma. With extensive disruption, all devitalized tissue should be removed, and an absorbable mesh wrapped around the spleen acting as a compressive dressing.

### POSTOPERATIVE ORDERS
**Admit to:**
**Diagnosis:** s/p laparoscopic splenectomy
**Condition:** stable
**Vital signs:** per routine
**Activity:** ad lib, early mobilization
**Allergies:**
**Nursing:** I&Os, IS, Pneumoboots
**Diet:** clear liquid diet
**IV fluids:** $D_5$/0.45% NS with 20 mEq KCl at 125 ml/h
**Medications:** vaccines if not already given
adequate analgesics
**Laboratory tests:** serum amylase and hematocrit on POD 1

## VI. COMPLICATIONS

Postsplenectomy complications include ongoing hemorrhage and sepsis. The risk for overwhelming sepsis is less than 0.3% in adults and 0.6% in children; however, the mortality of this condition is greater than 50%. Usual agents are the encapsulated organisms, *Streptococcus pneumoniae, H. influenzae,* and *Neissera meningitidis.* Treatment should include prophylaxis with vaccination before elective splenectomy or within a short time after urgent splenectomy.

## VII. DISCHARGE ORDERS

Patients are usually admitted to a regular surgical floor and are routinely in the hospital for 2 or 3 days. Patients are discharged once they are tolerating oral diet, ambulating without difficulty, and their pain is controlled with oral analgesics. Follow-up is within 7 to 10 days in the outpatient clinic. Patients need to be instructed that any signs of a fever should prompt a call to their physician for immediate workup.

# PART XII

## Cardiothoracic Surgery

# CORONARY ARTERY BYPASS GRAFTING

*Abeel A. Mangi*

Coronary artery disease is a manifestation of a systemic disease, athero-sclerosis, which results in progressive narrowing of arteries of the cerebral, coronary, and peripheral vascular trees. Although tremendous progress has been made over the last several years, approximately 1.5 million people in the United States have an acute myocardial infarction each year, and 500,000 die. It remains the leading cause of death in the Western world.

## I. PATHOPHYSIOLOGY

Ischemic cardiac pain, angina pectoris, is caused by an inability of the coronary vasculature to meet the metabolic demands of the heart. This is the result of atherogenic narrowing of the vessel lumen to about 70% of its baseline cross-sectional diameter. Complete occlusion of the vessel is brought about by rupture of an underlying plaque, with thrombosis of the vessel. This event will result in infarction of the affected part of the heart, unless recognized and immediately treated.

The population at risk for myocardial infarction is the population at risk for atherosclerotic disease. This includes patients with a family history of myocardial infarction before the age of 55, hypertension, hypercholes-terolemia, diabetes, and cigarette smoking.

## II. TYPICAL PRESENTATION

Patients with angina pectoris often describe an exertional heaviness, pres-sure, squeezing, or tightness in the chest that subsides after cessation of physical activity. Persistence of such symptoms for more than 30 minutes may represent myocardial infarction. The discomfort may radiate or be located primarily in the arms, neck, or jaw. They may also be diaphoretic, nauseated, and complain of dyspnea. Syncope and dysrhythmias may occur. In approximately 20% of patients, especially diabetics, myocardial infarction is associated with only mild symptoms or no symptoms at all.

The diagnosis is clinical and is suggested by the preceding symptom complex and certain electrocardiographic changes. Myocardial infarction is confirmed by elevations in serum levels of enzymes such as creatine kinase and cardiac troponin-I.

Further risk stratification is provided by radionuclide assessment of myocardial perfusion and coronary angiography. In general, most patients with symptoms of angina will undergo radionuclide stress testing. Those unable to exercise are stressed pharmacologically. The presence of a reversible defect on stress test indicates an area at risk.

These patients proceed to angiography. Contraindications to stress testing include acute myocardial infarction within the previous 2 days, crescendo-type angina despite maximal medical therapy, serious dysrhythmias, severe aortic stenosis, symptomatic heart failure, and acute aortic dissection. These patients will ordinarily proceed directly to cardiac catheterization and angiography.

The clinical picture and angiographic results then guide patients toward one of three arms—medical management, percutaneous transcatheter angioplasty (PTCA), or surgical revascularization. Candidates for coronary artery bypass grafting (CABG) include the following:

Patients with significant left main coronary artery disease
Patients with three-vessel disease and depressed left ventricular function
Patients with two-vessel disease and significant proximal left anterior descending disease
Abnormal left ventricular function
Data are conflicting as to whether PTCA or CABG is beneficial in two-vessel disease and normal left ventricular function
Patients with one- or two-vessel disease without significant proximal left anterior descending artery disease who have survived near cardiac death, sustained ventricular tachycardia, or who have inducible ventricular tachycardia on electrophysiologic testing
Patients who have had prior percutaneous revascularization fail
Diabetic patients
Patients with complications of myocardial infarction, for example, ventricular septal defects, acute mitral regurgitation, ventricular free wall rupture

## III. PREOPERATIVE WORKUP

### CAROTID AND PERIPHERAL VASCULAR DISEASE

The cardiac patient is at particular risk for vascular catastrophe because of the underlying disease process, atherosclerosis. Symptomatic carotid bruits need to be aggressively evaluated and treated. It is controversial as to whether the presence of asymptomatic carotid bruits presents an increased risk of perioperative stroke. In some institutions, all carotid bruits are evaluated with noninvasive Doppler ultrasonography studies, with the goal of concomitant carotid endarterectomy at the time of CABG, if deemed necessary.

Evaluation of the peripheral vasculature is necessary because of the potential need for intraoperative or postoperative intraaortic balloon pump support. In addition, saphenous vein harvesting techniques must be particularly meticulous in the patient with peripheral arterial insufficieny. Finally, any femoral arterial injury, for example, pseudoaneurysms, caused at the time of cardiac catheterization can be repaired at the time of CABG.

## RENAL FAILURE

Patients who are dialysis dependent can undergo cardiac surgery if particular attention is paid to optimizing the patient's fluid and electrolyte balance in the preoperative state. The patient's ability to tolerate potassium cardioplegia is another concern, and intraoperative adjustments may be required if this is a concern.

The patient with borderline renal function presents more of a management problem. Aortic cross-clamping may induce renal ischemia or may exacerbate renal insufficiency by embolic showers from an atherosclerotic aorta. With current technologies, off-pump CABG may be a consideration in this patient population.

## PULMONARY INSUFFICIENCY

Median sternotomy is usually well tolerated by pulmonary patients. If there is a history of severe chronic obstructive pulmonary disease, asthma, or smoking, preoperative pulmonary function tests and arterial blood gas analysis may provide insight into the ventilatory weaning and postoperative management of these patients. They may also benefit from intensive pulmonary rehabilitation preoperatively, for example, incentive spirometry, bronchodilators, and quitting smoking.

## CHRONIC STEROID USE

Chronic steroid use predisposes patients to problems with wound healing, infection, gastric ulceration, or exacerbation of diabetes. If surgery is elective, the need for steroid use should be reevaluated and steroids discontinued if at all possible. In the setting of emergency surgery, stress dose steroids should be used.

## DERANGED LIVER FUNCTION

Patients with right-sided heart failure usually have deranged liver function and may be seen with elevated prothrombin times. These patients may benefit from preoperative vitamin K. In addition, a history of hepatitis is beneficial for the purposes of protection of the operating team.

## HEMATOLOGIC ABNORMALITIES

Antiplatelet agents are common in the preoperative cardiac population. Ordinarily they need to be continued to the time of surgery.

The blood bank needs to be notified of the number of units of blood that may be required at the time of surgery.

Cardiac procedures can also be performed in patients with known hematologic conditions such as hemophilia and von Willebrand's disease, assuming appropriate preparation by the surgical team and blood bank.

## DIABETES

Patients on oral hypoglycemic agents should have their medication held the morning of surgery. Patients who are insulin dependent are given half their normal dose the night before surgery, and their insulin is withheld the morning of surgery. All patients receive dextrose-supplemented crystalloid the night of surgery. All patients have their blood glucose levels monitored in the preoperative period and postoperatively.

The stress of surgery may occasionally unmask severe postoperative hyperglycemia. Cardiopulmonary bypass and intraoperative hypothermia tend to decrease the efficiency of administered insulin. Aggressive management may result in hypoglycemia as the patient rewarms. Hyperglycemia, however, may result in a brisk osmotic diuresis and should also be avoided.

## PREOPERATIVE ORDERS

**Admit to:**
**Diagnosis:** CAD
**Condition:** stable
**Vital signs:** per routine
**Activity:**
**Allergies:** NKDA
**Nursing:** strict I&Os; hold all diuretics; shave and prep chin to ankles bilaterally; shower with pHisoHex after prep; paint neck, chest, legs with povidone-iodine solution after shower; NPO after midnight; call doctor for HR <55 or >90; RR <10 or >20; SBP <90 or >140 mm Hg; T >38.3°C (101°F), or chest pain
**Diet:** NPO after midnight
**IV fluids:** $D_5$/0.45% NS with 20 mEq K at 100 ml/h
**Medications:** cefazolin, 1 g IV on call to OR
patient to take beta-blockers per usual routine
lorazepam (Ativan)1 mg PO/IV q4h prn
**Laboratory tests:** ensure with blood bank that cross-match sample is adequate and that blood is set up

## IV. CONDUCT OF OPERATION

The patient is laid supine on the table, and a right radial arterial catheter and pulmonary artery catheter are placed through the right internal jugular introducer. In addition, patients have a left antecubital 14-gauge intravenous catheter placed. After the induction of general endotracheal anesthesia, Foley catheter, orogastric tube, rectal and nasopharyngeal temperature probes are placed, and the patient is placed in the frog-leg position. R2 adhesive defibrillator pads are also placed on the patient.

The median sternotomy is performed using an air-powered saw. An oscillating saw is used for redo sternotomy, with the groins prepped in case of the need to emergently institute bypass through the femoral vessels.

Simultaneously, a team is harvesting the greater saphenous vein from the patient's thigh. Care must be taken not to raise a subcutaneous tissue flap. Vein branches should be clipped away from the vein so as not to impinge on its lumen. Care must be taken not to avulse small branches off of the vein. These injuries will require repair stitches and may impinge on the lumen of the graft. If the internal mammary artery is to be harvested, it is done at this time.

The pericardium is opened and suspended to form a cradle, and attention is diverted to the ascending aorta. After systemic heparinization and achievement of an activated clotting time (ACT) of >400 seconds, the ascending aorta is cannulated through two concentric purse-string sutures. Venous cannulation is achieved either through the right atrium or through bicaval cannulation. Cardiopulmonary bypass is then instituted with membrane oxygenation and cooling of the patient to a rectal temperature of 25°C (77°F).

Attention is then diverted to myocardial protection. If the ventricle becomes noticeably distended, it should be vented by placing a catheter into the ventricle through a purse-string suture in the right superior pulmonary vein and draining it. Chemical protection is based on cardioplegia. There are two methods for delivering cardioplegia: antegrade and retrograde. After the aortic cross-clamp is applied, antegrade cardioplegia is administered through the ascending aorta into the root. Retrograde cardioplegia is administered through the coronary sinus, which has to be separately cannulated. A third alternative is direct cannulation of the coronary arteries. All three have their advantages and disadvantages. Traditional crystalloid cardioplegia solutions are cold, hyperosmolar, and hyperkalemic. There is also a school of thought that advocates warm blood cardioplegia, which may be of benefit in patients with severe embarrassment of myocardial reserve.

Once the aorta is clamped and the heart arrested, the sites for distal coronary anastomoses are selected on the epicardial surface of the heart, and these are performed first. The proximal vein graft anastomoses are then completed. Preparations are then made to separate from cardiopulmonary bypass and to decannulate the patient. The most important consideration is to ensure adequate deairing of the systemic chambers to prevent cerebral air embolization.

Once a stable rhythm has been attained, the patient has rewarmed, and the surgeon is satisfied with the suture lines, the patient is decannulated. Two atrial and two ventricular epicardial pacing wires are placed and brought out to the skin. The heparinization is then reversed by the administration of protamine. Then two mediastinal drainage thoracostomy tubes are placed, and pleural tubes are placed if the pleurae were opened. On occasion, placement of a left atrial catheter may be necessary. The sternal edges are then reapproximated by means of stainless steel sternal wires, and the skin closed in routine fashion.

The patient is transported to the recovery room intubated, with drips according to institutional protocol and surgeon preference. At our institution a standard cocktail might include fentanyl and midazolam (Versed) for sedation, nitroglycerin, lidocaine, and levophed or nitroprusside.

## VARIATIONS OF OPERATION

There are several variations along this basic theme. In the setting of extensive aortic plaque, when cross-clamping may not be attractive or feasible, it is possible to proceed with fibrillatory arrest. In this case, cardioplegia is not used, and there is no aortic clamp.

It is also possible to perform a "beating heart," or off-pump CABG. One of the main challenges in this technique is that to gain exposure, the heart needs to be displaced within the mediastinum without causing hemodynamic collapse. Ingenious techniques combining a gradual rotation of the heart using sponges, balloons, or even surgical gloves that are gently distended with positioning of the patient and the table allow this to be accomplished. Another major challenge is to stabilize the coronary vessel to allow the anastomosis to be performed. Again, the development of stabilizing devices such as the Octopus Tissue Stabilization System (Medtronic, Minneapolis, MN) allows this to be done. The drawbacks of this procedure are that there is no cardiac protection, and in fact, coronary flow needs to be arrested for the anastomoses to be safely performed.

There is also burgeoning interest in the field of minimally invasive CABG (Mid-Cab), which is performed while avoiding a full sternotomy, using port access techniques similar to those for laparoscopic and thoracoscopic approaches.

## POSTOPERATIVE ORDERS

**Admit to:** ICU
**Diagnosis:** s/p CABG
**Condition:** critical
**Vital signs:** per ICU protocol
**Activity:** bed rest
**Allergies:** NKDA
**Nursing:** PAC care; radial arterial catheter care; Foley to gravity; OGT to LCWS; NPO; vent settings: IMV 10, PS 10, PEEP 5, 100% $FIO_2$; chest tubes to 20 cm $H_2O$ suction; daily weights
**Diet:** NPO
**IV fluids:**
**Medications:** fentanyl/midazolam (Versed) drip per ICU protocol
              morphine $SO_4$ 1-5 mg IV q1h prn for pain
              ranitidine (Zantac) 50 mg IV q8h
              metoclopramide (Reglan) 10 mg IV q6h prn for nausea
              acetaminophen (Tylenol) 650 mg PO/PR q4h prn
              aspirin 325 mg PO/PR qd—first dose within 6 h of surgery
              norepinephrine (Levophed) per ICU protocol to keep MAP
                  65-75 mm Hg or SBP 90-100 mm Hg

nitroprusside per ICU protocol to keep MAP 65-75 mm
Hg or SBP 90-100 mm Hg
nitroglycerin at 1 $\mu$g/kg/min
lidocaine at 1 mg/h
cefazolin (Ancef) 1 g IV q8h

**Laboratory tests:** CBC, PT, PTT, BMP, ABGs on arrival to ICU, CXR
on arrival to ICU, 12-lead ECG on arrival to ICU

## V. COMPLICATIONS

### CARDIAC

**Low Cardiac Output.** Low cardiac output, the most common perioperative
issue, is related to the temporary decrease in ventricular function as the
heart recovers from arrest, hypothermia, and physical manipulation. Left
ventricular function usually is at its nadir around 4 hours after surgery and
will recover anywhere from 12 to 72 hours postoperatively. A cardiac index
of greater than 2 L/min/m$^2$ is desirable. To optimize it, an understanding of
basic cardiac physiology is critical.

Heart rate can be optimized by pacing the atria at 85 beats per minute.
The rhythm should be optimized too. Atrial or ventricular dysrhythmias
need to be recognized and controlled early, with pharmacologic or electrical
means. Ideally, drugs that depress contractility such as beta-blockers or
calcium channel blockers should be avoided in the early postoperative
period. Digoxin, adenosine, procainamide, and amiodarone are the drugs of
choice at our institution for the control of rapid atrial dysrhythmias in the
early postoperative period. Lidocaine and amiodarone are used for the
control of wide complex tachycardias.

Ventricular filling pressures need to be optimized. On average, a mean
pulmonary arterial pressure greater than 20 will suffice but may have to be
significantly higher in the setting of aortic stenosis or long-standing
hypertension, which result in a large, thick ventricle. If blood pressure
allows, reducing afterload pharmacologically may allow more effective
emptying of the ventricle, thereby boosting cardiac output.

Finally, failing all of the preceding measures, inotropes can be added to
enhance cardiac contractility. This class of drugs includes levophed,
dopamine (in doses greater than 3 $\mu$g/kg/min), epinephrine, milrinone,
dobutamine, and isoproterenol.

It is important to recognize that depressed cardiac output in the setting of
rising ventricular filling pressures indicates a tension pneumothorax or cardiac
tamponade. These conditions are readily recognized and fixed by a vigilant
observer and can rapidly result in the death of the patient if unrecognized.

**Hypotension.** The most common cause of postoperative hypotension is
rewarming. As the patient rewarms, vasodilation occurs. This temporary loss
of vascular tone results in hypotension. The resident needs to be vigilant

and ensure that the hypotension is not due to any of the causes listed earlier. If it is purely a tone issue, addition of a pressor (neosynephrine) or a pressor/inotrope (levophed) will maintain an adequate blood pressure.

**Hypertension.** There are several causes for hypertension in the postoperative patient. Pain, irritation from the endotracheal tube, emergence from anesthesia, disorientation, and uncontrolled preoperative hypertension can all contribute to this state. It is important to control because of all the vascular suture lines, which if they are disrupted can lead to uncontrollable bleeding or dissection. It can be controlled by the addition of vasodilators such as nitroglycerin or nitroprusside. Calcium channel blockers and beta-blockers are to be avoided, because they depress myocardial function.

## PULMONARY

Abnormalities of gas exchange are not unusual in the postoperative period but are usually minor. Hypoxia is usually the result of ventilation-perfusion mismatching as a result of postoperative *atelectasis*—most commonly seen in the left lower lobe. Vigorous pulmonary toilet is invaluable in this setting.

*Pneumothorax* must always be considered after surgery in the thoracic cavity. The combination of decreased breath sounds, hypoxia, and hypotension is suggestive of a tension pneumothorax, and unless prompt measures are taken, it can rapidly prove fatal in the patient on positive-pressure ventilation.

*Pleural effusions* must also be considered in this population. An early effusion represents unrecognized bleeding until proven otherwise, and unless aggressive measures are taken to evacuate the bleeding, it can result in a clotted fibrothorax.

## HEMATOLOGIC

Postoperative bleeding is distressingly common in the cardiac surgical population. At its best, it is easily recognized and quantified by chest tube output. "Normal" bleeding is generally 4 to 5 ml/kg/h for the first 4 hours, 2 to 3 ml/kg/h for 4 to 6 hours, and then less than 0.5 ml/kg/h thereafter. Bleeding in excess of this is a concern. At its worst, it presents as a gradual increase in filling pressures associated with decreased cardiac output—tamponade—which can quickly lead to arrest. When massive heparinization, the dilution of clotting factors, and postpump platelet dysfunction are added into the mix, the results can be disastrous if one is unprepared. The priorities in this setting should be correction of underlying abnormalities, such as coagulopathy, hypothermia, and acidosis. Fresh frozen plasma can be used with cryoprecipitate if needed to supplement clotting factors. Data suggest that administration of aminocaproic acid (Amicar) may limit pathologic fibrinolysis. Protamine may be readministered if deemed necessary. Deamino-D-arginine vasopressin (ddAVP) may help in platelet activation, and failing this, administration of banked platelets may become necessary.

## RENAL

Despite the hemodynamic perturbations associated with cardiac surgery, significant permanent renal failure is quite uncommon. If it does occur, it is ordinarily due to shower emboli, drug toxicity, or impaired renal perfusion. Most patients in whom renal failure does develop tend to have nonoliguric failure, which is easy to manage in the postoperative period. Oliguric renal failure, however, requires careful attention to hemodynamics, with administration of loop diuretics (furosemide) to augment urine output. This may be administered as a continuous drip. Occasionally, adding "renal-dose" dopamine may also help. However, on occasion even this maneuver may also prove unsuccessful, and the patient may become temporarily dialysis dependent. Most patients, however, will eventually regain renal function.

## INFECTIOUS

The risk of infectious complications is common to all surgical procedures. In cardiac surgery the most dreaded infectious complication is of mediastinal sepsis, which usually is associated with sternal dehiscence. Patients will often present with gram-positive sepsis and an unstable sternum on examination. The diagnostic test of choice is a contrast-enhanced computed tomography scan. The patient needs to be started on antibiotics and often will need to return to the operating room for sternal débridement, washout of the mediastinum, and flap coverage of the mediastinal space. This is accomplished either with a transposed omental flap or by bilateral pectoral advancement flaps.

## VI. DISCHARGE ORDERS

After routine uncomplicated CABG surgery, patients are ready to return home on the fourth or fifth postoperative day. Occasionally a short stay in a rehabilitation hospital may be necessary for conditioning and cardiac rehabilitation.

Patients are asked to take "sternal" precautions, that is, no heavy lifting and no using of the arms to prop up their body weight. They are asked to eat a low-fat, no added salt (an American Diabetic Association ADA 1800) diet if needed.

Patients are encouraged to ambulate early and to follow a regimen that includes stair climbing or riding a stationary bicycle within the first 3 weeks. However, before proceeding to a more rigorous program of exercise, the patient's cardiologist may choose to perform a stress test. This is usually done 2 to 3 months postoperatively.

Patients usually follow-up with their cardiologist within the first 2 weeks of surgery and with their surgeon after the first month, unless any wound-related issues arise.

# CARDIAC VALVE DISEASE

*Abeel A. Mangi*

Historically, rheumatic heart disease has been the predominant cause of valvular pathology. With the recognition and aggressive management of this entity, along with the aging of the population, this is less of a concern in affluent communities but continues to extract a toll from less affluent communities.

## I. PATHOPHYSIOLOGY

## 41

Mitral regurgitation is now commonly associated with ischemic cardiomyopathy, and in its most extreme form, it is associated with postinfarction papillary muscle rupture. Aortic stenosis, another common lesion, is commonly seen in the setting of valvular degeneration and calcification with age. It is also seen with early degeneration of a congenital bicuspid aortic valve. Rheumatic fever continues to be the most common cause of mitral stenosis. The inflammatory response induces fibrosis and calcification. This eventually results in retraction of leaflet tissue, resulting in a stenotic valve. Aortic regurgitation is most commonly associated with endocarditis.

## II. TYPICAL PRESENTATION

### MITRAL REGURGITATION

Chronic mitral regurgitation (MR) results in the transmission of a persistent regurgitant jet to the left atrium. The jet follows this pathway, as the low-pressure pulmonary circulation offers less resistance than the systemic circulation. A relatively hyperdynamic state is therefore established to maintain systemic perfusion. This in turn requires higher filling pressures (higher preload) for the left ventricle to satisfy systemic requirements. Both the left atrium and ventricle will eventually dilate in response to this chronic overload. The condition is often unrecognized for years and will come to attention late as the patient presents with fatigue, dyspnea, and peripheral edema. This occurs as the ventricular chamber decompensates. Patients may also present with atrial fibrillation due to atrial dilatation and may present for the first time after a thromboembolic event. The diagnosis is suggested by a midsystolic click and a holosystolic murmur. The diagnosis is established by Doppler echocardiogram. The indications for surgical management include the following:

Left ventricular (LV) dysfunction as manifested by decreased ejection fraction, increased LV end-systolic diameter, or volume
Pulmonary hypertension
Systemic emboli
Endocarditis
New York Heart Association (NYHA) class II or greater symptoms

## MITRAL STENOSIS

Mitral stenosis induces a pressure overload phenomenon predominantly on the atrial chamber as it attempts to eject into the ventricle across the high resistance offered by the stenotic mitral valve. There are two consequences of this. The first is that volume overload of the pulmonary circulation occurs with elevation of filling pressures. The patient can therefore experience dyspnea, and in the long term, severe pulmonary hypertension and right heart failure. The second is that LV filling is impaired, limiting the ability of the ventricle to provide adequate systemic flow. This is an important point to remember—that the ventricle itself is relatively healthy, as opposed to the situation in the three other valvular conditions. These patients have dramatically lowered exercise tolerance. This is because ventricular filling depends on diastolic filling. The patient becomes disproportionately tachycardic in response to increased systemic demand. This is because cardiac output cannot be increased by augmenting stroke volume. As the heart rate increases, the time spent in diastole is shortened, resulting in impaired ventricular filling. This condition can result in syncope. These patients may also present in atrial fibrillation. The diagnosis is suggested by physical examination, cardiac echocardiography, and again is confirmed by cardiac catheterization, which provides a more sensitive assessment of pressures in different chambers of the heart. The indications for surgery are as follows:

Mitral valve orifice area $<2$ cm$^2$
Pulmonary hypertension
Systemic emboli
Endocarditis
NYHA class II or greater symptoms

## AORTIC STENOSIS

The pathology of a stenotic aortic valve is quite different from those described earlier. As the left ventricle attempts to generate adequate forward flow, the afterload it faces as the result of a stenotic aortic valve exerts a pressure overload on the ventricle. It therefore compensates by a process recognized as concentric hypertrophy. This thicker ventricle is more able to eject against a stenotic valve. However, this does not come without a cost, and higher filling pressures are required to distend this thicker, less compliant ventricle. If the oxygen demand of this uncompliant ventricle increases and outstrips supply, for example, in an exercising patient, angina can occur. If forward cardiac output is embarrassed to a great extent, syncope can result, and the patient can become very dyspneic. These are the cardinal symptoms of aortic stenosis and are important to recognize, because there is a well-documented reduction in survival after the onset of symptoms. The diagnosis is suggested by physical examination (crescendo systolic murmur) and echocardiogram and is confirmed by cardiac catheterization. This is necessary, especially in eldery patients, to rule out the presence of concomitant coronary artery disease. The stenotic valve may result in poststenotic dilatation of the aortic root and aneurysmal change. This must be considered during the preoperative evaluation. The indications for proceeding to surgery include the following:

Any symptomatic patient, especially with syncope, angina, or congestive heart failure
Aortic valve area <0.7 cm$^2$

## AORTIC INSUFFICIENCY

Aortic insufficiency (AI) imposes a volume overload not dissimilar to that seen in MR. Incompetence of the valvular apparatus results in overfilling of the ventricle, which will undergo compensatory eccentric hypertrophy. The chamber retains its compliance, unlike in AS, and will often maintain a normal diastolic filling pressure until it begins to decompensate. AI is often well tolerated for several years, unless of course, it is acute. As the chamber decompensates, the LV end diastolic pressure is the first to rise, and because ventricular compliance is limited with decompensation, this is transmitted to the left atrium and the pulmonary vasculature. In this setting, dyspnea and fatigue are the usual modes of presentation. The diagnosis again is suggested by physical examination (diastolic murmur) and cardiac echocardiography. It is confirmed by cardiac catheterization, and the indications for surgery are as follows:

Any symptomatic patient with AI

## III. PREOPERATIVE WORKUP

## CAROTID AND PERIPHERAL VASCULAR DISEASE

The cardiac patient is at particular risk for vascular catastrophe because of the underlying disease process, atherosclerosis. Symptomatic carotid bruits need to be aggressively evaluated and treated. It is controversial as to whether the presence of asymptomatic carotid bruits presents an increased risk of perioperative stroke. Some institutions suggest evaluation of all carotid bruits with noninvasive Doppler studies, with the goal of concomitant carotid endarterectomy at the time of coronary artery bypass grafting (CABG), if deemed necessary.

Evaluation of the peripheral vasculature is necessary because of the potential need for intraoperative or postoperative intraaortic balloon pump (IABP) support. It should be pointed out, however, that IABP insertion does little to stabilize the cardiovascular status of patients with valvular pathologic conditions and may actually worsen their condition. In addition, saphenous vein harvesting techniques must be particularly meticulous in the patient with peripheral arterial insufficiency. Finally, any femoral arterial injury, for example, pseudoaneurysms, caused at the time of cardiac catheterization can be repaired at the time of CABG.

## RENAL FAILURE

Patients who are dialysis dependent can undergo cardiac surgery if particular attention is paid to optimizing the patient's fluid and electrolyte balance in the preoperative state. The patient's ability to tolerate potassium cardioplegia is another concern, and intraoperative adjustments may be required if this is a concern.

The patient with borderline renal function presents more of a management problem. Aortic cross-clamping may induce renal ischemia or may exacerbate renal insufficiency by embolic showers from an atherosclerotic aorta. With current technologies, off-pump CABG may be a consideration in this patient population.

## PULMONARY INSUFFICIENCY

Median sternotomy is usually well tolerated by pulmonary patients. If there is a history of severe chronic obstructive pulmonary disease, asthma, or smoking, preoperative pulmonary function tests and arterial blood gas analysis may provide insight into the ventilatory weaning and postoperative management of these patients. They may also benefit from intensive pulmonary rehabilitation preoperatively, for example, incentive spirometry, bronchodilators, and quitting smoking.

## CHRONIC STEROID USE

Chronic steroid use predisposes patients to problems with wound healing, infection, gastric ulceration, or exacerbation of diabetes. If surgery is elective, the need for steroid use should be reevaluated and steroids discontinued if at all possible. In the setting of emergency surgery, stress dose steroids should be used.

## DERANGED LIVER FUNCTION

Patients with right heart failure usually have deranged liver function and may present with elevated prothrombin times. These patients may benefit from preoperative vitamin K. In addition, a history of hepatitis is beneficial for the purposes of protection of the operating team.

## HEMATOLOGIC ABNORMALITIES

Patients with valvular pathology are often taking coumadin as a result of atrial fibrillation. They need to be brought into the hospital preoperatively, their international normalized ratio (INR) allowed to drift down, and heparinized before surgery if deemed necessary.

Antiplatelet agents are common in the preoperative cardiac population. Ordinarily, they need to be continued through to the time of surgery.

The blood bank needs to be notified of the number of units of blood that may be required at the time of surgery.

Cardiac procedures can also be performed in patients with known hematologic conditions, such as hemophilia and von Willebrand's disease, assuming appropriate preparation by the surgical team and blood bank.

## DIABETES

Patients on oral hypoglycemic agents should have their medication held the morning of surgery. Patients who are insulin dependent are given half their normal dose the night before surgery, and their insulin is withheld the morning of surgery. All patients receive dextrose-supplemented crystalloid the night of surgery. All patients have their blood glucose levels monitored in the preoperative period, as well as postoperatively.

The stress of surgery may occasionally unmask severe postoperative hyperglycemia. Cardiopulmonary bypass and intraoperative hypothermia tend to decrease the efficiency of administered insulin. Aggressive management may result in hypoglycemia as the patient rewarms. Hyperglycemia, however, may result in a brisk osmotic diuresis and should also be avoided.

## DENTAL EVALUATION

All patients under consideration for valvular surgery require preoperative dental evaluation, with extractions of diseased teeth if deemed necessary by the consultant. This is preferably done before valve surgery, as opposed to concomitantly, to avoid bacterial showers at the time of surgery and to avoid the complications of bleeding while on high doses of heparin for cardiopulmonary bypass.

## PREOPERATIVE ORDERS

**Admit to:**
**Diagnosis:** CAD
**Condition:** stable
**Vital signs:** per routine
**Activity:**
**Allergies:** NKDA
**Nursing:** strict I&Os; hold all diuretics; shave and prep chin to ankles bilaterally; shower with pHisoHex after prep; paint neck, chest, legs with povidone-iodine solution after shower; NPO after midnight; call doctor for HR <55 or >90; RR <10 or >20; SBP <90 or >140 mm Hg; T >38.3°C (101°F), or chest pain
**Diet:** NPO after midnight
**IV fluids:** $D_5$/0.45% NS with 20 mEq K at 100 ml/h
**Medications:** vancomycin 1 g IV on call to OR
 cefazolin 1 g IV on call to OR

> patient to take beta-blockers per usual routine
> lorazepam (Ativan) 1 mg PO/IV q4h prn

**Laboratory tests:** ensure with blood bank that cross-match sample is
adequate and that blood is set up

## IV. CONDUCT OF OPERATION

The patient is laid supine on the table, and a right radial arterial catheter
and pulmonary artery catheter are placed through the right internal jugular
introducer. In addition, our patients have a left antecubital 14-gauge
intravenous catheter placed. After the induction of general endotracheal
anesthesia, Foley catheter, orogastric tube, rectal and nasopharyngeal
temperature probes are placed, and the patient is placed in the frog-leg
position. R2 adhesive defibrillator pads are also placed on the patient.

The median sternotomy is performed using an air-powered saw. An
oscillating saw is used for redo sternotomy, with the groins prepped in case
of the need to emergently institute bypass through the femoral vessels. The
mitral valve can also be approached through a left or right thoracotomy.

The pericardium is opened and suspended to form a cradle, and
attention is diverted to the ascending aorta. After systemic heparinization
and achievement of an activated clotting time (ACT) of >400 seconds, the
ascending aorta is cannulated through two concentric purse-string sutures.
Venous cannulation is achieved through bicaval cannulation. Cardiopulmonary bypass is then instituted, with membrane oxygenation, and cooling
of the patient to a rectal temperature to 25°C (77°F).

Attention is then diverted to myocardial protection. If the ventricle
becomes noticeably distended, it should be vented by placing a catheter
into the ventricle through a purse-string suture in the right superior
pulmonary vein and draining it. Chemical protection is based on cardioplegia. There are two methods for delivering cardioplegia—antegrade and
retrograde. After the aortic cross-clamp is applied, antegrade cardioplegia is
administered through the ascending aorta into the root. Retrograde cardioplegia is administered through the coronary sinus, which has to be separately cannulated. A third alternative is direct cannulation of the coronary
arteries. All three have their advantages and disadvantages. Traditional
crystalloid cardioplegia solutions are cold, hyperosmolar, and hyperkalemic.
There is also a school of thought that advocates warm blood cardioplegia,
which may be of benefit in patients with severe embarrassment of myocardial reserve.

Mitral valve repair has been gaining favor, because the procedure uses
native tissue, decreases the requirement for long-term anticoagulation, and
maintains LV architecture. The goal in this procedure is to maintain valvular function. The fundamental functional anomaly that is amenable to
correction involves leaflet prolapse—that is, the free edge of the leaflet
overriding the plane of the anulus during systole. Mitral valve ring anulo-
plasty is required for most cases of MR and serves to reduce the size of the

dilated anulus. Prolapse is then corrected with a sliding leaflet technique. This entails performing a quadrangular resection of a portion of the valve leaflet.

For mitral valve replacement, the approach entails opening the left atrium through an incision parallel to the interatrial groove. This is then carried posterior to the vena cavae. The diseased valve is excised, and the valve ring is then sewn to the anulus. Valve choice is tailored according to the individual requirements of the patient. For example, younger patients require mechanical valves because of their greater durability. Older patients will usually receive tissue valves, because these valves do not require as intense a regimen of anticoagulation.

Aortic valve replacement is performed through a median sternotomy, with single atrial cannulation. After the patient is put on cardiopulmonary bypass, the aorta is entered through a transverse incision about 1 cm above the right coronary ostium. The diseased valve is excised, and the valve ring sewn to the anulus.

Preparations are then made to separate from cardiopulmonary bypass and to decannulate the patient. The most important consideration is to ensure adequate deairing of the systemic chambers to prevent cerebral air embolization.

Once a stable rhythm has been attained, the patient has rewarmed, and the surgeon is satisfied with the suture lines, the patient is decannulated. Two atrial and two ventricular epicardial pacing wires are placed and brought out to the skin. The heparinization is then reversed by the administration of protamine. Then two mediastinal drainage thoracostomy tubes are placed, and pleural tubes are placed if the pleurae were opened. On occasion, placement of a left atrial catheter may be necessary. The sternal edges are then reapproximated by means of stainless steel sternal wires, and the skin is closed in routine fashion.

The patient is transported to the recovery room intubated, with drips according to institutional protocol and surgeon preference. A standard cocktail might include fentanyl and Versed for sedation, nitroglycerin, lidocaine, and levophed or nitroprusside.

## VARIATIONS OF OPERATION

There is also burgeoning interest in the field of minimally invasive cardiac valve surgery, which is performed through a submammary intercostal approach, while avoiding a full sternotomy and using port access techniques similar to those for laparoscopic and thoracoscopic approaches.

## POSTOPERATIVE ORDERS

**Admit to:** ICU
**Diagnosis:** s/p CABG
**Condition:** critical
**Vital signs:** per ICU protocol

**Activity:** bed rest

**Allergies:** NKDA

**Nursing:** PAC care; radial arterial catheter care; Foley to gravity; OGT to LCWS; NPO; vent settings: IMV 10, PS 10, PEEP 5, 100% $Fio_2$; chest tubes to 20 cm $H_2O$ suction; daily weights; pacer: DDD at 85 bpm; continue antibiotics until all lines and tubes removed

**Diet:** NPO

**IV fluids:**

**Medications:** fentanyl/medazolam (Versed) drip per ICU protocol
morphine $SO_4$ 1-5 mg IV q1h prn for pain
ranitidine (Zantac) 50 mg IV q8h
metoclopramide (Reglan) 10 mg IV q6h prn for nausea
acetaminophen (Tylenol) 650 mg PO/PR q4h prn
aspirin 325 mg PO/PR qd—first dose within 6 h
 of surgery
norepinephrine (Levophed) per ICU protocol to keep
 MAP 65-75 mm Hg or SBP 90-100 mm Hg
nitroprusside per ICU protocol to keep MAP 65-75 mm
 Hg or SBP 90-100 mm Hg
nitroglycerin at 1 $\mu$g/kg/min
lidocaine at 1 mg/h
cefazolin (Ancef) 1 g IV q8h

**Laboratory tests:** CBC, PT, PTT, BMP, ABGs on arrival to ICU, CXR on arrival to ICU, 12-lead ECG on arrival to ICU

## V. POTENTIAL COMPLICATIONS

Many complications can occur with valvular surgery. Specifically, the general complications that are uniquely related to valvular surgery will be discussed here. For more details concerning general complications of cardiac surgery, please refer to the chapter on coronary artery bypass surgery.

*Issues germane to mitral regurgitation.* It is important to recall that the basic pathophysiologic mechanism behind this disease results in higher filling pressures. These patients will therefore require relatively higher filling pressures to maintain an adequate stroke volume.

*Issues gemane to mitral stenosis.* The ventricle in the patient with mitral stenosis is usually relatively healthy. Therefore, once the valve has been replaced, these patients should demonstrate a decrease in their filling pressures and require little, if any, volume in the postoperative period.

*Issues germane to aortic stenosis.* The patient with AS, much like the patient with MR, requires high filling pressures to maintain forward cardiac output. In addition, because of the size and thickness of the ventricle, we will often maintain their systemic blood pressures a little on the higher side to maintain ventricular perfusion.

*Issues germane to aortic regurgitation.* This patient population also requires higher filling pressures. They may also require long-term intravenous antibiotics selected according to which organism was responsible for the endocarditis lesion to begin with.

## INFECTIOUS COMPLICATIONS

The risk of infectious complications is common to all surgical procedures. In cardiac valvular surgery, the most dreaded infectious complication is of prosthetic valve endocarditis. Hence, all patients should remain on antibiotics until all invasive monitoring and catheters are removed. In addition, any fever should be aggressively investigated.

## VI. DISCHARGE ORDERS

After routine uncomplicated valve surgery, patients are ready to return home on the fourth or fifth postoperative day. Occasionally a short stay in a rehabilitation hospital may be necessary for conditioning and cardiac rehabilitation.

Patients are asked to take "sternal" precautions, that is, no heavy lifting and no using of the arms to prop up their body weight. They are asked to eat a low-fat, no added salt (an American Diabetic Association ADA 1800) diet if needed.

Patients are encouraged to ambulate early and to follow a regimen that includes stairclimbing or riding a stationary bicycle within the first 3 weeks. However, before proceeding to a more rigorous program of exercise, the patient's cardiologist may choose to perform a stress test. This is usually done 2 to 3 months after surgery.

Patients require particularly aggressive follow-up as the initial period of anticoagulation is obtained. Patients usually follow up with their cardiologist within the first 2 weeks of surgery and with their surgeon after the first month, unless any wound-related issues arise.

# LUNG CANCER

*Michael Rosen and Emad Zakhary*

Lung cancer accounts for more than 125,000 deaths annually in United States, accounting for more than a sixth of cancer deaths.

## I. PATHOPHYSIOLOGY

The two main classes are small-cell lung cancer (oat cell) and non-small-cell lung cancer.

1. *Small-cell lung cancers (SCLC):* Constitute 20% of all lung cancer, usually occur centrally near the hilum and occur exclusively in smokers. They have a rapid growth rate, characterized by early metastases with extensive mediastinal adenopathy. More than 70% of patients have metastases outside the thorax at the time of presentation. Bronchoscopy is typically positive. They are rarely amenable to surgery.

   Most cells exhibit neuroendocrine characteristics (amine precursor uptake and decarboxylation [APUD] cells) and may be associated with secretion of hormones such as adrenocorticotropic hormone (ACTH) causing Cushing's syndrome. Other paraneoplastic syndromes include the syndrome of inappropriate antidiuretic hormone secretion (SIADH) and carcinoid syndrome.

2. *Non-small-cell lung cancers (NSCLC):* Account for 80% of all lung cancers. There are three subtypes:

   a. ***Squamous cell carcinomas (SCC):*** The proportion has decreased from about 40% to 20% to 25% in North America. It is the classic lung cancer, central in location, endobronchial, sometimes with central cavitation, commonly associated with lobar collapse, obstructive pneumonia, or hemoptysis. It shows late development of distant metastases. Superior sulcus tumors (Pancoast tumor) are invariably squamous cancers and have a propensity for local invasion into ribs, the brachial plexus, and the cervical sympathetic plexus, producing Horner's syndrome (ptosis, myosis, and anhydrosis). SCC can secrete a parathormone-like substance causing hypercalcemia.

   b. ***Adenocarcinomas:*** The proportion has risen from 20% to 25% to about 40% in North America. It is not as strongly associated with smoking as SCC is. Adenocarcinoma is most often a peripheral lesion. Early development of metastases while the primary tumor is still an asymptomatic peripheral lesion is characteristic. Malignant pleural effusion is a common association. Bronchoalveolar carcinoma, a subtype, may be unifocal or multifocal.

   c. ***Large-cell carcinomas:*** Comprise about 10%, commonly large peripheral masses and sometimes with cavitation. They are poorly differentiated and are associated with early metastases to the mediastinum and brain.

## II. TYPICAL PRESENTATION

Lung cancer may be discovered on routine chest x-ray. The following clinical features may be present.

1. Bronchopulmonary symptoms include cough, dyspnea, hemoptysis, and postobstructive pneumonia.
2. Extrapulmonary thoracic symptoms include chest wall pain secondary to parietal pleural involvement. Superior sulcus tumors (Pancoast tumor) may produce shoulder pain, brachial plexopathy, or Horner's syndrome. Symptoms related to mediastinal spread include hoarseness with left-sided lesions caused by left recurrent laryngeal nerve injury, obstruction of superior vena cava with right-sided tumors, phrenic nerve paralysis, esophageal obstruction, or pericardial tamponade.
3. Symptoms related to metastases are common, particularly with adenocarcinoma. Sites of spread include the brain, pleural cavity, bone, liver, and adrenal glands.
4. Symptoms related to a paraneoplastic syndrome, Cushing's syndrome, SIADH, and carcinoid syndrome in small-cell cancer. Hypercalcemia caused by secretion of a parathormone-like substance occurs in squamous cell cancer. Tender gynecomastia and ectopic gonadotropin secretion occur in large-cell anaplastic carcinoma. Hypertrophic pulmonary osteoarthropathy, neuromyopathies, and myasthenia-like syndrome may occur. Various neurologic syndromes are seen in small-cell carcinoma.
5. Systemic effects such as anemia, weight loss, weakness, fatigue, and hypercoagulopathy are common. Dermatomyositis and membranous glomerulonephritis may be associated.

## III. PREOPERATIVE WORKUP

### Pulmonary Function Studies

Forced expiratory volume ($FEV_1$): the minimum acceptable predicted preoperative forced expiratory volume over 1 second is 800 ml for a patient to tolerate pulmonary resection.

Quantitative split ventilation-perfusion scan may be needed for better assessment of the contribution to the $FEV_1$ by each lung.

Blood gases: $Po_2$ less than 50 mm Hg or $Pco_2$ greater than 45 mm Hg without significant atelectasis is usually a contraindication for resection.

The diffusion capacity of carbon monoxide is a good predictor of morbidity and mortality from thoracotomy.

Exercise testing: physiologic information is obtained on both respiratory and cardiac function, and this test frequently can unmask cardiac ischemia. A cutoff of maximal oxygen consumption at 1 L/min is identified.

**Chest Radiograph.** Chest radiograph is the basic modality for diagnosis. The most common radiologic abnormalities are unilateral hilar enlargement, peripheral solid tumor mass, peripheral cavitating tumor mass, volume loss, apical Pancoast tumor, and pleural effusion.

**Computed Tomography Scan.** A computed tomography (CT) scan of the chest assesses hilar and mediastinal adenopathy and invasion of the tumor into adjacent structures. CT has 88% accuracy and negative predictive value of more than 90% to define enlarged mediastinal nodes. In the aortopulmonary window the accuracy is only 80% and the negative predictive value is 83%. Nodes less than 1 cm have a low probability of malignancy. Nodes more than 1 cm have between 50% and 70% chance of representing metastatic disease.

An abdominal CT scan should include cuts of the liver and adrenals to evaluate for metastatic disease. If there are neurologic symptoms, in advanced local disease (stage III) and in cases of adenocarcinoma before pulmonary resection, a CT or magnetic resonance imaging (MRI) scan of the brain is necessary.

> **Positron-emission tomography (PET)** is highly sensitive and specific for mediastinal staging.
> **Bone scans** are ordered for symptomatic bone pain.
> **Bone marrow aspiration** is routine in patients with small-cell cancer.

**Bronchoscopy.** Bronchoscopy is used to assess proximal bronchial disease (>2 cm from the carina for resection) and to rule out additional endobronchial lesions.

**Mediastinoscopy (Cervical or Left Parasternal).** The role of mediastinoscopy is controversial. Some centers routinely perform mediastinoscopy on all patients before thoracotomy. Other centers rely solely on chest CT.

All patients with mediastinal nodes larger than 1 cm on CT should be evaluated with mediastinoscopy by a cervical incision. This allows biopsy of paratracheal, tracheobronchial, and anterior subcarinal, regions. The aortopulmonary window, posterior subcarinal, and paraesophageal nodes are not accessible by this method. Sampling of all accessible nodal sites is required. Mediastinoscopy has a sensitivity of 93% and diagnostic accuracy of 96%.

**Video-assisted Thoracoscopy Surgery.** Video-assisted thoracoscopy surgery (VATS) is an evolving technique. It allows access to the pleural space and mediastinum, biopsy of peripheral lesions, and biopsy of contralateral lesions.

**Tissue Diagnosis.** Accurate tissue diagnosis is essential with the main differentiation being small-cell or non-small-cell carcinoma. Sputum cytologic examination may give a high yield for typically endobronchial tumors (eg, small-cell and squamous cell carcinoma), but the yield is poor for adenocarcinoma.

Fiberoptic bronchoscopy (direct biopsy, washing, and brushing) gives a high rate of diagnosis in excess of 90%. Percutaneous fine-needle aspiration is used for peripheral lesions and when bronchoscopy is inconclusive. It gives a yield of more than 85%. The risk of pneumothorax is about 20% to 35%, although only 5% of patients require a chest tube. Benign lesions are less reliably diagnosed with fine-needle aspiration biopsy. Biopsy can also be obtained by video-assisted thoracoscopy. With mediastinal disease or adenopathy tissue, diagnosis is made by means of mediastinoscopy. Ten to twenty percent of patients undergo thoracotomy without a proven diagnosis of cancer before operation.

## SOLITARY PULMONARY NODULE

Any asymptomatic solitary pulmonary nodule (SPN) needs evaluation. Half prove to be either primary or metastatic malignancies; the incidence rises to 60% to 80% above 50 years of age. The chance of malignancy increases with the size of the lesion, advancing age, and more extensive smoking. Lesions larger than 3 cm are almost always malignant. Increase in size over the past year favors malignancy. Specific types of calcification favor a benign diagnosis: central, lamellar, and popcornlike. Eccentric or stippled flecks can be seen with malignancy.

A logical approach to the SPN would include early thoracotomy for lesions in known risk populations: age older than 50, smoking history, absence of certain knowledge of a similar lesion on chest film for more than 2 years. A search for a primary tumor elsewhere is essential. If the patient is less than 35 and a nonsmoker, and the chance of malignancy is small, needle biopsy and bronchial brush biopsy are appropriate, with watchful waiting and close observation for growth or change.

## PREOPERATIVE ORDERS

Optimize respiratory status with inhalers and cessation of smoking at least 2 weeks before surgery
Pulmonary function tests
Bronchoscopy
Thoracic epidural is placed to allow early extubation and adequate postoperative pain relief

## STAGING OF LUNG CANCER

The aim of staging is to identify candidates for surgical resection with the potential for cure and to identify candidates for new aggressive multimodal treatments for locally advanced disease.

The TNM staging is less useful in patients with small-cell lung cancer (Table 42-1). Patients are classified into those with limited-stage disease

**TABLE 42-1**

AMERICAN JOINT COMMITTEE ON CANCER STAGING SYSTEM
OF LUNG CANCER

TUMOR STATUS (T)

**T1**  ≤3 cm without invasion of visceral pleura or proximal to lobar bronchus >3 cm
or any size with associated atelectasis or obstructive

**T2**  pneumonitis; may invade visceral pleura; proximal extent must be >2 cm from
carina.

Any size with direct extension into chest wall, diaphragm, mediastinal

**T3**  pleura without involvement of great vessels or vital mediastinal structures; cannot
involve carina.

Any size with invasion of heart or mediastinal vital structures or carina,

**T4**  malignant pleural effusion.

NODAL INVOLVEMENT (N)

**N0**  None

**N1**  Peribronchial or ipsilateral hilar lymph nodes.

**N2**  Ipsilateral mediastinal lymph nodes including subcarcinal

**N3**  Contralateral mediastinal or hilar lymph nodes, ipsilateral or contralateral scalene
or supraclavicular lymph nodes.

DISTANT METASTASES (M)

**M0**  None

**M1**  Distant metastases present.

42

LUNG CANCER

(about 33% of patients); those with tumor confined to one hemithorax,
including ipsilateral mediastinal and supraclavicular node groups, all of
which can be encompassed in a radiotherapy port; and those with
extensive-stage disease (remaining 67% of patients), with tumor outside
the limited stage boundaries and with distant metastases in most cases.
Bone marrow involvement occurs in 20% of patients.

## TREATMENT OF LUNG CANCER BY STAGE

### Treatment of Non-Small-Cell Lung Cancer

1. Stage I (T1N0, T2N0)
   a. Stage I cancers are treated whenever possible by surgical resection,
      with a 5-year survival in the range of 40% to 67% (Table 42-2).
   b. No role for adjuvant chemotherapy.
   c. Patients who are unfit for surgery are often candidates for primary
      radiotherapy with a 25% cure rate.
   d. Hyperfractionated accelerated radiotherapy is under investigation
      for improved local control.
   e. Prophylactic brain irradiation in patients with adenocarcinoma is
      not usually justified.
2. Stage II (T1N1, T2N1, T3N0)
   a. Stage II are routinely treated by surgical resection.

**TABLE 42-2**

FIVE-YEAR SURVIVAL ACCORDING TO AMERICAN JOINT COMMITTEE ON
CANCER STAGE GROUPS OF TNM STATUS

| Stage | TNM Classification | Five-year Survival (%) |
|---|---|---|
| Stage I | T1-T2, N0, M0 | 60-75 |
| Stage II | T1-T2, N1, M0 | 40-55 |
| Stage IIIa | T3, N0-N1, M0 | 20-30 |
| | T1-T3, N2, M0 | 10-15 |
| Stage IIIb | Any T, N3, M0 | <10 |
| | T4, Any N, M0 | <10 |
| Stage IV | Any T, Any N, M1 | 0 |

  b. Five-year survival is 25% to 55%, nonsquamous lower range.
  c. Adjuvant radiotherapy to patients with squamous cell cancer
   lowered local recurrence rate but did not affect survival.
  d. At present, the role of adjuvant chemotherapy is not established
   in stage II patients, although some reports have shown a slight
   increase in disease-free survival.
 3. Stage IIIA (T3N0-1, T1N2)
  a. Tumors locally invading chest wall, pleura, or pericardium, within
   2 cm of the carina. Nodes in the hilum (N1) or ipsilateral mediastinum (N2).
  b. These are marginally resectable.
  c. Treatment is multimodality protocol of combined chemotherapy,
   surgery, and radiotherapy. Resection alone proved unsatisfactory.
  d. The subgroup of patients with invasion of parietal pleura
   or chest wall or with superior sulcus tumor (but with negative
   nodes) (ie, T3N0), have been treated surgically, sometimes
   combined with radiotherapy. This finding led to the inclusion
   of such patients with T3N0 in stage II in the new staging
   scheme.
 4. Stage IIIB (any T, N3, M0, or T4, any N, M0)
  a. Direct extension to adjacent organs (pleura, heart, chest wall,
   diaphragm, or mediastinum). N3 = associated contralateral
   mediastinal or supraclavicular lymph node involvement.
  b. These tumors are unresectable.
  c. Multimodality therapy investigated. Induction chemotherapy
   before standard radiotherapy, simultaneous administration of
   chemotherapy and radiotherapy, or the use of intensified
   radiotherapy (continuous hyperfractionated accelerated
   radiotherapy).
 5. Stage IV
  a. Any tumors with distant metastases (M1).
  b. Forty percent to 50% of patients non-small-cell cancer present
   with metastatic disease.

c. With patients who maintain a good performance stage, chemotherapy is used. The new chemotherapy regimens (using docetaxel and gemcitabine) have shown better response rates. Palliative radiotherapy may be used for control of disease-related symptoms such as pain, hemoptysis, or obstructive symptoms.

**Treatment of Small-cell Lung Cancer.** Chemotherapy is the mainstay of treatment for small-cell lung cancer, and adjuvant radiotherapy is commonly used in patients with limited disease. Surgical resection is reserved for patients with pathologically documented stage I or II disease or as a part of a combined-modality clinical trial. The role of prophylactic cranial irradiation has been controversial; many clinicians suggest prophylactic cranial irradiation for patients with limited-stage cancer in complete remission.

## IV. SURGICAL ANATOMY

The lungs are divided into lobes. The left lung has an upper and lower lobe. The right lung has an upper, middle, and lower lobe. These lobes are further divided into segments based on bronchial anatomy. There are three segments in the right upper lobe, two in the right middle lobe, and five in the lower lobe. The left upper has four and the lower lobe has five segments. Each lobe has its own pulmonary circulation, consisting of a pulmonary artery, pulmonary vein, and bronchial artery.

## V. CONDUCT OF OPERATION

### MEDIASTINOSCOPY

Mediastinoscopy is used to diagnose N2 OR N3 nodal involvement. The patient is positioned supine with the neck extended. A small transverse incision is made a fingerbreadth above the sternal notch, and a plane is dissected down to the pretracheal fascia. Using finger dissection, a plane is developed along the anterior surface of the trachea posterior to the innominate artery. The mediastinoscope is inserted and lymph nodes are sampled. Care should be taken to aspirate all structures before biopsy to avoid inadvertent major vascular structures. On the left the recurrent laryngeal nerve should be avoided and on the right the pulmonary artery should be avoided as well.

### LOBECTOMY

The patient is placed in the lateral decubitus position. Anesthesia is induced, and a double-lumen endotracheal tube is placed. A muscle-sparing thoracotomy is performed 2 cm below the tip of the scapula, extending from the posterior edge of the serratus anterior to the anterior margin of the latissimus dorsi muscle. Next, a chest retractor is inserted, and the inferior

**42**

**LUNG CANCER**

pulmonary ligament is divided to allow for adequate mobilization. The appropriate pulmonary artery, vein, and bronchus of the segment or lobe to be resected are dissected and surrounded by vessel loops and divided by a vascular stapler. A chest tube is inserted through a separate stab, and the ribs are approximated with three to four interrupted Vicryl sutures. The muscles are closed with a running nonabsorbable suture.

## PNEUMONECTOMY

Historically total pneumonectomy has been the operation of choice; however, now it accounts for only 20% of all pulmonary resections. It is required when the tumor invades the mainstem bronchus or pulmonary arteries. The major disadvantage is that it removes a large volume of functional lung, which may lead to chronic respiratory failure.

Lobectomy, the most frequently performed lung resection, allows sparing of functional lung while still providing adequate margins and resection of N1 lymph nodes. Complete mediastinal lymph node dissection using frozen sections should always be performed at the time of lobectomy or pneumonectomy. If hilar N1 or N2 disease is confirmed by frozen sections, a radical lymph node dissection should be done to accurately stage and potentially cure the patient. The operative mortality of lobectomy for lung cancer is 2% to 3% and for pneumonectomy is 6% to 8%.

## VARIATIONS OF OPERATION

**Sleeve lobectomy** is used for tumors that involve the mainstem bronchus. They involve resection of the bronchus and sparing of pulmonary tissue.

**Segmentectomy** is used for resection of peripherally placed lesions. This usually involves metastatic tumors, small primary tumors, and patients with limited pulmonary reserve. This requires a thoracotomy and dissection of the segmental bronchus with removal of supplied lung tissue.

**Wedge resection** is the technique used for metastatic lesions. It can be performed through a standard thoracotomy incision or using a VATS technique. The involved segment of lung tissue is stapled across and removed.

**Chest wall resection:** For tumors involving the intercostal muscles and ribs, en bloc chest wall resection should be done with at least a 2-cm margin confirmed by frozen sections. Defects on the anterior chest wall or that involve more than two intercostal spaces should be reconstructed using Merlex mesh.

## SUPERIOR SULCUS TUMORS

Preoperative radiotherapy can downstage superior sulcus tumors and enable a margin-negative surgical resection in 25% of cases. A 50% survival rate can be expected for patients treated with preoperative radiotherapy and complete resection.

## POSTOPERATIVE ORDERS

**Admit to:** ICU
**Diagnosis:** s/p pulmonary resection
**Condition:** stable
**Vital signs:** per routine
**Activity:** bed rest and OOB to chair in AM
**Allergies:**
**Nursing:** Foley to gravity until epidural removed; routine epidural care; aggressive chest physiotherapy; IS q1h; Pneumoboots until fully ambulating; chest tubes: If pneumonectomy should be clamped overnight and removed on POD 1 after review CXR and no mediastinal shift. For routine lung resection, should remove when minimal drainage and no air leak after watersealed, usually POD 2 or 3; ventilator: most patients are extubated immediately postoperatively; if they are not, attempt early extubation and minimize positive-pressure ventilation
**Diet:** strict NPO with aspiration precautions once diet advanced on POD 1
**IV fluids:** should be kept on the dry side with $D_5$/0.45% NS with 20 mEq KCl at 60 ml/hr
**Medications:**
**Laboratory tests:** need CXR each AM

## VI. COMPLICATIONS

Supraventricular dysrhythmias occur in up to 30%. Hemodynamically stable patients can be treated with digoxin and calcium channel blockers. It is usually temporary and a result of atrial irritation from the thoracic surgery.

Mediastinal shift after pneumonectomy can result in hemodynamic changes and can be treated by chest tube drainage. It can be a sign of hemorrhage and can necessitate reexploration.

Bronchopleural fistula is a result of a breakdown of the bronchial stump closure. By definition the pleural space is infected. It requires reexploration, closure, and flap buttressing of the disrupted stump.

Pulmonary toilet is essential in these patients because retained secretions can lead to pneumonia. This includes aggressive chest physiotherapy and bronchoscopy as necessary.

## VII. DISCHARGE ORDERS

After major thoracic surgery, patients will often require a stay in a rehabilitation hospital. Patients should be given adequate pain medication to permit comfortable deep breathing and coughing to clear secretions. They require follow-up with an oncologist. They should be directed to return for a wound check in 7 to 10 days.

# LUNG VOLUME REDUCTION SURGERY

*Ikenna Okereke*

Chronic obstructive pulmonary disease (COPD) affects nearly 10 million people in the United States, ranging from the mild "smoker's cough" to severe incapacitation and chronic oxygen requirement. COPD is classically divided into chronic bronchitis and emphysema.

## I. PATHOPHYSIOLOGY

The most common risk factor associated with developing COPD is cigarette smoking. Up to 90% of people with COPD have some smoking history. Moreover, patients diagnosed with COPD who continue to smoke have an accelerated decline in respiratory function. Other risk factors include occupational exposures to dusts and minerals, asthma, age, history of recurrent childhood respiratory infections, and certain genetic impairments, for example $\alpha_1$-antitrypsin deficiency. All of these causes should be ascertained when evaluating a patient suspected of having COPD.

## II. TYPICAL PRESENTATION

Chronic bronchitis is a clinical diagnosis, in which the patient exhibits a productive cough for at least 3 months of a year and for at least 2 consecutive years. Emphysema is defined histologically and is characterized by destruction of the alveolar walls by inhaled irritants. This destruction leads to chronic hyperinflation of the airway, and inability to generate adequate expiratory pressures.

## III. PREOPERATIVE WORKUP

Diagnosis of COPD is largely based on the patient's symptoms and spirometry values. On presentation of a symptomatic patient to the primary care physician, spirometric values and chest roentgenograms should be obtained. Because COPD is mainly a limitation of expiratory airflow, $FEV_1$ values are significantly diminished, leading to a low $FEV_1/FVC$ ratio. Typically, these are less than 70% of normal levels.

Preoperative workup for potential lung volume reduction surgery (LVRS) patients is extensive. Standard imaging studies obtained include chest x-ray and computed tomography (CT) scan of the chest. Chest x-rays and CT scans will show hyperinflation of the lungs, increased anteroposterior diameter (barrel chest), and flattened diaphragms. Other complications of COPD, like apical bullae or interstitial infiltrate, may also be seen.

A ventilation-perfusion scan is performed. This scan permits determination of how much of the diseased lung parenchyma will be excised.

| TABLE 43-1 |
| --- |
| **INCLUSION CRITERIA FOR LVRS** |
| Age less than 75 |
| $FEV_1$ <40% |
| Total lung capacity >120% |
| Moderate to severe decrease in quality of life |
| Absence of severe pulmonary hypertension (mean PAP <35 mm Hg and systolic PAP <45 mm Hg) |

Cardiac clearance usually entails a resting and dobutamine stress echocardiogram. Cardiac catheterization is performed if needed.

The surgery team becomes involved in the management of the COPD patient when medical management fails to provide sufficient relief for the patient. In the past, surgical options were limited to bullectomy for large apical bullae and lung transplantation. In the last several years, lung volume reduction has become more readily performed. Currently, LVRS is offered to those who meet the inclusion criteria listed in Table 43-1.

## IV. PREOPERATIVE ORDERS

Routine laboratory work: CBC, BMP, PT, PTT, UA
Cardiac clearance
$\dot{V}/\dot{Q}$ scan
PFTs
Aggressive pulmonary toilet
Preoperative antibiotics
Inhalers prn

## V. CONDUCT OF OPERATION

LVRS was initially described in the 1950s by Otto Brantigan. Because the normal elastic recoil of the lungs is impaired by the diseased apical tissue, he postulated that removal of apical lung tissue could lead to restoration of this normal recoil force. The operation was initially performed with staged bilateral thoracotomies, performing the second thoracotomy 3 months after the first operation. The procedure was abandoned soon after its inception because of high postoperative morbidity and mortality. LVRS was repopularized in the late 1980s, when advanced technology allowed for better results and increased success.

LVRS can be performed either by means of an open approach or thoracoscopically. Before the operation, a thoracic epidural catheter is placed at the T6-T8 level. General endotracheal anesthesia is induced with a double-lumen endotracheal tube. When performed thoracoscopically, the patient is placed in the lateral decubitus position. Three 10-mm ports are placed in the eighth intercostal space. A 5-mm port is placed in the fourth intercostal space. The lung parenchyma is inspected, and the amount of diseased lung to be excised is determined. On average, one third to one fourth of the lung is removed using an endoscopic stapler. If bilateral LVRS is to be performed, the patient is turned onto the contralateral side, once again in the decubitus position, and the procedure is repeated. At the end of the procedure, two chest tubes are placed in each hemithorax.

## VARIATIONS OF OPERATION

Open LVRS is usually performed by use of a median sternotomy. Bilateral pleural tents are made by separating the parietal pleura from the chest wall. These tents serve as an extra layer of protection against air leaks from the staple line. The more severely affected lung is evaluated first. The upper lobe of the lung is isolated, and the lung tissue is palpated. The amount of lung excised is based on the preoperative ventilation-perfusion scan and by the actual feel of the lung. An advantage of the open technique versus the thoracoscopic approach is that the lung can be palpated, providing better tactile evidence of the extent of diseased lung.

## POSTOPERATIVE ORDERS

Most patients are able to be extubated in the operating room after completion of the case. Early extubation lowers the risk of barotrauma from prolonged positive-pressure ventilation. Chest tubes are placed on low continuous suction and are removed once the amount of drainage subsides and the pneumothorax is eradicated. Intravenous fluids are given judiciously to prevent fluid overload and pulmonary edema.

**Admit to:** ICU
**Diagnosis:** s/p LVRS
**Condition:** guarded
**Vital signs:** q1h
**Activity:** OOB to chair with assistance
**Allergies:**
**Nursing:** epidural care, Foley until epidural out, chest tube to 20 cm $H_2O$ suction, IS 10 puffs q1h while awake, aggressive formal chest PT, Pneumoboots, PAS until ambulating
**Diet:** clear liquids with strict aspiration precautions
**IV fluids:** $D_5$/0.45% NS with 20 mEq KCl at 60 ml/h Heplock when tolerating oral intake
**Medications:** routine antibiotics while chest tube in place
**Laboratory tests:** CBC, BMP, PT, PTT in AM, ECG on arrival in ICU, CXR on arrival in ICU

## VI. COMPLICATIONS

The most common complication of LVRS is persistent air leak, defined as the presence of a pneumothorax for longer than 7 days. A persistent air

43

LUNG VOLUME REDUCTION SURGERY

leak is witnessed in 30% to 50% of patients. Other complications include cardiac dysrhythmias, myocardial infarction, pneumonia, and prolonged gastrointestinal ileus.

## VII. DISCHARGE INSTRUCTIONS

Most series report total length of stay in the hospital to be 2 weeks. Routine postoperative follow-up should be scheduled within 2 to 4 weeks after discharge. Early results on the benefit of LVRS have been favorable. $FEV_1$ increases by approximately 50%. Six-minute-walk distance increases, and quality of life surveys show significant improvement in the first 12 months after surgery. The main limitation of most of these studies is the short-term follow-up.

# VIDEO-ASSISTED THORACOSCOPIC SURGERY

*Eric E. Roselli*

With the increasing use of minimally invasive surgical techniques has come the resurgence of thoracoscopic techniques first described by Jacobaeus in 1910. Recent advances in video and instrument technology have allowed for the development of the new surgical approach known as video-assisted thoracoscopic surgery, or VATS, to be used to perform increasingly more complex operations. These minimally invasive techniques can markedly reduce pain, hospitalization, and recovery, but these short-term benefits should never compromise the long-term goals of the intended procedure.

**44**

## I. PATHOPHYSIOLOGY

VATS techniques may be used to diagnose or treat pathology involving nearly all of the organs and structures within the thoracic cavity.

VATS has most commonly been used to treat disorders of the pleura. Pleural effusions of either a benign or malignant nature can be treated and diagnosed. Early empyema thoracis often related to pneumonia or trauma can be drained, and chylothorax can be diagnosed and treated by thoracic duct ligation. VATS also allows for the diagnosis, staging, and mechanical or chemical pleurodesis of malignant mesothelioma.

The other most common indications for VATS involve disorders of the lung. Benign disorders, including bullous disease, recurrent spontaneous pneumothorax, and persistent air leak, may be treated by means of bullectomy or pleurodesis. VATS is also useful as a mode of diagnosis of solitary pulmonary nodules (if they are <3 cm, surrounded by lung, and without parenchymal disease) and chronic interstitial lung disease by means of wedge resection or lung biopsy. Many reports in the literature describe the use of VATS as a mode of diagnosis to evaluate the lungs and diaphragm in trauma. Malignant lung disease, including both primary lung cancer and metastatic nodules, can be diagnosed by wedge biopsy (with subsequent lobectomy usually by thoracotomy) or treated as in the case of wedge metastectomy for potential survival benefit.

Mediastinal structures are also accessible with VATS. Benign tumor resection and malignant tumor diagnosis may be approached through this technique. Partial sympathectomy of the stellate ganglion provides relief of hyperhidrosis, Raynaud's syndrome, and reflex sympathetic dystrophy. Pericardial window for the treatment of pericardial effusion is an ideal indication for the use of VATS.

Esophageal malignancy may be diagnosed and staged using VATS. In the postoperative period, thoracoscopy may be used to evaluate the conduit for ischemia or breakdown. Benign esophageal indications include achalasia, reflux, and leiomyoma.

## II. PREOPERATIVE WORKUP

Contraindications to VATS surgery include pleural symphysis and acute respiratory insufficiency. Obliteration of the pleural space is most common in patients with a history of empyema, tuberculosis, or previous thoracotomy. Patients with low oxygen saturation and high airway pressures cannot tolerate single-lung ventilation.

Chest radiograph may reveal masses, nodules, increased interstitial markings, pneumothorax, or pleural effusion. A decubitus chest x-ray can help to delineate free-form loculated effusions.

Chest computed tomography (CT) provides excellent localization and characterization of intrathoracic structures, including mass lesions, lymph nodes, fluid collections, bronchi, and vascular structures to help plan the approach to an operation.

Bronchoscopy with biopsy or lavage is performed in patients with a suspicious lung nodule on chest x-ray to provide a histologic or cytologic diagnosis.

Fine-needle aspiration can also provide cytologic diagnosis of accessible suspicious lesions.

Mediastinoscopy is performed in patients with lung cancer to sample lymph node stations 2, 3, 4, and 7 for staging purposes.

Pulmonary function tests should be performed in patients undergoing pulmonary resection to determine tolerance.

### PREOPERATIVE ORDERS

NPO after midnight
IS teaching
PAS on call to the OR for cancer patients
Give steroid stress dose for COPD patients on chronic steroids
Use any usual COPD medications the morning of surgery

## III. SURGICAL ANATOMY

The bony structure of the thoracic cavity and the capacity for lung isolation by means of single-lung ventilation allow for excellent intrathoracic exposure without the need for insufflation. Ports should be placed at the superior surface of ribs to avoid injury to the neurovascular bundle.

## IV. CONDUCT OF OPERATION

Surgery is performed with the patient under general anesthesia with either double-lumen endotracheal intubation or the use of a bronchial blocker. The patient is placed in the lateral decubitus position. The whole chest is prepared and draped, allowing access to all the interspaces. A thoracotomy set should be in the room at all times for emergency thoracotomy if necessary. With the surgeon and assistant on opposite sides of the table, a small

12-mm oblique incision is made usually at the eighth interspace in the midaxillary line. After carefully entering the pleural space and palpating for adhesions, a 12-mm thoracoport is placed for the thoracoscope. The scope is preferably angled either at 30 or 45 degrees to allow full visualization of the intrathoracic structures. Because insufflation is not used, instrumentation includes many long-handled standard thoracotomy instruments and specialized thoracoscopic instruments with trigger grips. Standard electrocautery with an extended tip may be used. Several endoscopic stapling devices are now available. After placement of the thoracoscope and brief exploratory thoracoscopy, the pathology is identified, and the working port incisions are made under direct thoracoscopic vision. These working ports are often within the sixth interspace (in case of need for conversion to thoracotomy) or at desired chest tube insertion sites. Most procedures can be performed through three properly selected incisions. Pathologic specimens suspicious for malignancy are removed with the use of an Endobag retriever. At the conclusion of the procedure, a chest tube is inserted through one of the port sites and secured to the skin. Hemostasis is confirmed, and the incisions are closed by reapproximation of the subcutaneous tissue and skin with absorbable suture.

## VARIATIONS OF OPERATION

For lung wedge resections or biopsies, the procedure depends on the identification of the lesion in question and its location near the periphery of the lung. With a long ring forceps the area in question is grasped and elevated from surrounding lung parenchyma. Endostaples are then applied in a wedgelike fashion to include the tumor, and vessels are stapled and divided. The specimen is then handed off the field for frozen section evaluation. The lung is tested for leaks by submerging the margin then insufflating air to look for bubbles. If the frozen section is benign, a chest tube is placed, and the patient is discharged. If malignant, then further exploration and node sampling should take place. If N2 lymph nodes are negative, lobectomy may be performed. If the lesion is benign, the incisions are closed.

Apical bullae and blebs may also be resected by use of a stapling device. The rest of the operation proceeds as earlier, except the superior pleura is stripped from the inside chest wall using blunt dissection.

Pleurodesis after draining the effusion and lysis of restrictive intrathoracic adhesions can be performed by mechanical abrasion of the pleura or the insufflation of talc within the pleural space.

In VATS for spontaneous pneumothorax, it is always important to include inspection of the lung apices with a Valsalva maneuver.

## POSTOPERATIVE ORDERS

**Admit to:** thoracic surgery; telemetry for lung resections or mediastinal procedures; length of stay varies from 1-7 days depending on the procedure

**Diagnosis:** s/p VATS

**Condition:** stable

**Vital signs:** per routine with I&Os, record chest tube output every shift

**Activity:** bed rest, ambulate with assist in AM

**Allergies:**

**Nursing:** Encourage IS use; chest tube to −20 cm $H_2O$ suction; once there is no air leak and the chest tube output is sufficiently decreased (typically between 100 and 250 ml/d), the chest tube(s) may be placed to water seal and removed the following day; check CXR in recovery room to confirm lung expansion and to rule out fluid collection; consult respiratory therapy for patients with chronic lung disease

**Diet:** NPO if at risk for early postoperative hemorrhage and for esophageal procedures; then advance to a regular diet once recovered from anesthesia

**IV fluids:** $D_5$/0.45% NS + 20 mEq KCl at maintenance rate until tolerating oral intake

**Medications:** IV PCA while the chest tube(s) is in, then change to Percocet, 1 to 2 tablets PO q4-6h prn once chest tube removed

IV antibiotics with coverage directed at organisms characterized on stat Gram stain obtained from OR specimen for empyema

acetaminophen (Tylenol) 650 mg PO q4-6h prn T >38.5°C (101°F)

**Laboratory tests:**

## V. COMPLICATIONS

Intraoperatively, hemorrhage and inadvertent lung injury are the most common. These are usually controlled intraoperatively, occasionally requiring conversion to thoracotomy.

Postoperative air leaks, atelectasis, pneumonia, empyema, and dysrhythmias are the most common complications. Dissemination of malignancy to pleura and port sites is a controversial complication, with many reports of such in the literature. Because of the lack of long-term results and proven benefit over thoracotomy, lung resection for malignancy should only be performed by those very adept at VATS techniques for resection.

## VI. DISCHARGE INSTRUCTIONS

Discharge to home with home medications and oral narcotic analgesics. Most patients can return to full activity in 1 or 2 weeks. A follow-up appointment in 1 to 2 weeks for a routine port site check is made.

# PART XIII

Ear, Nose, and Throat

# NOSEBLEEDS (EPISTAXIS)

*Walter Lee*

Epistaxis (nosebleeds) will occur in 10% of the population at least once. Although most episodes may be treated with outpatient therapy, the potential for airway involvement makes diagnosis and treatment critical.

## I. PATHOPHYSIOLOGY

Epistaxis most commonly results from trauma after digital manipulation or fractures. Other common causes include extensive mucosal drying secondary to low humidity or chronic use of nasal decongestants and steroid sprays. In children, foreign bodies must be considered, especially when epistaxis is associated with purulent discharge. Chronic injury may result in damage to the septal perichondrium, resulting in cartilage ischemia and subsequent perforation.

Coagulopathies, such as idiopathic thrombocytopenic pupura, disseminated intravascular coagulation, and thrombotic thrombocytopenic pupura, often predispose patients to nosebleeds. Patients with platelet counts less than 20,000 mm$^3$ may have spontaneous epistaxis. Von Willebrand's disease (vWD) is the most common hereditary disorder that presents with epistaxis. Other causes of epistaxis include systemic conditions, including hereditary hemorrhagic telangiectasia (Osler-Weber-Rendu disease) (Table 45-1).

## II. PREOPERATIVE WORKUP

One should begin with an assessment of the ABCs (airway, breathing, circulation). Once the patient is stable, a thorough history should be obtained from him or her. Questions should determine the side of the nose where the bleeding began and the duration and estimated amount of blood loss. Medical history should include an investigation of any significant medical problems, liver disease, or coagulopathies. One should also ask whether there have been previous episodes of epistaxis and about the use of nasal sprays, nonsteroidal antiinflammatory drugs, and anticoagulants. A physical examination is then done using the following: head mirror/light source or nasopharyngoscope with light source, nasal speculum, bayonet forceps, suction/Frazier tip, cotton pledgets, gowns/face mask, nasal packs, nasal vasoconstriction sprays (phenylephrine 0.25%, oxymetazoline 0.05%), and lidocaine spray for anesthesia.

Laboratory values should include a complete blood count with differential, type and screen, prothrombin time, partial thromboplastin time, and international normalized ratio.

Although most nosebleeds are managed on an outpatient basis, some patients may be admitted for close observation of their airway.

| TABLE 45-1 |
| --- |
| ETIOLOGY OF EPISTAXIS |
| Trauma |
| Trauma, digital manipulation |
| Foreign body |
| Fracture |
| Coagulopathy |
| Arteriosclerotic disease with hypertension |
| Liver disease |
| Chronic nephritis |
| Leukemias |
| Nonsteroidal antiinflammatory drug use |
| Anticoagulation |
| Vascular disorders |
| Malignancy |
| Intranasal tumors |
| Local irritation |
| Low humidity/dry heat |
| Nasal sprays |
| Drug use (cocaine) |
| Irritants (smoke, environmental) |

## PREOPERATIVE ORDERS

**Admit to:**
**Diagnosis:** epistaxis
**Condition:** stable
**Vital signs:** per routine (include continuous pulse oximetry if nasal packing present)
**Activity:** ad lib
**Allergies:**
**Nursing:**
**Diet:**
**IV fluids:**
**Medications:** antibiotic if nasal packing present
**Laboratory tests:** T&S, CBC, PT, PTT, and INR

## III. SURGICAL ANATOMY

The blood supply from the nose derives from both the external and internal carotid arteries. The internal carotid gives rise to the anterior and posterior ethmoid arteries by means of the ophthalmic artery. The external carotid supplies the sphenopalatine, descending palatine, greater palatine, and superior labial arteries. These nasal vessels anastomose forming Kesselbach's plexus found on the anterior septum. Anterior bleeding, accounting for 90% to 95% of all cases, arises from Kesselbach's plexus.

Posterior epistaxis occurs more commonly in older patients with arteriosclerotic disease. Vessels of the posterior septum or lateral nasal wall (Woodruff's nasonasopharyngeal plexus) are responsible for this bleeding. Patients with posterior bleeding often complain of swallowing blood in contrast to anterior bleeding, in which the blood exits through the nares. Exsanguination by epistaxis is rare and usually involves facial trauma lacerating the maxillary artery.

## IV. CONDUCT OF OPERATION

All anticoagulation medication should be stopped. Reversal of bleeding time can be achieved with fresh frozen plasma or platelet transfusion and vitamin K. Once any underlying coagulopathies have been corrected and the patient is clinically stable, the source of bleeding is identified, using an anterior rhinoscope or rigid nasal endoscope. The patient should be seated upright and discouraged from swallowing the blood, because it is a strong emetic. The nose should be anesthetized, vasoconstricted and cleared of any obscuring blood.

Pressure to the caudal end of the nose for several minutes with the head upright may be effective, especially in children. Cauterization with silver nitrate is useful in anterior septal bleeding. Administration of lidocaine on cotton to the area before cauterization can decrease sensation and improve patient comfort. Electrocauterization can also be used to control epistaxis. Caution should be exercised, because aggressive electrocautery may lead to septal perforations. After cautery, absorbable packing (surgicel or Gelfoam) should be placed over the area to allow for local protection of the mucosa.

Persistent epistaxis should be treated with anterior packing. After the nose is well anesthetized, $1/2$-inch Vaseline gauze is carefully layered in the nasal cavity with bayonet forceps. The gauze should be grasped 4 to 5 inches from the end and placed onto the nasal floor. The next 4 to 5 inches is grasped and inserted on top of the previous piece of gauze. This is continued until the nasal cavity is packed. A rolled-2 × 2-inch sponge is taped at the nasal opening to secure the packing and collect secretions. A tag of gauze should be left for easy packing removal. Expandable packing (Gelfoam sponge, Merocel, or Surgicel) may be used instead of Vaseline gauze.

Posterior packing should be used when patients complain of bleeding into the throat, posterior bleeding is visualized, or when an anterior pack fails to stop the bleeding. Three lengths of 2-0 silk are tied around the middle of a 1-inch vaginal tampon ($1/2$-inch diameter) or rolled gauze of same dimensions. A 14 F catheter is passed along the nasal floor on the affected side and withdrawn from the mouth. Two of the silk ties are used to secure the pack to the catheter, and the pack is pulled into place when the catheter is withdrawn from the nose. The third silk tie should be seen in the oropharynx. A finger placed in the nasopharynx helps lodge the pack in place. The two silk ends should be tied around a nasal roll after an anterior pack is also placed.

45

NOSEBLEEDS (EPISTAXIS)

## VARIATIONS OF OPERATION

Angiography and embolization of the maxillary artery and its branches may be helpful in controlling persistent epistaxis. Success depends on anastomotic anatomy and the dominant vessel of the bleeding. Failure of angiography to stop bleeding results from either contralateral collateral maxillary artery branches or dominant ipsilateral facial arteries. Embolization may involve Gelfoam particles, polyvinyl alcohol, and coiled springs.

In cases of persistent bleeding, arterial ligation of the maxillary artery may be necessary to decrease intravascular pressure, facilitating clot formation. This procedure is most commonly done through a Caldwell-Luc approach. The maxillary sinus is entered, and a laterally based U-shaped incision is made in the posterior wall. The maxillary artery and its distal branches are identified in the pterygopalatine fossa and clipped. Other artery ligations involve the anterior and posterior ethmoidal arteries and also the sphenopalatine artery.

## POSTOPERATIVE ORDERS AND DISCHARGE INSTRUCTIONS

Avoid nose blowing
Open mouth when sneezing
Avoid anticoagulants (aspirin, warfarin)
Saline nasal spray may be used prn
First-generation cephalosporin or amoxicillin with clavulanic acid
    (prevent sinusitis and toxic shock syndrome)
Pain medication can be taken as needed: acetamenophen (Tylenol extra
    strength)
Nasal packs are removed in 3 to 5 days.

## V. COMPLICATIONS

All patients with posterior packing need to be admitted for airway observation. Close monitoring should include pulse oximetry. Patients with nasal packs also have a rare risk for toxic shock syndrome from colonization of *Staphylococcus aureus,* producing toxic shock syndrome toxin 1. Antibiotic coverage with a first-generation cephalosporin or amoxicillin with clavulanic acid should be given to all patients with nasal packing.

# TRACHEOTOMY

*Lee Akst*

A tracheotomy involves the operative placement of an artificial airway through the anterior portion of the second or third tracheal ring. In formal usage, "tracheotomy" refers to the operative procedure itself, whereas "tracheostomy" refers to the tracheocutaneous fistula, or stoma, that is created. In practice, these terms are used interchangeably. Tracheotomy becomes necessary when long-term access to the airway is required for ventilation or pulmonary toilet. Although it can be performed emergently for airway management, cricothyroidotomy is the preferred technique for patients who have lost their airway and cannot be intubated.

**46**

## I. TYPICAL PRESENTATION

### PROLONGED VENTILATION

The need for prolonged ventilation is the clinical setting for tracheotomy most commonly encountered by the surgical resident. In patients with respiratory failure, tracheotomy should be performed if intubation is expected to be prolonged for greater than 2 to 3 weeks. In these cases, tracheotomy provides greater patient comfort and mobility than laryngeal intubation does. In addition, the shorter tube length decreases the resistance of the ventilatory circuit and reduces the work of breathing. Some evidence suggests that early tracheotomy (<7 days of mechanical ventilation) is associated with more rapid weaning, decreased hospital stay, and lower incidence of pneumonia.

### UPPER AIRWAY OBSTRUCTION

Airway obstruction, from causes such as foreign bodies, tumors, congenital webs, hypoplasia, soft tissue swelling after maxillofacial trauma, laryngeal or tracheal fractures, and bilateral vocal cord paralysis may be treated with tracheotomy. Anticipated postoperative upper airway obstruction in many head and neck cases necessitates tracheotomy as part of the operative plan.

### MANAGEMENT OF SECRETIONS

In patients who need assistance in clearing lower respiratory tract secretions, a tracheostomy allows a portal for frequent suctioning. In patients with decreased neurologic function who cannot manage their oral or gastric secretions, the presence of a cuffed tracheostomy tube effectively separates the airway from the esophagus, preventing aspiration.

## II. PREOPERATIVE WORKUP

There are no absolute contraindications to tracheotomy, and no preoperative testing is required in an emergency setting. In elective tracheotomy, however, patient care can be optimized by ruling out coagulopathy with routine prothrombin time and partial thromboplastin time.

## III. SURGICAL ANATOMY

Five midline structures are palpable and help to guide tracheotomy. From superiorly to inferiorly, the chin, the hyoid bone, the laryngeal prominence of the thyroid cartilage (the "Adam's apple"), the cricoid cartilage, and the suprasternal notch mark midline. The cricothyroid membrane lies between the inferior portion of the thyroid cartilage and the cricoid cartilage—it lies close to the skin surface and is the site of airway access in emergency cricothyroidotomy. The tracheal rings begin inferior to the cricoid cartilage, and these become palpable as dissection is carried down toward the trachea. The isthmus of the thyroid and the pyramidal lobe of the thyroid (thyroid tissue that persists in the midline path of descent of the gland) usually lie over the second and third tracheal rings. Paired thyroid lobes are located paratracheally. Other lateral structures include the paired platysma muscles, which are deficient in the midline. The anterior and external jugular veins lie deep to the platysma and run in a superoinferior course. Neither superficial veins nor motor nerves of the neck cross or occupy the midline.

## IV. CONDUCT OF OPERATION

The patient is placed supine on the operating room table, and a shoulder roll is placed to obtain slight hyperextension of the neck. In a patient with known or suspected cervical spine injury in whom the neck cannot be extended, the shoulder roll is omitted. After proper patient positioning, the neck is prepped and draped sterilely. The cuff of the tracheostomy tube is tested. A midline skin incision is made midway between the cricoid cartilage and the suprasternal notch. Either a vertical or transverse skin incision may be used. Although a horizontal incision provides better cosmesis, a vertical incision allows for easier midline dissection and avoids an inferior flap under which secretions might accumulate. The skin incision is carried through the subcutaneous tissue and the platysma to reveal the paired sternohyoid and sternothyroid ("strap") muscles. These muscles are retracted laterally, and blunt dissection continues in the midline with a hemostat. With a small right-angled retractor on each side, subsequent levels of tissue are retracted laterally as the midline dissection is carried toward the trachea. The isthmus of the thyroid is often encountered lying over the second or third tracheal ring. If small, the isthmus can be retracted superiorly or inferiorly to expose the trachea. If large, the isthmus is doubly ligated and divided in the midline. The pretracheal fascia is dissected to provide a clear view of the trachea. A cricoid hook is placed between the cricoid cartilage and the first tracheal ring, and the trachea is elevated.

Several incisions may be made in the trachea itself. An H- or T-shaped incision made through the anterior portion of the second or third tracheal ring is generally sufficient. Once the airway is opened, lateral stay sutures are placed in the trachea and brought out of the wound to aid in localization of the trachea in case of accidental extubation. After the trachea is entered, the endotracheal tube (if present) is withdrawn slowly until it is just above the level of the tracheal stoma. A spreader is used to widen the stoma itself. The tracheostomy tube is lubricated and inserted into the trachea. The tube is inserted into tracheal stoma with its axis perpendicular to the midline. Once the tube is felt to "pop" into the trachea, the tube is "twisted" inferiorly so that it lies in the same plane as the trachea. The obturator is withdrawn, and the cuff is inflated. After the tube is connected to the airway circuit, the return of end-tidal carbon dioxide confirms tube placement within the trachea. The tube should be suctioned to remove blood and mucus from the airway. The tube should be secured by suturing the flange to the skin anteriorly and by tying tracheostomy tapes around the neck (placing two fingers beneath the tapes during tying will prevent it from being tied too tightly).

## VARIATIONS OF OPERATION

**Cricothyroidotomy.** Because the cricothyroid membrane is the most superficial part of the airway, cricothyroidotomy is the quickest and safest means of obtaining airway access in an emergency. Landmarks for cricothyroidotomy include the hyoid bone, the thyroid cartilage, and the cricoid cartilage. A right-handed surgeon stands on the patient's right side, stabilizing the thyroid cartilage with the left hand and palpating the cricothyroid membrane with the left index finger. Using a scalpel oriented transversely, a short stabbing incision is made through the membrane into the airway. Once the subglottic space is entered, the knife handle is inserted into the wound and twisted vertically, opening the window in the cricothyroid membrane and allowing for placement of a tracheostomy tube. Because cricothyroidotomy carries an increased risk for subglottic stenosis, it is unsuitable for long-term airway management and should be converted to a formal tracheostomy should a surgical airway be needed for more than 3 to 5 days.

**Pediatric Tracheotomy.** Tracheotomy in a child is similar to tracheotomy in an adult, with some minor modifications. If possible, an endotracheal tube or ventilating bronchoscope should always be placed before tracheotomy to help identify and provide rigidity to the supple trachea. In children, tracheal cartilage is never resected, and the trachea is entered with a vertical incision through the second, third, or fourth tracheal ring. Because infants have short, fat necks relative to adults, lateral stay sutures should always be placed to aid reintubation in the case of possible catastrophic dislodgment of the tracheostomy tube.

**Percutaneous Dilational Tracheotomy.** In this procedure, a needle is inserted anteriorly into the trachea through the first or second tracheal rings under bronchoscopic monitoring to confirm placement. A guidewire is passed through this needle into the trachea, and with this as a guide, the tracheostomy tract is dilated either by the passage of serial dilators or with a "tracheotome." Once the tract is dilated, the tracheostomy tube is inserted and the guidewire withdrawn. Proponents of percutaneous tracheotomy point to shorter operative time, ease of performance, and decreased cost as advantages of the technique. Despite these advantages, the procedure is neither safer nor more effective than standard tracheotomy. Because neither blood vessels nor the thyroid gland is visualized, and given the inability to place stay sutures, complications such as bleeding or accidental extubation are potentially more catastrophic after a percutaneous approach. For these reasons, it is rarely used.

**Bjork Flap.** In a Bjork flap, introduced in 1960, a transverse incision is made in the trachea, and a flap consisting of the second or third tracheal ring anteriorly is sewn to the inferior skin margin. Use of such an inferiorly based Bjork flap reduces the risk of accidental extubation and makes possible reintubation easier. However, the Bjork flap also increases the risk of tracheocutaneous fistula, and it is unsuitable for children or in cases in which the tracheostomy tube is to be left in place only a short time.

## POSTOPERATIVE ORDERS

Because pneumothorax or pneumomediastinum is always possible after tracheotomy, a chest x-ray should always be included in the postoperative orders. Routine care of the tracheostomy tube is also essential. Humidification of the inspired air, either through mechanical ventilation, trach collar, or a nebulizer, is necessary to prevent tracheitis and crusting. Routine suctioning is necessary to clear pulmonary secretions and prevent clogging of the tracheostomy tube. The tube itself should not be changed for at least 3 days, until a stable tract forms. After 3 days, stay sutures and the sutures securing the tracheostomy tube to the skin may be discontinued and the tube changed as necessary to a smaller, cuffless, or fenestrated tube to meet the patient's needs. There is no role for prophylactic antibiotic therapy after tracheotomy. The tracheostomy is always colonized by bacteria, and the use of antibiotics merely results in colonization by resistant organisms.

**Admit to:** surgery
**Diagnosis:** s/p tracheotomy
**Condition:** stable
**Vital signs:** per intensive care unit routine
**Activity:**
**Allergies:**
**Nursing:** routine tracheostomy care—humidify inspired air, suction tube prn

**Diet:**
**IV fluids:**
**Medications:**
**Laboratory tests:** CXR to rule out pneumothorax and confirm tube
position

## V. COMPLICATIONS

### INTRAOPERATIVE COMPLICATIONS

Intraoperative complications include pneumothorax or pneumomediastinum,
tracheoesophageal fistula, injury to either the left or right recurrent laryngeal
nerve, or hemorrhage. Although pneumomediastinum generally requires no
treatment, it may produce circulatory embarrassment or rupture into the
pleural space, creating a simple or tension pneumothorax. Pneumothorax is
more commonly caused by direct injury to the cupola of the lung and may
require the placement of a chest tube. Tracheoesophageal fistula results
from making a deep incision through the anterior trachea and carrying it
down through the posterior trachea into the esophagus. If a posterior
tracheal laceration occurs, immediate operative repair is required. The
recurrent laryngeal nerves run bilaterally in the tracheoesophageal grooves,
and injury to these can be prevented by careful midline dissection.
Similarly, hemorrhage can be prevented by meticulous hemostasis and by
careful midline dissection away from the great vessels. Frequently, however,
small-vessel bleeding may be noticed postoperatively as intravascular
pressure increases or coughing transiently increases venous pressures.
These cases of persistent oozing can be controlled by carefully packing
around the tracheostomy tube.

### EARLY POSTOPERATIVE COMPLICATIONS

Early postoperative complications after tracheotomy include mucous
plugging, tube displacement, and postobstructive pulmonary edema.
Mucous plugging can be prevented by humidification of inspired air, sterile
saline flushes, and suctioning of the tracheostomy tube. Displacement of
the tube occurs more frequently in the pediatric population because of the
softer neck tissues and more pliable tracheostomy tubes used in this
population. Accidental extubation requires immediate reintubation, either
through the tracheostomy or laryngeally. Extubation is prevented by
securing the tracheostomy tube in place, and reintubation is greatly aided
through the presence of either a Bjork flap or stay sutures. Postobstructive
pulmonary edema is diagnosed by the presence of frothy sputum after
tracheotomy, and it may occur in patients who have labored with airway
obstruction for a long time. These patients have developed extremely
negative intrathoracic pressures during inspiration and extremely positive
intrathoracic pressures during expiration so that they could move air around
the obstruction. The sudden normalization of intrathoracic pressures in

46

TRACHEOTOMY

these patients after tracheotomy leads to a dramatic increase in venous return and a hydrostatic pressure gradient across the alveolar membranes, which leads to pulmonary edema. If it occurs, pulmonary edema can be treated with positive end-expiratory pressure (PEEP) ventilation and possibly diuretics.

## LATE POSTOPERATIVE COMPLICATIONS

Late complications after tracheotomy include tracheal stenosis and tracheo-innominate artery fistula. Tracheal stenosis is the most common late complication. It may present at the level of the stoma, cuff, or tube tip. Clinical suspicion for tracheal stenosis is raised by the onset of stridor. Tracheal stenosis at the level of the cuff can be prevented by maintaining cuff pressures beneath 25 cm $H_2O$, because pressures greater than this may predispose to tracheal ischemia by occluding the submucosal capillaries. Stenosis at the level of the cuff tip can be prevented by making sure that the tracheostomy tube is properly sized and fitted so that it does not irritate the tracheal wall. Tracheoinnominate artery fistula is a potentially fatal complication (73% mortality rate) that can result from the placement of a tracheostomy tube beneath the third tracheal ring. At this low level, the tip of the tube may erode through the anterior tracheal wall into the innominate artery. This artery crosses the midline from left to right, with its upper margin just beneath the sternum. Although bleeding within the first 48 hours may be from the incision, bleeding 4 or 5 days after tracheotomy must be considered "sentinel" bleeding, which often precedes tracheoinnominate fistula. To manage tracheoinnominate artery fistula, a long tube should be inserted through the tracheostomy so that its cuff lies beneath the bleeding and protects the airway. Bleeding can also be controlled by inserting a finger into the trachea and pressing anteriorly to compress the innominate artery against the sternum. Definitive treatment of tracheoinnominate artery fistula requires emergency operative ligation of the innominate artery.

## VI. DISCHARGE ORDERS

For patients in whom long-term tracheostomy is required, continued use of the stoma will ensure its patency. In these patients, it may be possible to switch to a fenestrated tube. These tubes allow for diversion of airflow past the vocal cords to generate a voice. For patients with resolving respiratory failure, tracheostomy tubes can be sequentially downsized until the patient no longer requires a tracheostomy. At this point, decannulation and the application of a dressing across the stoma allows for stoma closure.

# PAROTIDECTOMY

*Christopher Discolo*

The bilobed parotid is the largest of the salivary glands. Its superficial location and anatomic relationships result in important surgical considerations, including the need for superficial versus deep lobectomy, cosmesis, and the preservation of the facial nerve. Surgery of the parotid gland remains a common and challenging task for the head and neck surgeon.

Most surgical diseases of the parotid gland should be approached with a superficial parotidectomy, with identification and preservation of the facial nerve. In most cases this is a diagnostic and curative procedure. Surgical biopsy of a parotid mass is not recommended. The use of enucleation or excisional biopsy results in high recurrence rates, especially for pleomorphic adenomas. The role of open biopsy is usually reserved for those patients with obvious malignancies who are believed to be inoperable. In this case the biopsy results can help guide palliative therapies.

## I. PATHOPHYSIOLOGY

### NEOPLASTIC DISEASE

Tumors are the most common indication for surgery of the parotid. Approximately 80% of all salivary gland neoplasms occur in the parotid. There are a variety of benign and malignant tumors that can affect the gland. Of these, 80% are benign. Salivary tumors are rare in children accounting for only 5% of cases.

**Benign Tumors.** Overall the most common neoplasm of the parotid, as with other salivary glands, is the pleomorphic adenoma. It is also known as a benign mixed tumor, because it contains both epithelial and mesenchymal components. It appears smooth and lobular. Although well defined, its capsule is often incomplete, and transcapsular growth is common. Thus, these tumors are prone to high recurrence rates, unless adequate resection margins are achieved. Other less common benign tumors of the parotid include Warthin's tumor (papillary cystadenoma lymphomatosum), oncocytoma, and monomorphic adenoma.

**Malignant Tumors.** The most common malignant tumor is the mucoepidermoid carcinoma. The low-grade variety has a high mucous/epidermoid cell ratio and tends to behave like a benign neoplasm. They are capable of local spread and metastasis, however. High-grade lesions may resemble squamous cell carcinoma and have a very high likelihood of metastasis. Other varieties of malignant lesions are adenoid cystic carcinoma, acinic cell carcinoma, adenocarcinoma, squamous cell carcinoma, sarcomas, and lymphomas.

## CHRONIC RECURRENT SIALADENITIS

Chronic recurrent sialadenitis refers to a localized condition of the salivary gland, most commonly the parotid, in which there are repeated episodes of pain and inflammation. These patients commonly have fever, chills, malaise, and leukocytosis. Eventually parenchymal degeneration and fibrous replacement of the gland occur. As the number of episodes increases, ductal ectasia with intervening areas of stenosis is caused by the irreversible damage to the architecture of the gland. A key component of this condition is the reduction of salivary flow. This then leads to contamination with ascending oropharyngeal bacteria, which causes acute suppurative sialadenitis. Most commonly, the reduction of flow is caused by sialolithiasis, but there are a number of other causes. These include side effects of medications, cachexia, dehydration, radiation therapy, chemotherapy, benign lymphoepithelial lesions, Sjögren's syndrome, stress, stricture of Stenson's duct, extrinsic compression, and foreign bodies. The conservative management of chronic recurrent sialoadenitis has failed to reveal any consistent and effective therapies. Parotidectomy is a safe and effective tool in the management of this disease.

## II. TYPICAL PRESENTATION

Parotid gland neoplasms most commonly present as a painless mass. These masses most often are found in the tail of the gland and tend to enlarge slowly. They may be painful in cases of hemorrhage, infection, or cystic degeneration. Malignant tumors more commonly cause pain secondary to neural involvement. Pain is a poor prognostic factor in malignant neoplasms of the parotid gland.

## III. PREOPERATIVE WORKUP

Any patient with a suspected neoplasm should undergo a thorough head and neck examination. The function of the facial nerve should be evaluated carefully. Facial nerve palsy can occur with benign neoplasms, especially rapidly growing tumors, but is most often associated with malignancy.

Fine-needle aspiration (FNA) is helpful in evaluating a parotid mass. It is both well tolerated and easy to perform in the office setting. It has very few complications, and seeding of the needle tract with tumor cells has not been reported. As with any FNA, the experience of the cytologist plays an important role in interpretation.

Computed tomography or magnetic resonance imaging of the parotid is unnecessary. It rarely differentiates benign from malignant tumors and typically does not alter the treatment algorithm. Imaging studies should be obtained in cases of very large masses, recurrences, or suspected involvement of the parapharyngeal space or carotid artery.

Occasionally, some normal anatomic structures can be confused with parotid gland enlargement. Most commonly these include the masseter muscle, the mandibular processes, and the transverse process of the atlas. Also, nutritional deficiency, inflammatory conditions, and infections can cause true enlargement of the parotid gland. A patient's clinical scenario must be taken into account when working up parotid enlargement.

## IV. SURGICAL ANATOMY

The parotid gland occupies a superficial location on the face. It may be palpated between the mastoid process and the ramus of the mandible. Only skin and dermis cover the lateral surface of the gland. Medially, the gland is in proximity to the styloid process and its associated musculature (stylohyoid, styloglossus, stylopharyngeal), the carotid sheath, and cranial nerves IX, X, and XII. The anterior border of the sternocleidomastoid muscle serves as the inferior boundary, and the zygomatic arch acts as the superior boundary.

The parotid gland is divided into two asymmetric lobes by the facial nerve. The larger of the lobes is superficial, and the smaller is deep to the nerve. There is a glandular isthmus connecting the two. This relationship becomes very important surgically. The facial nerve exits the skull at the stylomastoid foramen and then courses through the parotid to innervate the muscles of facial expression. The facial nerve divides into five branches as it courses through the gland. Ranging superiorly to inferiorly these are the temporal, zygomatic, buccal, marginal mandibular, and cervical branches. Identification and preservation of the facial nerve and its branches are crucial to successful parotid surgery. The only constant landmark for identifying the nerve is the stylomastoid foramen, from which it exits the skull base.

The parotid duct travels anteriorly along the masseter muscle until it abruptly turns medially to pierce the buccinator muscle and buccal fat pad to enter the oral mucosa. The buccal branch of the facial nerve travels with the duct. Stensen's duct, as it is also known, is visible opposite the second maxillary molar. The secretory function of the gland is controlled by cranial nerve IX. Histologically the parotid gland's acinar cells are mostly of the serous variety.

Various other structures also come in close proximity to or even enter and leave the parotid gland. These include the auriculotemporal nerve, superficial temporal artery and vein, retromandibular vein, and branches of the facial nerve as they prepare to travel in the submuscular plane of the face, posterior auricular artery, transverse facial artery, occipital artery, and the great auricular nerve. The great auricular nerve is a major branch of the cervical plexus and supplies cutaneous innervation over the region of the submandibular triangle and the mastoid.

## V. CONDUCT OF OPERATION

After induction of general anesthesia, the patient's face and neck are prepped and draped in a sterile fashion. A transparent drape is used to cover the face to allow for adequate visualization of the ear, neck, parotid, corner of mouth, and corner of eye during the procedure. Patients are placed in a 30-degree reverse Trendelenburg position.

An incision is made in the preauricular region and extended inferiorly along the line of attachment of the lobule and finally curving into a skin crease on the upper neck, usually two fingerbreadths beneath the lower border of the jaw. A skin flap is raised anteriorly, superficial to the parotid fascia, and carried to the posterior border of the masseter. Care must be taken to avoid the peripheral branches of the facial nerve while raising this flap. The tail of the gland is then dissected free from the sternocleidomastoid muscle. It is during this portion of the procedure when the greater auricular nerve must be sacrificed.

As the tail of the parotid is elevated, the digastric muscle comes into view. This is an important landmark for the facial nerve. The next plane of dissection is developed in the pretragal space by bluntly dissecting in a direction parallel to the course of the facial nerve. This serves to expose the tragal pointer (medial extension of auricular cartilage). Any remaining attachments of the gland to the mastoid are severed at this time. Bipolar cautery is used for the remainder of the case.

At this point the facial nerve is identified. The tragal pointer, posterior belly of the digastric muscle, and the mastoid process help to locate the facial nerve. The facial nerve usually lies about 1 cm medial and just inferior and anterior to the tip of the tragal pointer. Once the main trunk of the facial nerve is identified, following the nerve out peripherally identifies the individual branches. The superficial portion of the gland is then removed through this technique. Once removed, hemostasis is achieved, and the wound is closed over a Hemovac drain. A conforming pressure dressing is applied.

## VARIATIONS OF OPERATION

The main variation to this surgery is in the identification of the facial nerve. Although the nerve always exits from the stylomastoid foramen, its course through the gland is not fixed. Occasionally, large tumors distort the normal anatomy and make identification of the nerve extremely difficult. Other techniques for identifying the facial nerve do exist and rely on other anatomic landmarks. One such landmark is the tympanomastoid suture, although this is believed by some to be a poor predictor of nerve location. This is a groove that is palpable between the tympanic portion of the temporal bone and the mastoid. The nerve exits its foramen approximately 6 to 8 mm medial to this suture line. Yet another technique involves locating a peripheral branch of the nerve and tracing it back proximally to the main trunk.

Occasionally the deep lobe of the parotid gland must also be removed. Indications for deep lobe parotidectomy include a deep-lobe neoplasm, chronic/recurrent sialadenitis, and metastatic disease. The key to removing the deep lobe of the gland is meticulous dissection of the facial nerve from its underlying parotid tissue.

Malignant disease can invade the facial nerve, requiring its sacrifice during surgery. In these cases the nerve is transected proximal to its branching point (pes anserinus). Distally, the nerve is divided where appropriate, most commonly where it emerges from the gland. Here the nerve is resected en bloc with the parotid tissue. Nerve grafting is then carried out using a donor nerve, most often the anterior branch of the great auricular, the sural, or the lateral femoral cutaneous nerve.

## POSTOPERATIVE ORDERS

After parotidectomy, patients require little in the way of special orders. They may resume their normal diet as tolerated. Wound infections in this region are rare, and generally no antibiotic coverage is required once the drains are removed. Pain is usually well controlled with standard narcotic pain medication. Drains are removed on postoperative day 1 or when output falls to less than 30 cc/ml in 24 hours.

**Admit to:**
**Diagnosis:** s/p parotidectomy
**Condition:** stable
**Vital signs:** per routine
**Activity:** ad lib
**Allergies:**
**Nursing:** measure Jackson-Pratt drains every shift, I&Os
**Diet:** as tolerated
**IV fluids:** $D_5$/0.45% NS with 20 mEq KCl at 80 ml/h and Heplock when patient is tolerating oral intake
**Medications:** Percocet prn
**Laboratory tests:**

## VI. POTENTIAL COMPLICATIONS

**Facial Nerve Injury.** Temporary paralysis is reported to occur in up to 30% of patients. Permanent paralysis of one or all branches occurs in less than 3% of all superficial parotidectomies. The marginal mandibular branch is most susceptible to injury. Total parotidectomy, increasing age, overuse of the nerve stimulator, and reoperations all increase the risk of nerve injury. Temporary injury is expected to resolve in weeks to months postoperatively.

**Greater Auricular Nerve Hypoesthesia.** This is almost expected outcome of surgery. The nerve is sacrificed during the process of dissecting the tail of the parotid free from the sternocleidomastoid muscle. Patients have long-term sensory loss in the region of the parotid and the pinna. Patients are cautioned regarding potential thermal injury to this area by either hair dryers or curling irons.

**Wound Infection.** This rare complication after surgery is related to the rich vascular supply in this area. Careful handling of tissues and the use of aseptic technique decrease the risk of infection. Antibiotics, drainage, and local wound care are the treatments should infection develop.

**Hemorrhage/Hematoma.** This uncommon complication is caused by poor hemostasis at the time of surgery. Significant hematoma can compromise the airway. Treatment entails drainage of the hematoma and control of the bleeding vessels.

**Skin Flap Necrosis.** The distal tip of the postauricular skin flap is most vulnerable. During surgery this flap should not be curved too far posteriorly to minimize the risk of necrosis. Smoking contributes to this complication, and patients are cautioned to avoid smoking.

**Salivary Fistula and Sialocele.** Fistulas are a relatively common and self-limiting complication that occurs when the cut edge of the remaining salivary gland leaks saliva. This then collects beneath the flap or drains out through the wound. Management involves local wound care and pressure dressings. Sialoceles can require multiple aspirations and pressure dressings to overcome the secretory pressure of the gland.

**Frey's Syndrome (Gustatory Sweating).** Frey's syndrome occurs when severed parasympathetic fibers of the parotid regenerate themselves and come to innervate severed sympathetic fibers that supply the sweat glands. Dermal flushing or sweating occurs during salivary stimulation. Although in 30% to 60% of all parotidectomies some degree of Frey's syndrome develops, only 10% of these are symptomatic. The use of a thick skin flap or interposition of a superficial musculoaponeurotic system flap can prevent this complication. Treatment consists of topical antiperspirants/anticholinergics, botulinum toxin injections, and occasionally fascial graft interposition.

**Trismus.** Trismus is usually mild and related to inflammation and fibrosis of the masseter muscle. Trismus improves with jaw-opening exercises.

## VII. DISCHARGE ORDERS

Patients typically remain in the hospital overnight and can be discharged the following day. They do not require oral antibiotics and are usually sent home on pain medications. Activity can be resumed as tolerated by the patient.

If facial nerve injury has occurred (either temporary or permanent), patients may require the use of an artificial tears product or eye chamber to protect their eyes from traumatic injury, especially during sleep.

Patient follow-up is in a week to 10 days after surgery.

# PART XIV

## Transplant

# RENAL TRANSPLANTATION

*Wayne Kuang*
*Hazem Abou El Fettouh*

Renal transplantation is the treatment of choice for patients who receive chronic dialysis for bilateral end-stage renal disease. It has been shown to be cost-effective and is associated with decreased morbidity and mortality. More importantly, it has provided these patients with a higher quality of life. With continuing advances in organ preservation and immunosuppression, renal transplantation will be performed with increasing frequency and success.

**48**

## I. PATHOPHYSIOLOGY

The causes of end-stage renal disease include diabetes (36%), hypertension (30%), chronic glomerulonephritis (24%), and autosomal dominant polycystic kidney disease (12%). In pediatric patients, the predominant cause is congenital conditions (45%), such as obstructive hydronephrosis or congenital atrophy.

## II. TYPICAL PRESENTATION

Terminal renal failure is defined as a creatinine clearance less than 10 ml/min or a serum creatinine of greater than 8 mg/dl. Patients often have a history of uremia (uremic fetor, pericarditis, platelet dysfunction, asterixis, altered mental status, and neuropathy), constitutional symptoms (pruritus, fatigue, nausea, forgetfulness, and malaise), electrolyte abnormalities (hyperkalemia, metabolic acidosis, hypocalcemia with osteomalacia, and hyperphosphotemia), or anemia. Ultrasonography can identify the underlying cause and provide a means for percutaneous biopsies. Biopsy specimens often demonstrate nonspecific interstitial fibrosis and glomerulosclerosis.

Transplant candidates are often on chronic peritoneal dialysis or hemodialysis. These patients are at increased risk for infection, anemia, and atherosclerosis. Transplantation allows for a return to the normal physiologic state without the need for long-term dialysis.

## III. PREOPERATIVE WORKUP

### EXCLUSION CRITERIA

Risk factors that jeopardize the transplant or increase the chances of morbidity and mortality must be identified. Exclusion testing must identify any evidence of acute infection or active malignancy. Cancer screening involves mammography, prostate specific antigen testing, a Papanicolaou smear, and stool occult blood tests. After treatment for malignancy, a 2-year cancer-free period must pass before these patients are again eligible for consideration. Screening for infections includes serologic testing, a purified protein derivative test, urinanalysis, and a chest x-ray.

345

## INCLUSION CRITERIA

Inclusion testing requires full exploration of all possible comorbidities. Coronary catheterization is performed in patients with risk factors for coronary artery disease. The extent and severity of any systemic disease (systemic lupus erythematosus, amyloidosis, or vasculitis) should be determined. Peptic ulcer disease, inflammatory bowel disease, cholecystitis, and diverticulitis should be evaluated and treated before transplantation.

## RADIOLOGIC WORKUP

Vascular anatomy is investigated in patients with a history of either prior aortoiliac surgery or peripheral vascular disease. Computed tomography with three-dimensional reconstruction, abdominal ultrasonography, and angiography are used to delineate the underlying anatomy and the risk of steal syndrome.

## UROLOGIC WORKUP

A urologic evaluation is an integral component of the pretransplant evaluation. A voiding cystourethrogram evaluates lower urinary tract function and identifies vesicoureteral reflux. Urodynamic studies identify noncompliant bladders requiring augmentation. A baseline ultrasonogram will screen for renal cell carcinoma or acquired renal cystic disease that is a premalignant state. Indications for pretransplant nephrectomy (6 weeks before transplant) include uncontrolled hypertension, persistent pyelonephritis, calculi, malignancy, renal obstruction, and severe proteinuria. In patients undergoing retransplantation, transplant nephrectomy is indicated in cases of acute rejection while the person is on dialysis, infection, fevers, gross hematuria, myalgias, malaise, graft tenderness, or uncontrolled hypertension.

## DONOR EVALUATION

Candidates for kidney donation must be evaluated for any condition that puts them at risk for perioperative morbidity or that may impede the quality of their life or the function of their remaining kidney. Living related donors demonstrate a half-life that is extended by 5 years compared with cadaveric donors. Given the shortage of living related donors, living unrelated donation (eg, spouse) has become a viable option, demonstrating a 83% to 93% graft survival rate at 1 year. Cadaver donors must be evaluated for any disease, such as chronic hypertension, diabetes, cancer, or infections, that could affect the vascular integrity or perfusion of the allograft. Biopsy is often considered. Hemodynamically stable heart-beating donors between the ages of 2 and 60 are preferred, because the risk of acute tubular necrosis is minimized.

Histocompatibility leukocyte antigen (HLA) tissue matching is a widely accepted component of renal transplantation. HLA matching is inversely related to rejection episodes while directly related to allograft survival.

**PREOPERATIVE ORDERS**

**Nursing:** drain and cap CAPD catheter
**Diet:** NPO
**Medications:** cefazolin (Ancef) 1 g on call to OR
methylprednisolone 250 mg IV on call to OR
PAS on call to OR
**Laboratory tests:** CXR, EKG; blood work predialysis: CBC differential, CMP, PT, PTT; T&S (2 U of LPPC or CMV-negative blood); tissue typing (send both clotted and heparinized blood); hepatitis acute panel with hepatitis surface antigen; CMV buffy coat culture, viral IgG and IgM titers (CMV, HSV, EBV)
**Consult:** nephrology for preoperative dialysis

**48**

**RENAL TRANSPLANTATION**

## IV. SURGICAL ANATOMY

The descending right iliac fossa is the preferred location for a donor kidney. The external iliac vessels are more nearly horizontal with respect to each other making the anastomoses more feasible on this side.

## V. CONDUCT OF OPERATION

In a supine position, the patient receives general endotracheal anesthesia. After Foley catheter placement, antibiotic solution (neomycin-polymyxin B) is used to gravity-fill the bladder to capacity, and the catheter is clamped until the time of ureteroneocystostomy. The patient is shaved, prepped, and draped in the usual sterile fashion.

A Gibson incision (parallel to the inguinal ligament and lateral to the rectus border) is made in the right lower quadrant. The incision is carried down through the dermis, subcutaneous tissue, fascia, and muscles using both sharp dissection and electrocautery. Careful hemostasis is achieved, and the retroperitoneum is entered.

The inferior epigastric vessels are isolated, ligated, and divided with 0 silk free ties. The spermatic cord is circumscribed with a vessel loop and mobilized off the peritoneum to the level of the internal ring. The peritoneum is mobilized medially and superiorly. A self-retaining Bookwalter retractor is placed.

The external iliac artery and vein are skeletonized along their course and are circumscribed separately with vessel loops. All venules and lymphatics are isolated, ligated, and divided with 3-0 silk free ties.

After placement of the donor kidney within the operative field, a Satinsky clamp is placed on the external iliac vein, and a venotomy is made. The lumen is irrigated with heparinized saline. The venous anastomosis is performed end-to-side with 5-0 Prolene in a running quadrantlike fashion.

Attention is turned to the arterial anastomosis. A bulldog clamp is placed proximally. A pediatric renal artery clamp is placed distally, and an arteriotomy is made. The lumen is copiously irrigated. An aortic punch is used to expand the lumen in an elliptical fashion. The arterial anastomosis is performed end-to-end using 6-0 Prolene.

After a bulldog clamp is placed on the donor vein, the venous clamp is removed. Adequate hemostasis is achieved at the anastomosis. The remaining clamps are removed, and the kidney is rapidly warmed and well perfused.

The ureter is tailored to the appropriate length and widely spatulated. An extravesical ureteroneocystostomy is performed. By way of a submucosal tunnel, the ureter is passed into the bladder and secured to the bladder mucosa with 4-0 chromic catgut sutures. The bladder wall is then closed with two layers of 3-0 chromic catgut in a watertight fashion.

The fascia is closed with a running No. 1 polydioranone suture and intermittent interrupted 0 Ethibond stitches. The wound is copiously irrigated, and skin is closed with surgical clips. Sterile dressings are applied, and the Foley catheter is left in place.

## VARIATIONS OF OPERATION

For pediatric populations, a vertical or paramedian incision is used for adequate mobilization of the ascending colon and exposure of iliac vessels. The renal artery is anastomosed to the aorta in an end-to-side fashion. The renal vein is anastomosed to the inferior vena cava, still end-to-side. The kidney is often laid down behind the cecum.

Peritoneal dialysis catheters are removed in living related transplant recipients at the end of the operation. In recipients of cadaveric renal transplants, peritoneal dialysis catheters are removed only when good graft function has been established postoperatively.

In diabetics, the internal iliac arteries may be compromised, which may result in an increased risk of postoperative impotence. A renal-to-external iliac-artery end-to-side anastomosis is therefore performed.

## POSTOPERATIVE ORDERS

**Admit to:**

**Diagnosis:** s/p renal transplant

**Condition:** stable

**Vital signs:** q1h × 8 h, q2h × 8 h, then q4h; CVP: q1h in the PACU, then q4h × 24 h; notify transplant service if <12 or >16

**Activity:** bed rest until 6 AM on POD 1, then ambulate with assistance qid

**Allergies:**

**Nursing:** daily weights, Foley to gravity drainage (do not irrigate or clamp), IS q1h while awake, cough and deep breathe q4h, PAS × 48 h, call service for T >38.5°C, DBP >110 or <60, HR >120 or <60 bpm, and for sudden change in urine output

**Diet:** NPO except medications; advance as tolerated with return of bowel function

**IV fluids:** 0.45% sodium chloride with sodium bicarbonate 20 mEq/L at 30 ml/h plus previous hour's output up to 300 ml/h; if urine volume exceeds 300 ml/h, replace 300 ml plus two-third of the output exceeding 300 ml

**Medications general:** docusate sodium 100 mg PO tid
  fluconazole (Diflucan) 100 mg IV qd (if ureters are stented)
  TMP-SMZ (Septra) single strength PO qd
  Pepcid 20 mg PO qhs
  bisacodyl suppository 10 mg PR qd prn
  Fleet enema per rectum qd prn
  PCA × 24-48 h

**Medications immunosuppression:**

**Laboratory tests:** CXR in PACU, renal scan (technetium mag 3) on POD 1, CBC, BMP in PACU, serum $Ca^{2+}$ if urine output >400 ml/h × 4 h, daily AM CBC and differential, BMP, cyclosporine level (if applicable), CMP, every Monday, Thursday; antithymocyte globulin (ATG) or muromonab-CD3 (OKT3) monitoring every Monday, Wednesday, Friday

**Consults:** renal dietitian and transplant social worker

---

**TABLE 48-1**

IMMUNOSUPPRESSION (ANTIBODY INDUCTION AND TRIPLE-MAINTENANCE THERAPY WITH DELAYED CALCINEURIN INHIBITOR INSTITUTION)

**MAINTENANCE**

| | |
|---|---|
| Methylprednisolone (POD 0, 1, 2) | 250-500 mg PO bid × 3 days |
| Prednisone (started after methylprednisolone) | 60 mg PO bid |
| Mycophenolate mofetil | 1000 mg PO bid |
| Cyclosporine | 5 mg/kg PO bid |
| (If living-related, immediately started postoperatively) | |
| (If cadaver, started when creatinine <4 mg/dl or POD 7) | |

**ANTIBODY INDUCTION**

**(Single Agent from List Below Is Started Within 6 Hours of the Transplant)**

| | |
|---|---|
| Antithymocyte globulin (ATG) (POD 1-10) | 100 mg/kg PO qd |
| Muromonab-CD3 (POD 1-10) | 2.5-5 mg PO qd |
| Basiliximab (Simulect)* (POD 0, 4) | 20 mg PO qd |
| Thymoglobulin (POD 1-10) | 1-1.5 mg/kg PO qd |
| Premedicate: | |
| Diphenhydramine | 50 mg PO |
| Acetaminophen | 650 mg PO |
| Hydrocortisone | 100 mg |

*Simulect is often given on POD 0 and 4, whereas the remainder is given at most for 10 days postoperatively. If an adequate level of cyclosporine is attained (225 to 275 $\mu$g/L) before 10 days, then antibody induction is discontinued.

## VI. COMPLICATIONS

**Vascular Occlusion.** This occurs immediately after the transplantation (<1%) with kinked vessels, stenosis of a suture line, or thrombosis. In patients with a sudden decrease in urine output, emergency exploration is indicated once after renal obstruction has been eliminated as a possible cause.

**Delayed Renal Artery Stenosis.** This occurs in 1.5% to 8% of patients. Atheromas, faulty surgical technique or immunologic mechanisms may all contribute to its development. Patients present with poorly controlled hypertension, worsening renal function, or a bruit. These patients must be evaluated by renal ultrasonography or angiogram or both. Rejection and cyclosporine toxicity must be eliminated as possible causes. Percutaneous transluminal angioplasty and open surgical repair are therapeutic options.

**Urologic Complications.** These occur in 2% to 5% of cases. Clinically, patients present with decreased urine output and graft dysfunction. An anastomotic leak, ureteral or anastomotic stricture, ureteral obstruction, and ureterovesical disruption all can be assessed by ultrasonography or a renal scan. Leaks can be further delineated by retrograde cystourethrography.

**Hematuria.** If noted in the immediate postoperative period, hematuria can be localized to the ureteroneocystostomy or cystostomy site. First-line therapy is catheter irrigation. If hematuria persists, endoscopic fulguration followed by transvesical exploration is indicated. Infection, malignancy, calculus, or other renal processes must be excluded in cases of late hematuria.

**Lymphoceles.** Lymphoceles occur in 6% to 18% of patients. Most are asymptomatic and are treated conservatively. Symptoms include wound swelling, leg edema, and graft dysfunction due to regional compression. Ultrasonography can be used for diagnostic aspiration. Marsupialization and drainage into the peritoneal cavity by means of a laparoscopic approach is the treatment of choice.

**Acute Tubular Necrosis.** ATN occurs in 5% to 40% of patients (mostly in recipients of cadaveric kidneys). Predisposing factors include prolonged anastomotic times and cold-preservation ischemia. A renal scan can be diagnostic. Duplex ultrasonography should eliminate postrenal causes. Expectant and supportive therapy is indicated. Renal function should recover over several weeks.

**Infections.** Infections can occur any time in the postoperative period. Although conventional wound, lung, and urinary tract infections will present within the first month, opportunistic infections (eg, viral) emerge thereafter during the 2- to 6-month period after transplantation. Cytomegalovirus causes symptoms in 35% and death in 2% of the transplant recipients. Seronegative recipients of positive donor kidneys have the highest risk. They typically present with a flulike illness (fever, malaise, fatigue, myalgias, arthralgias). Without treatment, site-specific symptoms (pulmonary, urinary, or gastrointestinal) may develop. Laboratory examination will often demonstrate atypical lymphocytosis and elevated transaminases. Leukopenia and thrombocytopenia are common. Although active infection is confirmed by cell culture, early detection is possible with monoclonal antibodies. Therapy entails a reduction in immunosuppressive regimen, ganciclovir, and supportive care (antipyretics and intravenous hydration). Postoperative ganciclovir is often administered prophylactically for up to 3 months, depending on the serologic tests of donor and recipient.

**Malignancy.** Cancer occurs in 2.5% of patients. In this setting of immunosuppression, skin cancer, lymphoma, and Kaposi's sarcoma are most prevalent. Lymphoproliferative disorders (often Epstein-Barr virus–related) with cyclosporine will on average present at 15 months after transplant; however, 32% will be present within 4 months. Therapy requires either reducing or stopping immunosuppressive medications all together.

**Hyperacute Rejection.** Although hyperacute rejection is a rare occurrence (0.1%), a single episode of acute rejection occurs in 25% to 55% of patients. Presenting within weeks to months of the transplantation, these patients demonstrate worsening renal function and may complain of fever and tenderness over the graft. Most episodes will respond to immunosuppressive therapy. Treatment entails corticosteroids or antibody therapy (muromonab-CD3 [OKT3]/antilymphocyte antithymocyte globulins). High-dose steroids at 7 mg/kg are administered for 3 days. If steroids are ineffective, 5 mg OKT3 intravenously every day for 7 to 14 days is given. With prolonged or high-dose antibody therapy, patients will be at risk for posttransplant lymphoproliferative disorder. In addition, human anti-murine antibodies should be tested for in nonresponding patients. Chronic rejection occurs in 5% to 7% of cadaveric kidneys per year after the first year and tends to present within months or years of the transplant. No known treatment exists; consequently, these patients will return to chronic dialysis.

## VII. DISCHARGE ORDERS

**Diet:** low animal fat; no added salt
**Activity:** no heavy lifting for 1-2 mos; 6-8 weeks off work
**Medications:** prednisone taper, 60 mg PO bid, then 50 mg bid, then 40 mg bid, then 30 mg bid, then 30/15 mg bid, and then 30 mg qd. Thereafter decrease qd dose by 2.5 mg every month until the 7.5 mg PO qd maintenance dose is attained.

| | |
|---|---|
| mycophenolate mofetil | 1000 mg PO bid |
| cyclosporine | 5 mg/kg PO bid |

**Follow-up:** 2, 4, 8, 12 weeks, then 6, 9, 12, 16, 20, 24, 30, and 36 months.

**Laboratory tests:** CBC, BMP, and cyclosporine level at 2×/wk until 3 months, every week until 6 months, every other week until 9 months, every month until 1.5 years, then every other month until 2 years, and 4×/y thereafter if doing well.

# TRANSPLANTATION OF THE PANCREAS

*Kevin L. W. Banks*
*Venkatesh Krishnamuthi*

In general, pancreatic transplantation is performed to establish a normo-glycemic state and reverse or arrest secondary end-stage complications associated with severe type 1 diabetes. The end-stage complications of diabetes include advanced retinopathy, end-stage nephropathy, disabling neuropathy, and extensive macrovascular and microvascular disease. There are three settings in which the pancreatic transplantation can be applied: simultaneous transplantation with a kidney graft (most common), sequentially after successful renal transplantation, and transplantation of the pancreas alone in the preuremic patient. Absolute contraindications to pancreatic transplantation are malignancy and active infection.

**49**

## I. PATHOPHYSIOLOGY

The pancreas is a complex organ that has both endocrine and exocrine functions. The exocrine function of the pancreas plays a central role in the process of alimentary tract function and digestion, but has no bearing on the pathophysiology necessitating pancreatic transplantation, and for the purposes of this discussion will be ignored. The best-known endocrine function of the pancreas is glucose homeostasis through the production and release of insulin and glucagon from the beta- and alpha-cells located in the islets of Langerhans. Type 1 diabetes is caused by an autoimmune process in which the alpha-cells of the pancreas are destroyed. Despite advances in science and technology, the relation between genetic and environmental factors triggering the autoimmune response in type 1 diabetes is not known. Pancreatic transplantation is performed to provide a physiologic insulin replacement in type 1 diabetes. Insulin is essential for carbohydrate metabolism, and its deficiency results in hyperglycemia. The exogenous administration of insulin, regardless of how finely tuned, cannot prevent intermittent wide variations in glucose levels. It is believed that this wide variation in glucose levels is responsible for the occurrence and progression of end-stage complications seen in diabetics. Pancreatic transplantation allows physiologic control of glucose levels within a normal range, which ultimately arrests the progression of end-stage diabetic complications.

## II. TYPICAL PRESENTATION

### RECIPIENT INCLUSION CRITERIA
Recipient inclusion criteria can be categorized on the basis of the degree of nephropathy, because most pancreas transplantations are performed simultaneously with kidney transplantation.

1. Type 1 diabetes with evidence of secondary complications. Nephropathy is the most frequent secondary complication of diabetes and the most common cause necessitating renal transplantation
2. Previous kidney transplantation with evidence of diabetic changes
3. Severe glycemic lability with hypoglycemic unawareness

## III. PREOPERATIVE WORKUP

Following is a list of pretransplant evaluation parameters. Significant coronary artery disease may be present in diabetics in the absence of angina, making cardiac evaluation the most important portion or the pretransplant workup.

### PRETRANSPLANT EVALUATION

1. Cancer screening: mammogram, prostate specific antigen, Papanicolaou smear, and stool occult blood test.
2. Infection screening: PPD, urinalysis, chest x-ray, and serologic tests for CMV, HSV, EBV, HBV, HCV, RPR, HIV, and *Toxoplasma*.
3. Cardiac screening: electrocardiogram, cardiac stress testing (dobutamine or thallium stress test), coronary angiography if stress test is positive.
4. Urologic evaluation: serum creatinine, creatinine clearance, renal ultrasonography, and voiding cystourethrogram (for bladder drainage).
5. Vascular evaluation: vascular evaluation is based on physical examination of peripheral pulses (mainly femoral). If the physical examination is abnormal, further evaluation is performed with magnetic resonance or contrast angiography.
6. Miscellaneous studies: C-peptide level and glycosylated hemoglobin.

### PREOPERATIVE ORDERS FOR SIMULTANEOUS KIDNEY-PANCREAS TRANSPLANTS

**Admit to:** kidney/pancreas transplant service
**Diagnosis:** type 1 diabetes mellitus, ESRD
**Condition:** good
**Vital signs:** q4h
**Activity:**
**Allergies:**
**Nursing:** I&Os q4h, height and weight on admission, NS enemas until clear, Hibiclens shower, Accuchecks q4h
**Diet:** NPO except medications
**IV fluids:** D$_5$NS at 80 ml/h
**Medications:** Zosyn 3.375 g IV on call to OR
        if penicillin allergic, cefoxitin 1 g IV plus gentamicin
        1.7 mg/kg on call to OR

if penicillin and cephalosporin allergic, clindamycin
    900 mg IV on call to OR
methylprednisolone (Solu-Medrol) 500 mg IV on call to OR
basiliximab (Simulect) 20 mg IV on call to OR
glucagon 0.5 to 1 mg SC or $D_{50}W$ one-half ampule for
    suspected hypoglycemia

**Laboratory tests:**

## IV. SURGICAL ANATOMY

For the purposes of transplantation the pancreas can be grafted either as a whole organ graft (including the first, second, and a variable length of the third portion of the duodenum) or a segmental graft (tail and body only). In the United States, whole organ pancreas grafts are the preferred method of transplantation and account for most pancreas transplantations performed. For the purposes of discussion, all general references to pancreatic transplantation will imply whole organ grafts in setting of simultaneous kidney transplantation.

In general, arterial supply for whole organ pancreas transplantation requires preservation of the splenic and superior mesenteric arteries. During the "backtable" reconstruction, these arteries are anastomosed to the donor iliac Y graft. Specifically, the splenic artery is anastomosed to the internal iliac and the superior mesenteric to the external iliac. Venous drainage of the whole organ graft requires preservation of the splenic and portal veins.

Segmental pancreatic transplantation requires only preservation of the splenic artery and its branches, including the dorsal pancreatic artery. Venous drainage of the segmental pancreas transplant requires preservation of only the splenic vein. In the living pancreatic donor, only segmental pancreatic transplantation is possible.

Exocrine function of the transplanted pancreas is managed by one of the following methods:

1. Urinary/bladder drainage: The duodenal segment is anastomosed to the dome of the bladder.
2. Enteric drainage: The duodenal segment is anastomosed to bowel by a variety of different enteric anastomoses.
3. Duct injection (only for segmental grafts): A selected polymer is injected into the pancreatic duct, resulting in obliteration to the pancreatic ductal system.

## V. CONDUCT OF OPERATION

General endotracheal anesthesia is induced with the patient in the supine position. A Foley catheter is placed and the bladder is filled with antibiotic solution. The patient is then prepped and draped in the normal sterile fashion. Pancreas transplantation can be performed through either a lower quadrant extraperitoneal incision or through a midline intraperitoneal approach. With a retroperitoneal approach, it is recommended that the peritoneum be opened to facilitate absorption of peripancreatic secretions. In general, a midline intraperitoneal incision is preferred, because this approach allows for maximum flexibility and for the performance of concomitant procedures such as simultaneous kidney transplantation, peritoneal dialysis catheter removal, nephrectomy, and appendectomy. After routine exposure of the abdomen, lymphatics overlying the iliac artery and vein are divided. The right iliac artery and vein are preferred sites of implantation, because there is more favorable anatomy in the right iliac venous system.

The preferred method of venous drainage remains controversial. Systemic venous drainage (SVD), the method used in more than 90% of reporting centers, is an established surgical technique that is associated with excellent long-term results. A theoretical disadvantage of SVD drainage, however, relates to the high levels of insulin in the peripheral circulation. Hyperinsulinemia has been shown in experimental systems to be associated with insulin resistance and altered lipid metabolism. Portal venous drainage (PVD), a more physiologic method that eliminates hyperinsulinemia, is gaining interest among pancreas transplant centers. Although follow-up is limited, several centers have shown excellent graft survival rates and a reduced number of surgical complications with PVD.

The technique of SVD involves anastomosis of the donor portal vein to the recipient iliac (common or external) vein or vena cava. During the backtable preparation, the donor portal vein should be mobilized to the confluence of the splenic and superior mesenteric branches. This often involves division of several pancreaticoduodenal branches. In addition, the recipient common and external iliac veins should be fully mobilized by dividing all internal iliac and lumbar branches, effectively placing this vein anterolateral to the iliac artery on the right side and medial to the external iliac artery when performed on the left side. This maneuver decreases tension on the venous anastomosis, allows it to be performed under improved exposure, and reduces the risk of venous thrombosis. In cases of SVD, we perform an end-to-side anastomosis directly between the portal vein and the iliac vein using fine (6-0 or 7-0) polypropylene suture. Several authors have described the use of venous extension grafts to facilitate the venous anastomosis. We, along with others, believe the use of extension grafts is to be avoided because of the increased incidence of venous thrombosis.

PVD remains our preferred technique of venous drainage. In this technique, the transverse colon is reflected cephalad, exposing the small bowel mesentery. In many instances the superior mesenteric vein (SMV) or large-caliber tributary may be immediately visualized. When this is not the case, the peritoneum in the root of the mesentery is incised, the mesenteric lymphatics are divided between ligatures, and the SMV is exposed. A sufficient length (3 to 4 cm) of the SMV is then circumferentially mobilized. This may require division of small draining branches. In preuremic recipients we administer intravenous heparin (50 U/kg) before clamping the vein. An end-to-side anastomosis between the portal vein and the SMV is then performed using 7-0 polypropylene suture. Once the venous anastomosis is complete, we occlude the donor portal vein with a bulldog clamp and restore the venous drainage of the bowel. At this point, a tunnel is made in the small bowel mesentery adjacent to the venous anastomosis and through which the arterial graft is passed to the retroperitoneum.

In addition to its potential physiologic advantages, PVD may be technically easier to perform compared with the SVD procedure. Complete mobilization of the iliac vein can be time consuming and technically challenging, particularly in a deep pelvis. With PVD, a large tributary of the SMV can be isolated quickly, and the anastomosis is generally performed in a well-exposed area of the operative field. In addition, anastomosis to a mesenteric vein does not seem to increase the risk of thrombosis.

## VARIATIONS OF OPERATION

**Pancreatic Islet Cell Transplantation.**  Pancreatic islet cell transplantation has great promise, but limited numbers of clinical trials have not produced significant long-term insulin independence. Donor islet cells are separated from exocrine tissue then planted beneath the renal capsule into splenic parenchyma or injected into the portal vein for engraftment into the liver. This technique has the potential to obviate the need for surgery and possibly immunosuppressive therapy.

Further scientific investigation is needed before this technique gains wider clinical applicability.

## POSTOPERATIVE ORDERS

    **Admit to:** transplant service, Dr. _____

    **Diagnosis:** simultaneous pancreas-kidney transplantation

    **Condition:** stable

    **Vital signs:** q1h × 8 h, q2h × 8 h, then q4h

    **Activity:** ambulate >2 times per day

    **Allergies:**

    **Nursing:** I&Os, daily weights, Foley to gravity, PAS while in bed, ventilatory settings per ICU, IS q1h when extubated, NGT to LCWS, Accuchecks q1h, notify house officer if blood sugar >200 mg/dl, check bilateral lower extremity pulses q1h × 24 h

    **Diet:** NPO except ice chips

    **IV fluids:** $D_5$/0.45% NS at 150 ml/h

    **Medications general:** PCA for pain control × 48-72 h
                        TMP-SMZ disulfide (Bactrim) 1 tablet PO qd
                        nystatin swish and swallow qid
                        famotidine (Pepcid) 20 mg PO/IV bid
                        docusate sodium (Colace) 200 mg PO bid
                        aspirin 325 mg PO/PR qd
                        Zosyn 2.25 g IV q6h × 48 h

49

TRANSPLANTATION OF THE PANCREAS

**Medications immunosuppression:**
  methylprednisolone (Solu-Medrol) 250 mg IV POD 1 and 2, then
    start taper on POD 3
  mycophenolate mofetil (CellCept) 1g PO/NG q12h
  basiliximab (Simulect) 20 mg IV on POD 4
**Laboratory tests:** CBC, BMP, $PO_4$, Mg, AST, ALT, alkaline, phosphate,
  amylase, lipase, PT, PTT, INR on arrival to SICU then q6h × 24 h
  then qAM; tacrolimus (FK506) level with daily AM labs, muromonab-
  CD3 (OKT3)/ATG monitoring with daily AM labs; CXR and ECG in
  SICU

## VI. COMPLICATIONS

The following complications pertain to simultaneous pancreas-kidney
transplantation.

### GRAFT REJECTION

Graft rejection remains a major cause of graft loss. The histologic sequence in which pancreatic rejection occurs causes substantial difficulty
in early diagnosis. The early phase of mononuclear cell infiltration
involves primarily acinar tissues, making substantial graft destruction
possible before later stage islet cell damage is reflected in glucose levels.
In isolated pancreas transplantation, urinary amylase has been shown to
be the most useful clinical measure of rejection. This fact supports the
use of urinary drained grafts over enteric or injected grafts when the
pancreas is transplanted alone. Suspected episodes of rejection must be
confirmed with tissue biopsy. Fortunately, most pancreatic transplantations are performed simultaneously with renal transplantation. Renal
transplant rejection with its accompanying rise in creatinine supercedes
pancreatic rejection almost exclusively and may be the most sensitive
marker of pancreatic rejection.

### GRAFT THROMBOSIS

Thrombosis usually occurs in the immediate postoperative period and is
marked by a sudden loss of graft function (ie, rising blood sugars requiring
exogenous insulin). The cause of graft thrombosis is believed to be due to
a technically poor vascular anastomosis, vessel kinking, or low flow. Segmental pancreatic transplantation represents a low-flow state, and thrombotic complications are more likely than with whole pancreas transplantation. Clinical and ultrasonographic findings suggestive of thrombosis
mandate immediate exploration. Confirmation of thrombosis generally results in removal of the graft. When thrombosis is suspected, a technetium
scan or Doppler ultrasonography should be obtained.

### REFLUX PANCREATITIS

Pancreatitis is associated with mild to moderate elevations in serum amylase, urinary amylase, and abdominal pain. Pancreatitis can be seen in

approximately 10% of pancreatic transplant patients. This complication is rarely severe or hemorrhagic. Effusions can commonly be seen surrounding a pancreatic graft, most of which resolve spontaneously.

## BLADDER/DUODENAL SEGMENT LEAK

Spillage of pancreatic secretions into the peritoneum can cause ascites. Patients may experience fever, abdominal pain, abdominal tenderness, hyperamylasemia, leukocytosis, and in extreme cases abdominal compartment syndrome. Bacterial and fungal peritonitis must be ruled out with cultures followed by computed tomography scanning of the abdomen. Ascites can be managed conservatively with electrolyte correction and bowel rest, but infection requires exploration, explantation of the graft, and discontinuation of immunosuppression.

## LYMPHOCELE

Lymphoceles are not common with intraperitoneal transplants but can be found in up to 20% of extraperitoneal transplant patients. Most lymphoceles are asymptomatic and will resolve spontaneously over time. Symptoms of lymphoceles warranting intervention are a result of regional compression, which include graft dysfunction and lower extremity edema. Treatments of symptomatic lymphoceles include ultrasound-guided drainage and operative marsupialization.

## HEMATURIA

Hematuria can be seen in approximately 50% of bladder-drained transplants, occurring most commonly in the immediate postoperative period. Most posttransplant hematuria can be traced to the cystotomy site(s). Initial management should consist of gentle catheter irrigation. If bleeding persists or is substantially heavy, cystoscopy with fulguration can be used.

### VII. DISCHARGE ORDERS

**Diet:** low animal fat, no added salt
**Activity:** lifting nothing heavier than 25 pounds for 6 weeks
**Return to work:** 12 weeks
**Medications:** tacrolimus 0.05 mg/kg PO bid
mycophenolate mofetil 1000 mg PO bid
prednisone taper
**Laboratory studies:** CBC, BMP, amylase, lipase, and tacrolimus levels thrice weekly for 3 months, then biweekly for 6 weeks, then every other week for 3 months, then monthly for 9 months, then every other month for 6 months, then 4 times per year thereafter
**Follow-up:** 2 weeks, then 1, 2, 3, 6, 9, 12, 16, 20, 24, 30, and 36 months

# LIVER TRANSPLANTATION

*Justin S. Wu*
*David P. Vogt*
*Michael J. Henderson*

Liver transplantation has become the accepted definitive therapy for many types of end-stage liver disease (ESLD). The overall 1-year survival rate for liver transplantation ranges from 75% to 85%; 85% to 90% of the survivors are medically rehabilitated. The factors responsible for the successful evolution of liver transplantation over the last decade include better recipient selection, optimal donor management, improved organ preservation, standardized operative techniques including venovenous bypass, more efficacious immunosuppression, and the training of new transplant teams.

**50**

## I. PATHOPHYSIOLOGY

The general indications for hepatic transplantation are ESLD, life-threatening complications associated with liver disease, and correction of inborn errors of metabolism. The most common diseases for which orthotopic liver transplantation (OLT) is performed are listed in Table 50-1.

As liver transplantation has evolved, the list of contraindications has become smaller, rather than larger. There are few absolute contraindications to liver transplantation: advanced cardiac or pulmonary (nonhepatic in origin) disease, irreversible neurologic impairment, active alcohol or other chemical dependence, active infection outside the biliary tract, extrahepatic cancer, the inability to comply with postoperative medications and follow-up, and insufficient personal or social resources to be a transplant recipient.

Portal vein thrombosis is only a relative contraindication to liver transplantation, because techniques are available to bypass the obstructed vein depending on the extent of the thrombosis. Renal insufficiency, either acute or chronic, increases the morbidity of hepatic transplantation but is not a contraindication. Renal transplantation can be performed concurrently for patients with end-stage renal disease as well.

## II. TYPICAL PRESENTATION

The most common manifestations of ESLD include, intractable ascites, spontaneous bacterial peritonitis, multiple episodes of encephalopathy, and easy bruising indicating poor synthesis of coagulation factors. Esophageal-gastric variceal bleeding may or may not be associated with ESLD. Jaundice, fatigue, and muscle wasting are also common.

## III. PREOPERATIVE WORKUP

Patients are referred to transplant centers either urgently or electively. The evaluation determines the need, the urgency, and the technical feasibility

---

**TABLE 50-1**

**DISEASE FOR LIVER TRANSPLANTATION**

| | |
|---|---|
| **INBORN ERRORS OF METABOLISM** | Congenital hepatic fibrosis |
| Wilson's disease | Primary sclerosing cholangitis |
| Hemochromatosis | Familial cholestasis |
| $\alpha_1$-antitrypsin deficiency | **HEPATOCELLULAR LIVER DISEASE** |
| Primary amyloidosis | Alcoholic liver disease |
| Cystic fibrosis | Chronic hepatitis B |
| Glycogen storage disease types I and IV | Chronic hepatitis C |
| Primary hyperoxaluria type I | Autoimmune hepatitis |
| Type IV hyperlipidemia | Cryptogenic hepatitis |
| Hemophilia A and B | Drug-induced liver disease |
| Tyrosinemia | **HEPATIC NEOPLASM** |
| **BUDD-CHIARI SYNDROME** | Hepatocellular carcinoma |
| Hepatic vein thrombosis | Hepatoblastoma |
| Veno-occlusive disease | Multiple hepatic adenomas |
| **CHOLESTATIC LIVER DISEASE** | Epitheloid hemangioendothelioma |
| Biliary atresia | **MISCELLANEOUS** |
| Primary biliary cirrhosis | Adult polycystic liver disease |
| Secondary biliary cirrhosis | Caroli's disease |

---

of OLT. The core team consists of surgery, hepatology, transplant coordinators, social worker, psychiatry, anesthesiology, and bioethics. Consults may be indicated depending on the situation; these include chemical dependency, infectious disease, cardiology, pulmonary, nephrology, and neurology.

## ELECTIVE TRANSPLANTATION

Under elective conditions the potential candidate undergoes a multidisciplinary evaluation. This is based on history, physical examination, laboratory evaluation, result of endoscopic procedures, cardiac and pulmonary evaluation, and radiologic examination (Table 50-2). The focus of the evaluation is (1) medical necessity, (2) medical contraindication, and (3) psychosocial suitability. A search must be made to exclude infection promptly, and transplantation should be postponed until the infections are resolved. Patients with spontaneous bacterial peritonitis require antibiotic treatment, and transplantation should not be performed when the polymorphonuclear count of the ascitic fluid is greater than 250/ml.

Patients may be approved for immediate listing; approved but not listed because they are too well or not psychologically ready; not approved; or postponed to a future meeting if further evaluation is necessary. The decision of when to list a patient for transplant must factor in the average wait of 9 to 18 months for a donor organ. After approval, the patient is

---

**TABLE 50-2**

EVALUATION OF POTENTIAL LIVER TRANSPLANT RECIPIENTS

History

Physical examination

Laboratory analyses

Microbiology analyses: cultures from ascites

Electrocardiogram

Chest x-ray

Doppler ultrasonography: assess vascular patency

CT scan or MRI of the abdomen

Liver biopsy, when indicated

Esophagogastroduodenoscopy: assess varices, peptic ulcers

Cholangiography (ERCP, PTHC, or T tube) with brushings for cytology: for sclerosing
    cholangitis (10% coincidence of cholangiocarcinoma)

Dobutamine stress echocardiography

Cardiac catheterization: age 50 with risk factors or age >55

Pulmonary function tests

Head CT scan: for signs of fixed neurologic deficit or fulminant liver failure

Psychosocial evaluation

---

notified, given a pager, and listed with the United Network for Organ Sharing (UNOS), which is the national organization that strives to ensure equitable organ distribution for transplant candidates. Data important in the listing process includes the patient's weight, blood type, and medical status.

The opportunity to receive an organ for liver transplant depends on listing status. Status 1 patients—who have fulminant liver failure (no chronic disease)—will receive an organ offer within 2 to 5 days. Status 2A patients—who have acute decompensation of their chronic disease, are in an ICU, and are judged to have less than 1 week to live—have a 50% to 70% chance of an organ offer within that week. Status 2B patients—who have to have a life-threatening event such as spontaneous bacterial peritonitis, severe encephalopathy, or major variceal bleeding and is Childs class C11 or worse—will receive an organ offer within 3 to 12 months. Status 3 patients—who do not fulfill any of the above criteria—are unlikely to receive an organ offer.

## URGENT TRANSPLANTATION

Selected patients with acute or fulminant hepatic failure can also be candidates for OLT. The pretransplantation evaluation is conducted in a fashion similar to that for the elective patient but needs to be completed within 12 to 24 hours. However, rapid determination of neurologic status, hemodynamic instability, infection, or renal failure may limit the candidacy.

A careful neurologic examination must be done in this setting, and the coma grade should be determined. Patients with grade IV (unresponsive) coma should have continuous perioperative monitoring of the intracranial pressure (ICP), as untreated severe elevations in ICP can result in permanent brain injury and possibly death. The goal is to maintain cerebral perfusion pressure (mean arterial BP minus ICP) above 70 mm Hg. After volume resuscitation, vasopressors are used to treat low mean arterial blood pressure. High ICP is treated with hyperventilation, mannitol, and elevation of the head of bed.

## DONOR SELECTION

Potential cadaver organ donors are brain dead patients who are being maintained on a ventilator. Trauma and spontaneous intracerebral bleeding are the usual causes of brain death. An "ideal" donor meets the following guidelines:

1. Between 3 months and 55 years of age
2. Short hospitalization (2 to 3 days)
3. Hemodynamically stable requiring no or minimal pressor support
4. Normal liver studies including transaminases, bilirubin, and prothrombin time
5. No acidosis
6. No hypoxemia
7. No history of drug or alcohol abuse
8. Absence of sepsis or transmissible disease (HIV, hepatitis)

## PREOPERATIVE ORDERS

**Admit to:** liver transplant service
**Diagnosis:** ESLD due to _____
**Vital signs:** every shift
**Nursing:** bowel prep, 1 L of GoLYTELY (in selective cases when time allows; check with staff); void on call to OR; If PT >18 sec, administer 2 U FFP
**Diet:** NPO
**IV fluids:** $D_5$/0.45% NS at KVO
**Medications:** antibiotics on call to OR: ceftizoxime (Cefizox) 1 g
**Laboratory tests:** CMP, GGT, CBC, PT, 10 cc red top tube to tissue typing for crossmatch, T&C 10 U PRBCs, 20 U FFP, 20 U platelets; CXR, ECG

## IV. SURGICAL ANATOMY

The segmental anatomy of the liver divides the liver into eight segments on the basis of the ramifications of the portal triad structures. With few exceptions the ramifications of these three structures (portal vein, hepatic artery, and biliary apparatus) accompany each other through the liver parenchyma.

The venous drainage of the liver, via the hepatic veins, drain each of these segments.

The liver is attached to the diaphragm by a series of peritoneal reflections termed ligaments. As the peritoneal leaves of the falciform ligament reach the liver, they diverge to left and right to form the triangular ligaments that surround the bare area of the liver. On the right the ligament consists of anterior (superior) and posterior (inferior) layers that are widely separated from each other, and on the left the anterior and posterior layers are quite close. Division of the right and left triangular ligaments is necessary to mobilize the liver and expose the hepatic inferior vena cava.

The major structures within the hepatoduodenal ligament include the common hepatic/bile duct anterior-right, the common/proper hepatic artery anterior-left, and the portal vein posteriorly. The common hepatic duct is formed by the confluence of the right and left ducts at the porta hepatis. This union may be intrahepatic or extrahepatic. The arterial supply is probably the most variable. Typically the common hepatic artery divides into the left and right branches at the porta hepatis before entering the liver parenchyma. The right hepatic artery usually courses posterior to the common hepatic duct; however, it can cross anteriorly and does so 10% of the time. The right hepatic artery frequently arises from the superior mesenteric artery (15% of cases), and the left hepatic artery can arise from the left gastric artery (10% of cases). The portal vein usually divides into left and right branches extrahepatically.

## V. CONDUCT OF OPERATION

### CADAVERIC DONOR LIVER HARVEST

The operation is usually part of a multiple organ harvest and begins with a median sternotomy and midline laparotomy. The aorta is cleared for cannulation at its bifurcation and cross-clamping at the diaphragm. The portal vein is usually cannulated via the inferior mesenteric vein. Then the surgeon identifies and preserves all of the hepatic hilar structures, including the common bile duct, portal vein, hepatic artery, and any aberrant arterial blood supply such as a left hepatic artery from the left gastric artery or a replaced right hepatic artery from the superior mesenteric artery. When the other organ teams are ready to cross-clamp, the liver is flushed and cooled with University of Wisconsin (UW) preservation solution through the portal vein and the aorta cannulas. Then the liver is removed with its diaphragmatic attachments, a cuff of aorta surrounding the celiac axis and the superior mesenteric artery, and a portion of the suprahepatic and infrahepatic vena cava. The liver is stored in cold UW solution and packed on ice during transportation. The remainder of the liver dissection is performed on the back table under cold storage conditions. With the advent of UW solution, donor livers can be preserved for up to 20 hours before revascularization.

## HEPATIC TRANSPLANTATION

OLT has become a relatively standardized, although demanding operative procedure. The operation may be thought of in three stages: (1) hepatectomy of diseased liver, (2) implantation of donor liver, and (3) reperfusion of donor organ. The first phase involves the dissection of the recipient's diseased liver, which can be the most demanding portion of the procedure because of coagulopathy and portal hypertension, especially in patients who have had prior right upper quadrant surgery. After the portal structures are skeletonized, the liver including the retrohepatic vena cava is mobilized from the diaphragm to just above the renal veins.

The second phase, known also as the anhepatic phase, refers to the period starting with devascularization of the recipient's liver and ending with revascularization of the newly implanted liver. Many centers routinely use venovenous bypass during the anhepatic stage of the operation. Heparin-bonded tubing is inserted into the femoral and portal veins; the blood is returned to the axillary vein by a centrifugal pump. Another option is to perform a temporary portacaval shunt and not clamp the inferior vena cava. The rationale for both techniques is that maintenance of venous return from the kidneys and lower extremities during the anhepatic phase results in a smoother hemodynamic course and less blood loss, allows time for a more deliberate approach to hemostasis in the right upper quadrant, reduces visceral edema and splanchnic venous pooling, and decreases the incidence of postoperative renal dysfunction. The hepatic artery is ligated, and vascular clamps are placed on the vena cava both above and below the liver if venovenous bypass is used. The liver is then excised, often leaving the vena cava in situ for a piggyback implantation of the allograft.

The liver allograft is implanted by anastomosing the suprahepatic vena cava if a piggyback technique is used or both the suprahepatic and infrahepatic vena cava if the recipient vena cava was divided while on venovenous bypass. During the caval anastomosis the preservation solution is flushed from the graft with 500 ml of room temperature lactated Ringer's solution through the portal vein cannula. This maneuver prevents hyperkalemia and possible cardiac arrest when the clamps are removed. Next the portal vein anastomosis is performed, and blood flow to the liver is reestablished. The patient is taken off venovenous bypass, and the hepatic arterial anastomosis is performed. If the recipient hepatic artery is not suitable for anastomosis, a donor iliac arterial graft can be used as a conduit from the infrarenal or suprarenal aorta. When hemostasis is adequate, biliary reconstruction is carried out, the gallbladder is removed, and a cholangiogram is obtained. Biliary continuity can be performed via a duct-to-duct anastomosis over a T tube or a choledochojejunotomy. A duct-to-duct anastomosis is preferable; however, it is not possible when there is a donor-recipient bile duct size discrepancy or a diseased recipient bile duct (eg, with primary sclerosing cholangitis, biliary atresia, or secondary biliary cirrhosis). Drains are placed in the subphrenic space and in the subhepatic space. The abdomen is closed, and the patient is transported directly to the intensive care unit.

## POSTOPERATIVE ORDERS

**Admit to:** SICU, transplant surgery service
**Diagnosis:** s/p liver transplant
**Condition:** guarded
**Vital signs:** q1h
**Activity:** bedrest until extubated; then up in a chair q shift as tolerated
**Allergies:**
**Nursing:** I&O q1h, call house officer if urine output <30 ml/h, Foley to gravity, abdominal drains to bulb suction, T tube to bile bag, respiratory care per SICU; do not give FFP for PT <20 seconds; do not give platelets for platelet count >20,000/mm$^3$; keep 4 U of RBCs and FFP on hold for 48 hours
**Diet:** NPO, NGT to gravity drainage or LCWS
**IV fluids:** lactated Ringer's at 125 ml/h
**Medications:** sucralfate (Carafate) 1 g per NGT/PO q6h

    norfloxacin (Noroxin) 400 mg per NGT/PO bid

    mystatin (Mycostatin) 20 ml per NGT or swish and swallow qid

    Renal dose dopamine × 24 h

    ceftizoxime (Cefizox) 1 g IV q6h × 48 h (tailor on basis of intraoperative cultures)

    methylprednisolone (Solu-Medrol) 50 g IV q6h × 4, then
        40 mg IV q6h × 4, then
        30 mg IV q6h × 4, then
        20 mg IV q6h × 4, then
        20 mg IV q12h × 2, then
        20 mg IV qd

    ganciclovir 1 g per NGT/PO tid × 2 weeks, then convert to acyclovir for 6 months (If donor organ is CMV+ and recipient is CMV−, use IV ganciclovir 5 mg/kg q12h × 14 days; adjust for creatinine clearance.)
**Laboratory tests:** on admission to SICU and q6h first 24 hours, then daily: CMP, GGT, CBC, PT, PTT, Mg; ECG and CXR on admission to SICU; duplex ultrasound of hepatic vessels tomorrow AM

### POD 1

**Nursing:** D/C NGT, start sips of clear fluids
**Medications:** tacrolimus (FK506) 1-2 mg PO bid
**Laboratory tests:** tacrolimus level qAM.

50

LIVER TRANSPLANTATION

**POD 7**
> **Nursing:** transfuse platelets if platelet count <50,000/mm$^3$
> **Tests:** duplex US of hepatic vessels, US-guided liver biopsy, T tube
> cholangiogram to r/o obstruction or leak, HIDA scan if no T tube

## VI. COMPLICATIONS

### PRIMARY LIVER DYSFUNCTION OR NONFUNCTION

The use of UW solution for organ preservation has decreased the incidence of primary nonfunction. However, for poorly understood reasons, 5% of transplanted livers immediately fail postoperatively. Primary nonfunction is characterized by hemodynamic instability, poor quantity and quality of bile, renal dysfunction, failure to regain consciousness, increasing coagulopathy, persistent hypothermia, and lactic acidosis in the face of patent vascular anastomosis (as demonstrated by Doppler ultrasonography). Death ensues without retransplantation.

### HEPATIC ARTERY THROMBOSIS

Hepatic artery thrombosis (HAT) can occur early (within the first postoperative week) or late. Its incidence is approximately 8% (5% adults, 15% children). Technical errors such as using a recipient vessel with inadequate inflow, development of an intimal flap, and a substandard anastomosis may result in HAT. However, nontechnical factors including rejection, which causes graft edema and diminished arterial flow, a hematocrit above 45%, and vessels 3 mm or less in diameter also predispose recipients to arterial thrombosis.

HAT presents with equal frequency in one of three ways: (1) asymptomatic and found incidentally by ultrasound, (2) ischemic cholangiopathy, and (3) relapsing bacteremia. Fulminant liver necrosis presents an average of 16 days after transplant; fever, markedly elevated transaminases, and multiorgan system failure are the clinical manifestations. Urgent retransplantation is the only recourse; approximately 25% of patients survive. Ischemic cholangiopathy manifests approximately 1 week to 1 month postoperatively either with necrosis of the donor bile duct and a bile leak or with biliary strictures that have a radiographic appearance analogous to primary sclerosing cholangitis. Therefore, studies to assess hepatic artery patency are required urgently in a patient who develops either a biliary leak or stricture. The initial therapy for a leak consists of controlling it by external drainage, either percutaneously or surgically; strictures are stented either endoscopically or percutaneously. Although urgent revascularization may salvage some grafts, retransplantation is required in 75% to 80% of patients. Relapsing bacteremia is the most insidious presentation of HAT. It does not become symptomatic until 4 to 6 weeks after transplant. The liver function remains normal, and antibiotics are temporarily effective in controlling the recurrent sepsis. Duplex ultrasonography or arteriography is necessary to confirm the diagnosis. Retransplantation is required in most patients.

## BILIARY COMPLICATIONS

Bile duct leaks are caused by hepatic artery thrombosis until proven otherwise. Leaks tend to occur within a week or two following transplantation and can result from a technically poor anastomosis as well as a thrombosed hepatic artery. Duplex ultrasound assessing the hepatic artery is essential. If the ultrasound results are equivocal, an arteriogram is required. Bile duct obstruction is diagnosed by cholangiography, and a single short bile duct stricture may be treated by either percutaneous or retrograde balloon dilatation. However, a long stricture or failed dilatation necessitates revision of the biliary tract anastomosis.

## INFECTION

Bacterial and fungal sepsis, often related to surgical factors, can cause hyperbilirubinemia in liver transplant patients within the first few weeks postoperatively. Herpes simplex, herpes zoster, and cytomegalovirus (CMV) may directly infect the graft and cause severe dysfunction. CMV typically occurs at the end of the first posttransplantation month and can mimic rejection. The diagnosis is made by liver biopsy, with CMV inclusion bodies being found with light microscopy or by polymerase chain reaction in peripheral blood (buffy coat). Treatment consists of decreasing baseline immunosuppression and administering ganciclovir (5 mg/kg q12h via central venous access for 3 weeks). Viral hepatitis B and C can recur in the hepatic allograft, but both are uncommon in the early posttransplantation period. The clinical presentation includes elevation of liver function tests, and the diagnosis is made with liver biopsy.

## REJECTION

Acute or cell-mediated rejection is common after liver transplantation, occurring in 40% to 50% of the recipients. However, rejection is a less common cause of graft loss than is primary nonfunction or hepatic artery thrombosis. Rejection commonly occurs between the fifth and the fourteenth day postoperatively. Most often rejection is asymptomatic. However, rejection can be characterized by fever, increased ascites, decreased bile quality and quantity, and elevation of total WBC, bilirubin, and transaminase levels. Liver transplantation rejection is diagnosed by percutaneous liver biopsy. In the early posttransplantation period a technical cause of hepatic dysfunction is ruled out by Doppler ultrasonography to assure vascular patency, and a T-tube cholangiography is obtained to rule out a bile duct obstruction or leak. Typical biopsy findings consistent with acute rejection include a triad of portal lymphocytosis, subendothelial deposits of mononuclear cells, and bile duct infiltration and damage. The first-line treatment for acute rejection is to increase tacrolimus levels by increasing the dose. If this does not work or if levels are already high, then a bolus of corticosteroids (Solu-Medrol, 1 g IV) is given. If the rejection responds appropriately, the patient undergoes steroid recycling (Solu-Medrol, 50 mg IV qid × 4 doses; 40 mg IV qid × 4 doses; 30 mg IV qid × 4 doses; 20 mg IV qid × 4 doses; 20 mg IV bid × 2 doses; and finally prednisone 20 mg PO qd). This regimen reverses 90% of acute rejection episodes. If rejection persists, however, further immunosuppression may be indicated, such as azathioprine (Imuran), mycophenolate mofetil (CellCept), or antilymphocyte preparations (Atgam or muromonab-CD3 [OKT3]).

## VII. DISCHARGE INSTRUCTIONS

The usual hospital stay is 10 to 14 days.

**Activity:** ambulate, otherwise as tolerated; no heavy lifting or driving for 4 weeks

**Medications:** immunosuppression (usually tacrolimus, prednisone 20 mg/d), Percocet prn

**Diet:** regular

**Call transplant service** for fevers, chills, HR >120 or <60 bpm, SBP >160 or <90, DBP >100, abdominal pain, wound discharge, or diarrhea

**Laboratory tests:** once per week as outpatient

**Check daily:** weight, temperature, pulse, blood pressure; record in diary

**Follow-up:** q week × 1 month, then q 2 weeks × 1 month, then q month for 1 year, then annually

# PULMONARY TRANSPLANTATION

*Eric E. Roselli*

Since the first successful human lung transplant in 1983, lung transplantation has become the preferred treatment for end-stage pulmonary disease. As of 1998, 7033 lung transplantation procedures have been performed, 4192 single and 2841 double. Overall survival at 1 year is 70%, 3 years 57%, and 5 years 46%.

## I. PATHOPHYSIOLOGY

End-stage pulmonary diseases amenable to pulmonary transplant can be categorized as obstructive, restrictive, and pulmonary hypertension. Emphysema is an obstructive process and includes bullous or nonbullous variations. Emphysema due to smoking affects the lung in a proximal acinar pattern, and $\alpha_1$-antitrypsin deficiency affects the lungs in a panacinar fashion. Septic lung diseases include cystic fibrosis and bronchiectatic diseases such as Kartagener's syndrome.

Restrictive disease warranting transplant is caused by idiopathic pulmonary fibrosis (IPF). It is important to differentiate this disease process from other similar diseases that may respond to corticosteroids.

The final category of disease processes for which transplant is indicated is pulmonary hypertension. In the primary form of the disease, right ventricular hypertensive heart disease develops with eventual heart failure. The increased right-sided pressures further lead to decrease cardiac output by altering left-sided compliance due to increased pressures across the septum. Secondary pulmonary hypertension is often associated with Eisenmenger's complex due to cardiac defects with a dominant right ventricle and thus a right-to-left shunt.

## II. TYPICAL PRESENTATION

To be listed for transplant patients should have evidence of progressive deterioration with the preceding diseases and a life expectancy of less than 24 months. Patients with chronic obstructive pulmonary disease (COPD) should have a forced expiratory volume in 1 second ($FEV_1$) of less than 25% predicted that is not reversible with bronchodilators. Furthermore, patients often present with increasing oxygen requirements and hypercarbia with a $PaCO_2$ of greater than 55 mm Hg. Patients with septic lung disease also present for transplant with progressively worsening lung disease manifest as rapidly decreasing $FEV_1$, increasing requirement for hospitalizations, massive hemoptysis, and weight loss. These patients also have increasing oxygen requirements and hypercarbia. IPF patients should be transplanted when they become symptomatic. They often are seen with rapidly worsening dyspnea and diffuse infiltrates on chest x-ray. Finally, those with pulmonary hypertension show both pulmonary and cardiac effects of the disease process. They present with both a decreased cardiac output and hypoxemia due to redistributions in pulmonary blood flow.

## III. PREOPERATIVE WORKUP

Patient and organ selection are two of the most important elements of having a successful operation.

### DONOR EVALUATION

The process begins with the choice of appropriate donor organs. Considerations include an age of less than 60, ABO compatibility, and no history of lung or cardiac surgery. If the donor smoked, it should be less than 20 pack years. It is important to remember that brain death puts the donor at risk for aspiration and that head injury is a risk factor for pulmonary edema. A mean arterial pressure greater than 70 and the delivery of large crystalloid volumes are also a risk for pulmonary edema as is the avoidance of inotropes, a management technique preferred by cardiac transplant teams. Chest radiographs should be performed to rule out infiltrates and hyperinflation. Bronchoscopy with lavage should also be performed to directly examine the lungs and rule out purulent secretions, aspiration, or masses. The presence of major pulmonary contusions may eliminate a potential donor. The final preoperative determinant of the adequacy of the lungs for donation is the $O_2$ challenge: on a $FIO_2$ of 100% and with positive end-expiratory pressure (PEEP) of less than 5 mm Hg, the $PO_2$ must be greater than 300. Finally, direct intraoperative visual inspection is performed to rule out severe adhesions or masses. This strict selection process further stresses an already limited pool of donors. In one study of 174 referrals, 128 (74%) donors were refused, and only 32 (18%) were retrieved.

### RECIPIENT EVALUATION

Once the severity of the patient's lung disease warrants transplant, he or she is thoroughly investigated to assess his or her overall medical condition and the severity of the lung disease. Evaluation begins with a thorough history and physical examination, routine blood work including complete blood count and coagulation, complete metabolic profile, thyroid function tests, hepatitis screen, blood typing, tissue typing, CMV, EBV, VZV, and HSV titers, rapid plasma reagin, toxoplasmosis, C-reactive protein, Westergren sedimentation rate, carcinoembryonic antigen, chest x-ray, pulmonary function tests, a ventilation-perfusion scan, chest computed tomography (CT), mammogram and Papanicalaou smear for women, and a serum prostate specific antigen and prostate examination for men. It is important to assure that patients do not have any contraindications to immunosuppression (ie, an active malignancy or infection). Patients with a history of malignancy, other than basal and squamous cell skin cancer and bronchoalveolar lung cancer, must be cancer free for at least 2 years.

Spine and hip x-rays are performed, as well as a CT head, stool guaiac with or without sigmoidoscopy, if warranted. Further preoperative testing should include an electrocardiogram, and a cardiac catheterization for women less than 40. Patients are closely followed by a transplant pulmonologist, nurse clinician, transplant coordinator, social worker, psychologist, and a support group. Other important lifestyle changes include the cessation of smoking for at least 6 months. Furthermore, weight loss is encouraged in obese patients, as persons with body mass indexes greater than 27 have a worse long-term prognosis.

A relative contraindication includes an age greater than 65 years old. Other contraindications include active drinking and the use of recreational drugs. Patients must also be free of coronary artery disease, and systemic diseases must be well controlled or in remission. Patients are also fully assessed to confirm adequate psychosocial support and the absence of psychiatric disorders.

## PREOPERATIVE ORDERS

**On Day of Transplant**
> **Admit to:** ICU
> **Diet:** NPO
> **Medications:** place IV and arterial lines preoperatively
>> cefuroxime 1.5 g IV to OR, or clindamycin and gentamicin if penicillin allergic
>> heparin 5000 SC, PAS bilaterally
>> cyclosporine 10 mg/kg PO prior to OR
>> alprostadil (Prostin VR) 500 $\mu$g/100 ml $D_5W$ to OR
>> methylprednisolone 1g IV to OR with patient
>
> **Laboratory tests:** CXR, CBC, CMP, PT, PTT, HIV Ab, hepatitis, CMV IgM and IgG, T&C for 6 U PRBCs (leukocyte poor) with or without CMV negative, and 6 U of FFP; tissue typing; sputum for Gram's stain and culture and fungal culture

## IV. CONDUCT OF OPERATION

### DONOR LUNG OPERATION

Once brain death has been confirmed and all the organ harvest teams have been coordinated, the donor operation is performed. The technique allows for the simultaneous harvest of the heart and lungs. Approach is by means of a median sternotomy. The pericardium is incised, and stay sutures are placed to tack it open. Preparation of the heart is performed by isolation of the venae cavae and dissection of the aorta and pulmonary artery. Next the aorta and superior vena cava are retracted laterally, and the posterior pericardium over the right pulmonary artery is incised to expose and encircle the trachea. The patient is then heparinized, and the aorta and pulmonary artery are cannulated for the delivery of cardioplegia and pulmonary flush. The lungs are then flushed through the pulmonary artery with prostaglandin $E_1$ (for vasodilatation) and then with 50 to 75 ml/kg of a crystalloid solution (either Euro-Collins or Wisconsin) at 4°C.

The heart is then removed, leaving an adequate left atrial cuff. The trachea is then divided above the carina with a TA-30 stapler, and the pulmonary artery is divided proximal to the bifurcation. If the lungs are traveling separately, they are divided on the back table. The lungs are then immersed in cold solution. Ischemic time is best if less than 6 hours, but successful transplant has been reported with times of up to 10 hours.

## SINGLE-LUNG TECHNIQUE

The least perfused recipient lung is transplanted. Foley, nasogastric, central venous pressure, arterial line, and Swan-Ganz catheters are placed. Transesophageal echocardiography is performed. A double-lumen endotracheal tube is placed, and a cardiopulmonary bypass pump is prepared. For children, routine cardiopulmonary bypass is used.

Once word has arrived from the donor site that the lung has passed final inspection and the team is about 1½ hours away, a standard posterolateral thoracotomy is begun. Hilar mobilization of the main pulmonary artery, both superior and inferior pulmonary veins, and the mainstem bronchus is performed. Once the donor lung is within the vicinity, a standard pneumonectomy is completed.

The bronchial anastomosis is performed first, with a running 4-0 prolene along the membranous portion of the bronchi, and interrupted periannular sutures are used for the rigid portion of the bronchus. The pulmonary artery anastomosis is performed next with running prolene sutures. Then the left atrial cuffs are anastomosed. The bronchial anastomosis is often wrapped with pericardial fat, if available. Finally the clamps are removed, and flow is reestablished.

An ipsilateral chest tube and an intrathoracic Jackson-Pratt drain are placed. The thoracotomy is closed in standard fashion.

## VARIATION OF OPERATION

**Double-Lung Technique.** This technique is indicated for septic lung disease, cystic fibrosis, and is possibly better for pulmonary hypertension, but this is still controversial. Preparation of the patient is as just described. Exposure is achieved through a clam-shell incision. Bilateral sequential replacement of the lungs is the favored technique. This can most often be achieved without bypass, unless the patient cannot tolerate single lung ventilation or if the indication is pulmonary hypertension. The least functional lung is replaced first. The same surgical technique as a single lung transplant is performed and then repeated for the other side. The second lung often exhibits compromised function initially, but then normalizes within 24 to 48 hours. This is probably due to the slightly increased ischemic time.

## POSTOPERATIVE ORDERS

**Admit to:** ICU intubated with all lines, plus drains; anticipate transfer to regular nursing floor on POD 3 or 4; average hospital stay is 2 to 3 weeks

**Diagnosis:** s/p lung transplant

**Condition:**

**Vital signs:** telemetry for duration

**Activity:** bed rest, elevate head of bed 30 degrees when hemodynamics are stable, up to chair on POD 3, ambulating by POD 5

**Allergies:**

**Nursing:** chest tubes at −20 cm $H_2O$ suction; remove if no leak and minimal drainage (POD 3-5). Jackson-Pratt drain is maintained to bulb suction until close to discharge date. Foley to gravity. NGT to LCWS; D/C after extubated. Vent: wean to extubation postoperatively asap, usually by POD 1. Incentive spirometry and respiratory therapy follow closely, including daily measurements of $FEV_1$ to screen for early rejection

**Diet:** NPO usually until POD 2 or 3; start clear liquids 1 day after extubated, then advance as tolerated to regular diet

**IV fluids:** $D_5$/0.45% NS + 20 mEq KCl at 50 ml/h; change IV tubing q48h; Heplock after tolerating oral intake (~POD 3)

**Medications:** epidural PCA until patient tolerating oral intake, then started on oral analgesics and medications POD 3 and 4

cyclosporine IV drops at 120 mg/d then PO daily to keep level ≥300

methylprednisolone 125 mg IV q8h × 6 doses, then 40 mg IV qd, then PO prednisone

azathioprine (Imuran) 120 mg IV/PO daily

Regular human insulin drops to keep blood sugar <200

perioperative cefuroxime (Zinacef) 1.5 g × 3 doses

ganciclovir 320 mg IV bid

amphotericin B inhaled 10 mg in 2 ml bid

furosemide (Lasix) 20 mg IV q8h begin POD 1

renal dose dopamine

heparin 5000 U SC bid

vitamin K 10 mg SC qd × 3 days

vitamin A 25,000 IU PO × 7 days

resume home medications once transferred to the regular floor

**Laboratory tests:** CXR on arrival then bid for 5 days, then qd; CBC and CMP every Monday, Wednesday, and Friday, cyclosporin level daily

## V. COMPLICATIONS

**Intraoperatively,** the most common complications are injuries to the phrenic and recurrent laryngeal nerves and myocardial infarction.

**Early postoperative (within 90 days)** complications include bacterial infection, donor organ failure, heart failure, rejection (6%), hemorrhage (6%), and airway dehiscence (6%). Anastomotic complications occur because of technical errors or because of ischemia and necrosis at the suture line. These complications are becoming less common because of improved surgical techniques related to performing the anastomosis and harvest techniques. If the cause of the leak is technical, it is treated with surgical repair. Ischemic leaks will often heal by granulation if properly drained. If occurring along the membranous portion, this often heals without further compromise, but if at the cartilaginous portion, the airway may become stenotic or malacia may develop. Long term, bronchial stenosis or bronchomalacia can often be treated with serial balloon dilatations.

**Infection** most commonly involves *Staphylococcus aureus.* Other common organisms include *Enterobacter,* and *Candida albicans.* Cytomegalovirus (CMV) is also common (~50%). Ganciclovir reduces the mortality of CMV from 40% to 10%.

**Rejection** is common to all transplants, but lungs are particularly sensitive. It is prevented by means of triple-drug immunosuppression with cyclosporin, imuran, and methylprednisolone. Rejection typically occurs at 5 to 7 days with fever, perihilar infiltrates, a decrease in $Po_2$, and a decrease in $FEV_1$. Differentiation of rejection from infection is difficult and is usually made clinically by the response to steroids. Diagnosis can be confirmed by transbronchial biopsy, but this is used variably. Treatment involves a steroid pulse with methylprednisolone (Solu-Medrol) 1000 mg intravenously each day for 3 days, and then a return to the maintenance dose.

**Obliterative bronchiolitis** is described as a progressive small airway destruction seen in 20% of patients. This complication is most common after 1 year. It is diagnosed by a decline in $FEV_1$.

## VI. DISCHARGE INSTRUCTIONS

Medication proficiency should be demonstrated before discharge. Patients are instructed to be vigilant about observing signs of infection. There are no dietary restrictions, but healthy living is emphasized. Limited strenuous activity is recommended for 6 weeks. Patients are instructed on following daily vital signs and pulmonary function tests ($FEV_1$).

Avoid close exposure to pets; no birds are allowed as pets.

Good hygiene is emphasized.

Do not go into crowds for 3 months.

Avoid sun exposure.

Wear Medic Alert tags.

Follow-up visits are weekly for 1 month, then every other week for 1 month, then variably tapered as the patient's condition improves.

Bronchoscopy and biopsy are performed 3 weeks, 6 weeks, 3 months, 6 months, 9 months, and 1 year after transplant.

51

PULMONARY TRANSPLANTATION

# CARDIAC TRANSPLANTATION

*Eric E. Roselli*

Since first performed in 1967, cardiac transplantation has dramatically changed. With the introduction of cyclosporine in the 1980s, cardiac transplantation became a very realistic option in the treatment of end-stage heart disease. Further refinements in surgical technique, immunosuppression, medical therapy, and the use of mechanical ventricular assist devices have significantly improved survival for cardiac transplant patients in the 1990s. Cardiac transplantation offers a dramatic improvement in quality of life and the only chance for survival for many patients with end-stage heart disease, who otherwise have an expected survival of less than 1 year.

**52**

## I. PATHOPHYSIOLOGY

Patients with advanced heart failure who are most symptomatic and at the highest risk for death constitute most of those who are considered for transplantation. The myocardial injury that leads to heart failure can be caused by many diseases. Coronary artery disease and cardiomyopathy comprise 85% of transplant patients. Other causes of end-stage heart disease include valvular heart disease, congenital heart disease, disorders of the pericardium, amyloidosis, and failed cardiac transplant. It is important to recognize that although cardiac transplant offers a solution to replace the failing cardiac pump, there are profound metabolic, humoral, and inflammatory consequences of end-stage heart failure that may persist for long periods of time after transplant.

## II. TYPICAL PRESENTATION

Most patients with heart failure referred for transplantation have severe congestive symptoms, including orthopnea, anorexia, abdominal discomforts, and dyspnea on minimal exertion. Furthermore, most of the patients have had little improvement of symptoms despite previous therapy with digoxin, vasodilators (angiotensin-converting enzyme inhibitors), and diuretics.

Others present with severe disabling angina without options for coronary artery revascularization or refractory life-threatening dysrhythmias.

## III. PREOPERATIVE WORKUP

### GENERAL

All potential patients are followed by a team composed of a transplant cardiac surgeon, a transplant cardiologist, a nurse clinician, a transplant coordinator, a social worker, a psychologist, and a support group. An extensive preoperative workup is aimed at characterizing the severity of the patient's heart failure to uncover any comorbidities that may compromise the transplant's success and to identify any potentially reversible causes of the patient's heart failure. Following are a description of these different parts of the workup, including the cardiac workup, and exclusion criteria that include contraindications to surgery and tests aimed at uncovering other comorbidities.

Listed patients are prioritized by category. Status 1 is defined as being in an intensive care unit on intravenous inotropes or requiring other life support devices, including intraaortic balloon pumps, ventricular assist devices, or the ventilator, or patients less than 6 months old. Status 2 is defined as all those at risk but not meeting the preceding criteria. Patients on home dobutamine are included in the latter group. Listed patients are reevaluated every 6 months.

## CARDIAC WORKUP

The cardiac workup includes a thorough history and physical examination, electrocardiogram, chest x-ray, lipoprotein screen, echocardiogram, MUGA (multiple gated acquisition) scan, cardiac catheterization, and endomyocardial biopsy if appropriate (for retransplant patients).

## EXCLUSION CRITERIA

Relative contraindications include age greater than 65 years old, but this has become quite variable from center to center. An uncured malignancy is another relative contraindication, and tests included to rule out occult malignancy include mammogram in women older than 40, prostate specific antigen for men older than 40, stool for guaiac or colonoscopy, and gynecologic evaluation with Papanicolaou smear. Other tests are aimed at detecting ongoing infection, including a hepatitis screen, CMV, EBV, VZV, HIV, HSV, toxoplasmosis, histoplasmosis, coccidioidomycosis, and rubella titers. Also skin testing for purified protein derivative with controls is performed. Transplant is contraindicated with ongoing infection unless the patient has an infected left ventricular assist device (LVAD). Other studies aimed at evaluating systemic disease or other high-risk reversible diseases include thyroid function tests, pulmonary function tests (transplant is contraindicated with severe pulmonary hypertension with pulmonary vascular resistance (PVR) >6 to 8 Wood's units), a dental consultation, a carotid duplex scan, abdominal ultrasonography to evaluate the gallbladder and aorta, pulse volume recordings, spine and hip x-rays, computed tomography (CT) of the head, and an eye examination.

Other contraindications include patients with a recent stroke, a pulmonary embolism within 6 weeks, an active ulcer, poorly controlled diabetes with end organ involvement, and active smoking, drinking, and recreational drug use.

Other important general data are collected with a psychosocial evaluation, blood typing, complete blood count, coagulation factors, and a complete metabolic profile. Finally, weight loss is encouraged in obese patients.

## DONOR CONSIDERATIONS

Acceptable donors are less than 55 years old (some exceptions are made), have negative serologic tests for human immunodeficiency virus and hepatitis, have no active infections or malignancy, have no evidence of cardiac disease or trauma and a low probability of coronary artery disease (high-risk donors may undergo coronary catheterization), acceptable left ventricular function without aggressive inotropic support (usually less than 10 $\mu$g/kg/min of dopamine), a compatible blood type, a negative preformed cytotoxic T-cell cross-match, a body weight index within 75% to 125% that of the recipient, and an anticipated ischemic time of less than 4 hours.

## PREOPERATIVE ORDERS

**Admit to:** ICU
**Diagnosis:** end-stage heart disease
**Condition:**
**Vital signs:** per routine
**Activity:** bed rest, family to wait in surgical waiting room
**Allergies:**
**Nursing:** clip chest hair, povidone-iodine scrubs × 2, T&C for 6 U of leukocyte-depleted PRBCs and 4 U of FFP, obtain informed consent
consult cardiothoracic anesthesia
insert invasive lines including central access and arterial line
check CXR once line placed
check CMP and CBC
**Diet:** NPO

## IV. SURGICAL ANATOMY

Anastomoses to all four chambers of the heart are performed in the transplant operation. It is crucial in both the donor harvest and the recipient explant to leave adequate tissue at both atria and the aorta and pulmonary artery to perform the anastomoses.

## V. CONDUCT OF OPERATION

### DONOR OPERATION

After declaration of brain death and evaluation as described earlier, the donor is brought to the operating room and prepared and draped in the usual sterile fashion. This operation is often coordinated with other organ harvest teams. After performing a median sternotomy, the pericardium is opened widely. The heart is visually inspected and palpated for great vessel palpable thrills, epicardial coronary lesions, and myocardial contusion. The aorta and pulmonary artery are dissected out superiorly to the level of the innominate vein and bifurcation, respectively. The venae cavae are then isolated. The superior vena cava is dissected to the level of the azygous vein and encircled with a tape. The donor is then fully heparinized. A cardioplegia cannula is placed in the aortic root. The superior vena cava is divided, and then the inferior vena cava is divided at the level of the diaphragm. The heart is allowed to beat until it is empty (approximately five beats), then the aorta is cross-clamped at the innominate artery. Two liters of cold potassium cardioplegia solution is delivered, or 15 to 20 ml/kg in children. Next, the pulmonary veins are divided at the level of the pericardium. Finally, the pulmonary artery is divided at the bifurcation, and the aorta is divided at the arch beyond the innominate artery. The heart is stored in cold saline at 4°C.

## ORTHOTOPIC TECHNIQUE

The native heart is exposed in much the same way as described in the preceding donor operation. Cardiopulmonary bypass is instituted. The recipient heart is then excised along the atrioventricular groove starting in the right atrium. The great vessels are divided above the sinuses of Valsalva. Simultaneously, the donor heart is examined. The atrial septum is closely inspected for patent foramen ovale, which is closed if found, and the pulmonary veins are connected to form an atrial cuff. Classically, the left atrial anastomosis is performed first, followed by the right atrial anastomosis. Care is taken to avoid injury to the sinus node or coronary sinus. Next, the pulmonary artery end-to-end anastomosis and the aortoaortic end-to-end anastomosis are performed. The aortic cross-clamp is removed. Epicardial pacing wires are placed, and the sternotomy is closed with wires.

As of 1994, 26,704 transplants from 251 centers have been performed.

| Survival | Overall | Cleveland Clinic Foundation ('84-'95) |
|---|---|---|
| 1 y | 80%, since 1983 86% | 87.8% |
| 5 y | 65%-75% | 73.4% |
| 10 y | 70% | — |

Fifty percent of patients return to full-time employment, and in recent years 1-year survival is close to 90%. Comparatively, the survival in patients referred but not receiving heart transplantation is 15% at 3 years.

## VARIATION OF OPERATION

The preferred ischemic time is less than 4 hours; sometimes this mandates that the left atrial and aortic anastomoses are performed first.

A bicaval anastamosis (vs a right atrial) may reduce perioperative atrial fibrillation and demonstrate earlier return of atrial systole.

**Heterotopic Technique.** Heterotopic technique is rarely used but may be indicated in patients with high irreversible pulmonary resistance or when the donor heart is too small. In this operation, the native heart is left in situ, and the donor heart inferior vena cava and the right pulmonary veins are oversewn. The recipient aorta is cross-clamped. Then, the left atrial anastomosis is performed, followed by the right atrial anastomosis. An aortoaortic end-to-side anastomosis and a pulmonary artery end-to-side anastomosis are then completed, the latter often with the use of an interposition graft. Survival with the heterotopic technique is significantly less that that of the orthotopic.

LVAD are more widely available as a bridging mechanism to transplant, with 55% to 80% of patients surviving to transplant, depending on the device chosen. LVAD removal at the time of transplant requires longer preparation.

Other surgical options include high-risk revascularizations, ventricular volume reduction, or the modified Dor procedure.

More complex reconstructions may be necessary in congenital heart diseases.

## POSTOPERATIVE ORDERS

**Admit to:** ICU intubated with all lines, plus drains; anticipate transfer to regular nursing floor on POD 3; average hospital stay is 2 to 3 weeks

**Diagnosis:** s/p heart transplant

**Condition:**

**Vital signs:** telemetry for duration, daily weights

**Activity:** bed rest, out of bed to chair on POD 2

**Allergies:**

**Nursing:** chest tubes at $-20$ cm $H_2O$ suction; remove if no leak and minimal drainage (usually POD 2-3). Foley to gravity, usually discontinued by POD 3-4. Swan-Ganz catheter for patients with elevated PVR; PVR responds well to pulmonary vasodilators (milrinone, nitrates, prostaglandin $E_1$). Vent: wean to extubation postoperatively asap, usually by POD 1. Incentive spirometry and respiratory therapy

**Diet:** NPO usually until POD 2 or 3; start clear liquids 1 day after extubated, then advance as tolerated to low fat, low salt diet

**IV fluids:** $D_5$/0.45% NS + 20 mEq KCl at 150 ml/h. Heplock once patient tolerating oral intake (~POD 3)

**Medications:** pressors and inotrope drops titrated prn to keep MAP 65-85 and CI 2.2 or better, wean by 72 hours
epidural PCA used for analgesia until taking PO. Start on oral analgesics about POD 3-4
Regular human insulin drops to keep blood sugar <200 mg/dl
(Zinacef) 1.5 g × 3 doses
(bactrim) (or pentamidine inhaler) and acyclovir prophylaxis
furosemide (lasix) 20 mg IV q8, begin POD 1
renal dose dopamine

52

CARDIAC TRANSPLANTATION

heparin, 5000 U SC bid

resume home medications once transferred to the regular floor

**Laboratory tests:** CBC and CMP qd in unit, cyclosporine level daily, CXR on arrival and qd in unit, ECG and cardiac enzymes on arrival, echocardiogram on POD 3-10 to evaluate RV and LV function, endomyocardial biopsy performed POD 7-10, before discharge, PICC line placed, pacer wires discontinued, and full teaching confirmed

## IMMUNOSUPPRESSION: TRIPLE-DRUG PROTOCOL

Cyclosporine

Preoperatively: 6-10 mg/kg PO

Maintenance level: ~200 ng/ml first 6 months, then ~100 ng/ml

Azathioprine

Preoperatively: 2.5 mg/kg

Maintenance: 2-2.5 mg/kg/d

Corticosteroids

Intraoperatively: methylprednisolone 500 mg then 125 mg q8h × 3, then maintenance

Maintenance: prednisone 1 mg/kg/d, taper to 0.4 mg/kg/d at 1 month, and then 0.3 mg/kg/d at 3 months

## VI. COMPLICATIONS

### REJECTION

After 6 months, rejection is usually symptomatic. Before that time, it must be screened for by means of myocardial biopsy. Biopsies are typically performed on postoperative day 7 to 10, then every week for 1 month, then every 2 weeks for the next month, then every month for the first year, then annually. The severity of rejection is graded on the basis of the histologic findings. Grades 0 to 2 are without myocyte necrosis. Grades 3 and 4 show moderate multifocal to severe myocyte necrosis.

Treatment is initiated with a pulse dose of methylprednisolone at 1 g/d intravenously for 3 days. Repeat biopsy is then performed. If the specimen shows continued rejection, therapy is advanced to muromonab-CD3, or polyclonal antibody for 7 to 14 days.

### GRAFT ATHEROSCLEROSIS

Graft atherosclerosis is a major cause of graft failure with selective involvement of the graft arterial tree. It is a direct result of chronic vascular rejection. Some of the known risks of this complication are an older donor, the presence of cytomegalovirus infection, elevated triglycerides, and the occurrence of two or more acute rejection episodes.

Treatment is directed at correcting the lesions with percutaneous transluminal coronary angioplasty or coronary artery bypass grafting for isolated lesions. Retransplantation is the definitive treatment option with a 1-year survival of only 54%.

## VII. DISCHARGE INSTRUCTIONS

Stay on a low-fat, low-cholesterol, low-sodium diet.

Do not smoke cigarettes.

Exercise daily but no lifting >10 pounds for 6 weeks.

Do not drive for 6 weeks.

Avoid crowds for the first 3 months, as well as people with colds or infections.

Avoid gardening for the first 6 months.

Always use sunscreen when outside because of the risk of malignancy with immunosuppression.

Wash all cuts well and watch for signs of infection.

Wash all fresh fruit and vegetables well.

Do not change kitty litter or bird cages.

Check daily: weight, temperature, pulse, and blood pressure and record in diary.

Call transplant team if T >100.5°F, HR >140 or <55, SBP >160 or <90, DBP >100.

Follow up every week × 1 month, then every 2 weeks × 1 month, then every month for 1 year, then annually.

# PART XV

## Palm Pilots

# DIGITAL PERIPHERAL BRAINS

*Adheesh A. Sabnis*

The day-to-day practice of medicine has changed drastically. The days of notecards are gone. Likewise, medical students and doctors carrying libraries of books in their pockets for quick reference on the wards is over. This is rapidly changing with the growing use of personal digital assistants (PDA) in the medical professions.

The advantages of PDAs are numerous but so are the types to choose from. How does one go about choosing the right PDA? A number of factors can help sort through the dilemma of choosing the right PDA. The purpose of this chapter is to help determine what systems are available and how they will assist each user.

**53**

## I. SYSTEM CHARACTERISTICS

### MEMORY

Windows CE, handheld PCs, and EPOC machines all have significantly more memory than Palm OS machines. However, these devices require the larger memory for their operating systems and for the other features they offer. Palm OS machines have a streamlined operating system that uses less memory.

In determining how much memory is required, it is useful to identify the quantity of information one wishes to store. The Internet or colleagues can help to estimate how much software and information storage capability one might require. Also, some Palm OS devices (eg, HandSpring and TRG) offer the ability to expand the system's memory. There are limitations to the Palm OSs maximum memory, and to bypass this limit requires additional software and steps to access the expanded memory.

### SIZE

What good is a powerful computer if it cannot fit in the pocket of scrubs and laboratory coats? However, the compact size comes at a premium. Prices for smaller and sleeker units might be 33% greater than larger units with similar functions. Again, the benefits of price to size must be considered with respect to the intended use. In general, Windows CE products are larger than the Palm OS products. The handheld PCs and EPOC machines are significantly larger and heavier than Palm or Windows product.

### OPERATING SYSTEM

If the Windows operating system is preferred, then the simple decision is to use Window CE products, which use a stripped-down version of the familiar Windows operating system. The advantage is primarily in ease of use and quicker learning of PDAs running Windows CE. However, performance is compromised with this operating system. Palm OS and EPOC machines use operating systems that are more streamlined. There is no advantage of one operating system over another with respect to linking data between the PDA and the desktop computer.

## SOFTWARE AVAILABILITY AND PEER SUPPORT

With respect to quantity, the depth and breadth of software for the Palm OS is unmatched. With more than 6500 programs, there is little that cannot be done with the Palm OS. Core programs such as databases, document readers, and drug guides are available on all platforms; however, as more specialized software is sought, Palm OS becomes the clear choice. Lastly, peer support plays an important role here. It is advantageous for people in a medical team to have similar operating systems and software to ease the transfer of information (eg, cross-cover lists, reference material, phone numbers) from one PDA to another. This cuts down on data entry time for the team as a whole and allows more efficient use of information.

## COLOR

Advantages of color devices include the ability to gain more information from similar data than without color. Color can be used to differentiate priority with respect to appointments, laboratory values, to-do lists, etc. Besides price, disadvantages of color devices include larger weight/size and shorter battery life.

## OTHERS/EXTRAS

Battery life is ever changing. Differences in units from the same company can vary greatly. Some PDAs are rechargeable in their synchronization cradles and can last a couple days on a full charge. Others use a pair of AAA batteries for more than a month. Another feature is the ability to upgrade the device. Palm OS devices such as the TRG Pro and Handspring offer expansion slots for adding functionality to the PDA. With rapid advances in technology, one must evaluate whether it is worth upgrading a PDA or simply replacing it. Last, the issue of wireless capability should be addressed. Most PDAs have the ability to exchange data by means of an infrared (IR) port. However, some of the newer units also offer wireless connectivity to the Internet. Again, this feature requires evaluation of one's need for such capability, service charges, and per-minute air time charges.

Choosing the right PDA is important and should custom suit each individual's needs. Additional information can be found on the web at *http://pdamd.com*. Because Palm OS devices are currently more popular and have a rich variety of software, further information in this section will be devoted to the Palm OS.

## II. HARDWARE MANUFACTURERS

Palm
URL: *http://www.palm.com*
Handspring
URL: *http://www.handspring.com*
TRG Products
URL: *http://www.trgpro.com*
Sony Corporation CLEI
URL: *http://www.sony.com*

Consult the manufacturers' Websites for up-to-date product and pricing information. This is not a complete list of Palm OS PDA manufacturers. Some wireless telephone manufacturers are also including the Palm OS in their products, and other consumer electronic companies are considering marketing their own PDAs using the Palm OS.

## III. REVIEW OF SOFTWARE

Following is a brief list and review of software products for the Palm OS. For information regarding more software, please refer to the following sites:

PDA Surgery: *http://www.pdasurgery.com* (has up-to-date information pertinent to surgery)
PDA-MD: *http://www.pdamd.com* (has information on Windows CE and EPOC machines)
Palm Gear: *http://www.palmgear.com*

### PATIENT TRACKING

#### Patient Keeper

Developer: The VIRTMED Corp.
Website: *http://www.patientkeeper.com/*
Approximate price: $35.00.
Description: PatientKeeper stores everything from names and medical record numbers, to problem lists and laboratory values. It can generate history and physical examination, subjective, objective, assessment, and plan (SOAP) notes, checkouts, and more.
Pertinent positives: great for keeping laboratory data and test results, summarizes important facts on one screen for presentation, logs procedures and events in a patient's history, customizable pop-up lists, able to beam patient to others for cross-coverage.
Pertinent negative: setup for medicine rather than surgery, lacks easy way of tracking specific intake and output measurements, lacks ability to synchronize patient data between team members.

### HandDBase

Developer: DDH Software, Inc.

Website: *http://www.handbase.com/*

Approximate price: $19.99.

Description: powerful engine allows multiple relational databases to be linked in several ways.

Pertinent positives: allows multiple database linking, many programs already available, with additional software can link and synchronize with Microsoft Access, very customizable.

Pertinent negative: requires initial time to setup a database, customization requires knowledge about basic database functions.

### J-File

Developer: Land-J Technologies.

Website: *http://www.land-j.com/jfile.html*

Approximate price: $24.95.

Description: JFile is a fast, efficient, and user-friendly database program for the PalmOS platform.

Pertinent positives: more user-friendly than HandDBase, because it has fewer features; desktop program available to work on data on PC rather than handheld; useful for tracking procedure logs.

Pertinent negative: rather limited functionality when combining databases.

## DRUG REFERENCES

### ePocrates qRx

Developer: ePocrates, Inc.

Website: *http://www.epocrates.com/*

Approximate price: Free.

Description: ePocrates contains pertinent medical information on more than 1600 medications, including indication-specific dosing, contraindications, and drug-drug interactions. qRx is updated regularly and has an intuitive user interface. qRx enhancements will include mechanism of action, advanced multiple-drug interactions, packaging and tablet/caplet descriptions, and retail pricing. Future ePocrates products and services will also include formulary decision support tools, up-to-date medical and general news, and other transactional-based services such as electronic prescribing.

Pertinent positives: free, stays up-to-date with frequent synchronizations, relatively small memory requirement.

Pertinent negative: current version lacks mechanism of action, pharmocokinetics, etc.; requires scheduled synchronization for program to run.

### LexiDrugs

Developer: Skyscape.com, Inc.

Website: *http://www.skyscape.com/skyscape/index/index.html*

Approximate price: $64.95.

Description: LexiDrugs is specifically designed for all medical professionals, at any level of training or experience, requiring quick access to concise and comprehensive data concerning clinical use of medications. It contains a complete database covering more than 3900 medications and more than 1250 drug monographs; it spans about 500 different therapeutic classes.

Pertinent positives: comes in a few different sizes (memory), has information on mechanism, pharmocokinetics, etc.; shortcut keys to ease daily use.

Pertinent negative: upgraded less frequently than e-Pocrates.

### Physician's Drug Handbook

Developer: Handheldmed, Inc.

Website: *http://www.handheldmed.com/*

Approximate price: $75.00.

Description: the *Physician's Drug Handbook* offers the following categories of information on more than 5000 brand and generic drugs—how supplied, indications, route, dosage, pharmacodynamics, pharmacokinetics, contraindications, interactions, effects on diagnostic tests, adverse reactions, overdosage, special considerations, information for the patient, geriatric use, pediatric use, and breast feeding. In addition, the *PDH* also offers capsule summaries of appropriate drug use for more than 100 commonly encountered disease states.

Pertinent positives: with promotional offers, this program is sometimes free.

Pertinent negative: some find format of information presentation a bit inefficient, not as streamlined as e-Pocrates or LexiDrugs.

## MEDICAL MATHEMATICS

### MedMath

Developer: Phillip Cheng.

Website: *http://dolphin.upenn.edu/~pcheng/medmath/*

Approximate price: free.

Description: MedMath is a medical calculator for the Palm, written by a physician for rapid calculations of common formulas in adult internal medicine. Features more than 20 formulas sorted by category, with selectable units and onscreen numeric keypad. Runs on all Palm platforms without external libraries.

Pertinent positives: gives background data (ie, journal citations) on formulas, ease of data entry, displays formula.

Pertinent negative: only 20 formulas in current version, user cannot add additional formulas.

## Med Calc

Developer: Mathias Tschopp.

Website: *http://netxperience.org/medcalc/*

Approximate price: free.

Description: MedCalc is designed for rapid calculation of common equations used in internal medicine. Main features: available for free * available in English and French versions * easy to use * formulas sorted by categories * full-featured medical calculator (more than 40 formulas).* Most units are available either in S.I. or regular units.* Exclusive: results can be saved in a Palm OS database for later retrieval.

Pertinent positives: 40+ formulas with citations and information, changes between units for ease of data entry, can store data on specific patients.

Pertinent negative: user cannot add additional formulas.

## SynCalc

Developer: Synergy Solutions, Inc.

Website: *http://www.synsolutions.com/software/syncalc/*

Approximate price: $19.95.

Description: fully algebraic infix calculator. Support for unlimited number of nested parentheses and function calls. Up to 100 user-defined shortcuts may be added or imported. Real-time input and output functions. Add new functions by means of the Synergy Plug-in Architecture. Includes Math, Base Convertor, and Logic Plug-ins. Fully functional drag-and-drop editing. Double- and triple-tap editing features simplify editing of expressions. Twelve-memory locations are accessible by means of the drag-and-drop interface. Twenty-six numeric variables. Calculation log/printer tape feature. Added support for Plug-ins, macros. Comes with three plugins: MathPlugin, LogicPlugin, and BaseConvertorPlugin.

Pertinent positives: programmable for additional formulas.

Pertinent negative: cannot easily see formula, requires time to learn programming (simple but time consuming).

## ABG Pro

Developer: StacWorks.

Website: *http://www.stacworks.com/*

Approximate price: free.

Description: a program that will completely analyze arterial blood gases (ABGs) for you. No longer will you be confused by ABGs. The program not only will tell you whether you have a metabolic or respiratory acidosis or alkalosis but also will calculate expected $Pco_2$

and expected $HCO_3$ when needed and will then tell you whether there is a concomitant acid-base disorder. It will even calculate anion gap and delta-delta if necessary. Compiled into fast, efficient machine code using Quartus Forth.

Pertinent positives: free, quickly changes between units and validates with Henderson Hasselbach equation, output diagnosis with explanation using expected values.

Pertinent negative: time consuming if you already know how to interpret ABGs.

## DOCUMENT VIEWER

### TealDoc

Developer: TealPoint Software.
Website: *http://www.tealpoint.com/softdoc.htm*
Approximate price: $16.95.
Description: TealDoc is a full-featured reader for standard Palm Pilot docs, with quality, intuitive interface, and affordability. Supports embedded TealPaint pictures, bookmarks, headers, and hyperlink buttons. Other features include changeable fonts, convenient forward and backward searches with advanced search options, adjustable display options, and multispeed forward and backward autoscroll.

Pertinent positives: hypertext and bookmarks to ease presentation, allows for graphics to be displayed.

Pertinent negative: cannot edit within the program.

### SmartDoc

Developer: Cutting Edge Software, Inc.
Website: *http://www.cesinc.com/smartdoc/smartdoc.html*
Approximate price: $19.95.
Description: SmartDoc is the text document editor and reader application available for Palm Computing handhelds. It allows you to work with text documents on your Palm organizer. SmartDoc can be used as a supercharged MemoPad or using one of the many third-party document converters available today, you can read and edit MS Word documents directly on your device. There are thousands of useful documents, books, and reference materials ready to download for free.

Pertinent positives: can create documents and edit existing ones.

Pertinent negative: no hypertext or bookmarks.

## OTHER SOFTWARE

### DateBk4

Developer: Pimlico Software, Inc.
Website: *http://www.pimlicosoftware.com/datebk4.htm*
Approximate price: $24.95.

Description: replaces the built-in Datebook, Todo, and Memopad applications on all models of the Palm Organizer with a considerably more powerful, integrated program that maintains the general look and feel of the original applications. Runs on *all* models of the Palm Organizer from V-2.0 on up.

Pertinent positives: great for linking data between to-do lists, memo, and phone book; adds additional views to calendar function; adds icons to ease interpretation of schedule; color support; very similar to built in DateBook so there is no time wasted learning a new application.

Pertinent negative: none.

## PalmPrint

Developer: Stevens Creek Software.

Website: *http://www.stevenscreek.com/palm/palmprint.shtml*

Approximate price: $39.95.

Description: print from your PalmPilot to a wide variety of printers, using either IrDA or the serial port. PCL, Epson-compatible, and PostScript printers are supported. PalmPrint prints memos, to-do lists, and anything on the clipboard. It also supports printing from other applications. Modified versions of the standard Palm Address Book, which prints envelopes, and of the standard Palm Mail application, which prints e-mails, are distributed with PalmPrint. A free Satellite Forms extension (SFX) allows applications written in Satellite Forms to print using PalmPrint.

Pertinent positives: allows quick "beaming" to IR capable printers, no PC needed.

Pertinent negative: text formatting (eg, bold, italics, underline) and graphics not fully supported.

## TealPhone

Developer: TealPoint Software.

Website: *http://www.tealpoint.com/softphon.htm*

Approximate price: $17.95.

Description: TealPhone is a replacement for the standard system address/phonebook application. It offers an improved interface and many convenient enhancements over the standard Palm application, including a quick-seek index bar, one-screen integrated display, sorting by first name, last name, or company, separate sorting options for each category, on-the-fly switching of sorting options, city and country history buffers, and powerful search features.

Pertinent positives: larger display than original address program, great search function, number pad to ease entry of phone numbers, pop-up lists for frequently entered data (eg, city, state), can set up to beam multiple business cards.

Pertinent negative: can adversely affect other programs.

### WordComplete

Developer: Communication Intelligence Corp.

Website: *http://www.shopcic.com/*

Approximate price: $24.99.

Description: WordComplete supports the most popular text entry systems, including the Graffiti, Jot, and the pop-up keyboard. WordComplete is like shorthand for your Palm-connected organizer. This utility helps to speed text entry time and accuracy by offering a pop-up pick list of words once you have entered a few letters. To complete your word entry, just tap on the word that you want and it is automatically entered where your cursor is. WordComplete's dictionary provides a quick and easy way to check the spelling of a word and can be customized, so that frequently used words appear at the top of the pop-up list.

Pertinent positives: greatly reduces time of entering long medical words, supports pop-up lists and custom dictionaries.

Pertinent negative: conflicts with search capability on other programs.

## IV. ACCESSORIES

There are numerous accessories for the personal digital assistants out in the market. Examples include the following.

### CASES

These not only store your PDA but serve other functions as well. Some cases hold everything from pens and business cards to cash and credit cards. Other cases offer tough padding and are constructed of rubber to resist damage caused by dropping your digital investment. Still other cases offer the benefit of being waterproof to guard against splashes at the scrub sinks.

### KEYBOARDS

For those people who find graffiti inefficient for lengthy text, there are keyboards available that make data entry easier and quicker. Some of the keyboards fold down to just slightly bigger than the PDA itself. Besides increased speed, keyboards also offer multiple shortcut keys to common applications on the PDA. The major disadvantage of using a keyboard is that it detracts from the simplicity and compactness of most PDAs.

## PRINTERS

To produce a document, a printer is necessary. With software such as PalmPrint, documents can be easily "beamed" to an IR printer without worrying about cumbersome connections to PCs. Another alternative to the purchase of a printer is using an IR upgrade and connecting it to existing printers. This would allow software beaming to the printers as explained previously. Last, portable printers exist specifically for laptop computers and PDAs. Many of these can be reviewed at the PalmPrint Website.

# PART XVI

## Bedside Procedures

# CHEST TUBES

*Michael Rosen*

Chest tubes are used to drain air, fluid, or blood from the pleural space. These can accumulate in the pleural space spontaneously or secondary to trauma, intrathoracic operations, malignancies, and infections.

## I. PATHOPHYSIOLOGY

The pleural space is typically under negative pressure to aid in lung expansion during inhalation. When fluid, air, or blood accumulates in this space, it can compress the adjacent lung tissue. This can result in atelectasis, entrapment, and eventual infection. Moreover, as the fluid or air accumulates in the hemithorax, it can begin to compress the mediastinum, resulting in a mediastinal shift and prevent adequate venous return with resultant hemodynamic collapse.

## II. TYPICAL PRESENTATION

Many disease processes that require chest tube insertion have a variety of classical presentations. Most commonly, trauma patients can present with either hemothorax or pneumothorax. These patients can present with life-threatening hemodynamic instability or simply shortness of breath, pleuritic chest pain, and occasionally subcutaneous emphysema on examination. A high level of suspicion is warranted in patients with multiple rib fractures. Of note, any trauma patient with any size pneumothorax who will require positive-pressure ventilation will need a tube thoracostomy secondary to the risk of tension pneumothorax.

Patients undergoing elective pulmonary surgery also receive chest tubes postoperatively. These tubes function as monitors for any postoperative hemorrhage and relieve postoperative air leaks until the lungs have time to heal.

## III. PREOPERATIVE WORKUP

It is imperative that the chest x-ray of the patient be reviewed before tube placement. Particular attention should be paid to the level of the hemidi-aphragms for safe and adequate tube placement. A lateral decubitus film may be necessary to differentiate a loculated effusion from a free-flowing one. This distinction is important to accurately direct the placement of the chest tube. If the indication for tube placement is an isolated pneumothorax, an anterior apical tube should be placed. Alternatively, if fluid drainage is required, a posteroinferiorly directed tube is appropriate. Generally, a 28-F chest tube is adequate to drain both fluid, blood, and air. However, occasionally in trauma with large amounts of bleeding, smaller chest tubes can clot and become blocked. Thus, some advocate at least a 36-F tube. A thorough history and physical examination should be performed, with attention to any prior thoracic cavity surgeries or lung resections that could alter the usual anatomy.

## PREOPERATIVE ORDERS

Review CXR.
Confirm coagulation status of patient.

## IV. SURGICAL ANATOMY

The intercostal neurovascular bundle runs on the inferior aspect of the rib. This relationship is important when placing chest tubes so as not to inadvertently damage these structures. These can be safely avoided by directing the chest tube over the superior aspect of the rib. Chest tubes are typically placed in the anterior axillary line formed by the lateral border of the pectoralis major muscle. In the male, the nipple typically lies over the fourth intercostal space. In the female, the inframammary fold intersects the anterior axillary line over the fifth intercostal space. The parietal pleural reflection at the anterior axillary line is at the eighth thoracic vertebra, and the risk of injuring the spleen, liver, or diaphragm is low with tube placement in the fifth intercostal space.

## V. CONDUCT OF OPERATION

The patient receives 1 g of cefazolin (Ancef) before chest tube insertion. The patient can be positioned in the supine position with an axillary role for elevation or be placed in the decubitus position, with the affected side elevated if necessary. The arm should be abducted and raised over the head to enlarge the intercostal space. The area is prepped and draped in a sterile fashion. A subcutaneous wheel of lidocaine is then injected. This lidocaine is then dispersed along the proposed tract of insertion. The needle should be advanced into the intrathoracic space while withdrawing until either blood or air is obtained, confirming location before placing the chest tube. Then, the needle should be slowly withdrawn, taking care to adequately anesthetize the parietal pleura, which is most sensitive.

An incision large enough to accommodate an index finger is made approximately 1 to 2 cm below the proposed rib of entry site to allow formation of a tunnel. This is particularly important in elderly, thin patients with malignant effusions to allow a tract to seal after chest tube removal. Also, this will allow the subcutaneous tissue to fall together, permitting the tract to seal and prevent air from being sucked in when the tube is removed. The incision is carried through the dermis. The direction that the tube is desired to lie in is determined by the trajectory of the tunnel. The two points of fixation are the skin and the entry site into the pleural space and thus care should be taken to direct the tunnel appropriately. With a blunt-tipped instrument and repetitive slow spreading motions the subcutaneous tissue and muscle are dissected until the pleura is entered on the superior aspect of the rib. The instrument is spread on removal to enlarge the space.

Before placing the chest tube, it is imperative that a finger is inserted into the thoracic space. This will confirm accurate location, and any adhesions can be gently swept away. If adhesions cannot be gently removed, the procedure should be aborted and a radiologically guided tube should be placed. Once the adhesions have been swept away, the chest tube can be inserted with a blunt-tipped clamp or freely into the pleural space. Of note, if resistance is met, advancement should stop. This usually means that the tube is either abutting the mediastinum or in the fissure. The major fissures follow the course of the sixth rib from the root of the spine of the scapula posteriorly to the sixth costochondral junction anteriorly. The tube should be withdrawn and redirected. After adequate placement of the chest tube, it should be secured to the skin with a purse-string or U stitch and an airtight dressing applied. The tube should then be attached to a watertight suction device. Finally, a chest x-ray is ordered to confirm correct placement with the last side port inside the thoracic cavity.

**54**

**CHEST TUBES**

## VARIATIONS OF OPERATION

Pleural effusions that are loculated can require a radiologic-guided tube placement. This can be accomplished under computed tomography or ultrasonographic guidance.

## POSTOPERATIVE ORDERS

**Nursing:** redress wound with sterile dressing and Vaseline gauze every day. Place chest tube to 20 cm of $H_2O$ suction and adjust wall suction to allow slow bubbling throughout respiration, check for air leaks, monitor amount of drainage and characteristics of fluid

**Medications:** cefazolin (Ancef) 1 g IV q8h is continued while the chest tube is in place

**Laboratory tests:** upright CXR should be taken after placement and every AM while tube is still in place; send initial fluid for appropriate tests: amylase, cell count, cytology, pH, microbiology, lactate dehyrogenase, protein, glucose, and specific gravity

### VI. COMPLICATIONS

Postexpansion pulmonary edema: Occasionally, after rapid drainage of large pulmonary effusions, postexpansion pulmonary edema can develop. This requires aggressive treatment with diuresis and supplemental oxygen.

Empyema can result from contamination of the chest tube and thoracic cavity. Residual pneumothorax can result from air entering the thorax at the time of chest tube removal. This usually can be managed conservatively with serial x-rays.

## VII. DISCHARGE ORDERS

There is no set standard for when to remove a chest tube. Some loose guidelines include 24-hour drainage of less than 100 ml, no air leaks, and drainage of fluid with no pneumothorax on chest x-ray. The technique for removing a chest tube is important to prevent air from entering the thoracic cavity. A generous portion of petroleum gauze is placed on several 4 × 4's, and an outer layer of tape is fashioned. The securing stitch is cut. The patient is instructed to take a deep breath and hold it for 5 seconds. Next, the dressing is placed in one hand partially covering the chest tube, and the other hand rapidly withdraws the tube. The dressing is then placed firmly down, and the patient is allowed to breathe normally. Alternatively, a stitch previously placed can be secured when the tube is withdrawn; however, this usually requires an assistant. A follow-up chest x-ray is obtained to confirm the absence of a pneumothorax. The dressing can be removed in 48 hours, and any stitches can be removed in 14 days.

# THORACENTESIS

*David Sharp*

Thoracentesis is indicated for determining the cause and performing therapeutic drainage of pleural effusions. Thoracentesis is a bedside procedure that allows pleural fluid sampling, quantitation, and microscopic evaluation. Along with clinical presentation, it allows the accurate diagnosis of a pleural effusion in approximately 75% of cases.

## I. PATHOPHYSIOLOGY

Pleural fluid is an ultrafiltrate of plasma. A pleural effusion forms when a process interrupts the steady-state condition, in which pleural fluid absorption is equivalent to pleural fluid formation. Several physiologic processes can result in pleural fluid accumulation. For instance, increased hydrostatic pressure (congestive heart failure), increased capillary permeability (pneumonia), decreased plasma colloid oncotic pressure (hypoalbuminemia), increased negative intrapleural pressure (atelectasis), and impaired drainage of the pleural space by obstruction of lymphatics (tumor) are associated with pleural effusions.

Traditionally, pleural effusions are defined as *exudates* or *transudates*. One or more of the following criteria characterize exudative effusions:

Pleural fluid protein to serum protein ratio >0.5
Pleural fluid lactate dehydrogenase (LDH) to serum LDH ratio >0.6
Pleural fluid LDH >200 U/ml (or >two-thirds the upper limit of
    normal LDH)

Forty-three percent of pleural exudates are due to malignant disease, and 83% of transudates are caused by congestive heart failure. The differential diagnosis of pleural effusions is listed in Table 55-1.

## II. TYPICAL PRESENTATION

Pleural effusions may or may not be symptomatic and can be a sign of systemic or pleural disease. Large effusions may compress the adjacent lung tissue, resulting in atelectasis and dyspnea. Infectious or malignant effusions may irritate the parietal pleura and cause pleuritic chest pain.

## III. PREPROCEDURE WORKUP

Thoracentesis is performed after review of old and new chest radiographs. Lateral decubitus films should be evaluated for signs of a loculated effusion. Coagulation laboratory values should be reviewed, with prothrombin time or partial thromboplastin time >1.3 ratio or platelets <50,000 being contraindications. Thoracentesis should also not be performed in the setting

---

**TABLE 55-1**

**DIFFERENTIAL DIAGNOSIS OF PLEURAL EFFUSIONS**

**TRANSUDATIVE PLEURAL EFFUSIONS**

Congestive heart failure
Pericardial disease
Cirrhosis
Nephrotic syndrome
Peritoneal dialysis
Superior vena cava obstruction
Myxedema
Pulmonary emboli
Sarcoidosis
Urinothorax

**EXUDATIVE PLEURAL EFFUSIONS**

Neoplastic diseases
  Metastatic disease
  Mesothelioma
Infectious diseases
  Bacterial infections
  Tuberculosis
  Fungal infections
  Viral infections
  Parasitic infections
Pulmonary embolization
Gastrointestinal disease
  Esophageal perforation
  Pancreatic disease
  Intraabdominal abscess
  Diaphragmatic hernia
  Postabdominal surgery
  Endoscopic variceal sclerotherapy
Collagen vascular diseases
  Rheumatoid pleuritis
  Systemic lupus erythematosus
  Drug-induced lupus erythematosus
  Immunoblastic lymphadenopathy
  Sjögren syndrome
  Wegener granulomatosis
  Churg-Strauss syndrome
Postcardiac injury syndrome
Asbestos exposure
Sarcoidosis
Uremia
Meigs syndrome
Yellow nail syndrome

*Continued*

---

**TABLE 55-1**

DIFFERENTIAL DIAGNOSIS OF PLEURAL EFFUSIONS—cont'd

EXUDATIVE PLEURAL EFFUSIONS—cont'd

Drug-induced pleural disease
    Nitrofurantoin
    Dantrolene
    Methysergide
    Bromocriptine
    Procarbazine
    Amiodarone
Trapped lung
Radiotherapy
Electrical burns
Urinary tract obstruction
Iatrogenic injury
Ovarian hyperstimulation syndrome
Chylothorax
Hemothorax

From Greenfield LJ, ed. Surgery. 2nd ed. Philadelphia; Lippincott-Raven, 1997:1454.

of pleural varices from portal hypertension. The effusion may be further characterized if necessary by ultrasonography or computed tomography (CT) scan as clinically appropriate.

## IV. CONDUCT OF OPERATION

The patient should be positioned seated in the upright position, slightly leaning forward, and with arms resting on a bedside table. The patient's back is percussed to identify the bottom of the unaffected lung field and the meniscus of the affected lung field. These landmarks are marked on the patient's skin. The site of thoracentesis may be selected as a position just above a posterior rib, two interspaces below the top of the identified effusion, but not below the eighth intercostal space. Alternatively, the seventh intercostal space may be used generally and is localized as the site two fingerbreadths inferior to the tip of the scapula. Prepare and drape the patient. A local anesthetic (eg, 1% lidocaine) is used to raise a wheal in the epidermis. Local anesthetic is also instilled over the periosteum of the inferior rib and the parietal pleura in the intercostal space. This is done by guiding the needle over the superior margin of the rib and remaining perpendicular to the rib. This is important so as not to injure the neurovascular bundle, which passes in the intercostal groove of each rib under its inferior margin. The needle is carefully advanced while continuously infiltrating with lidocaine. Once over the rib, the needle is slowly advanced into the chest while aspirating the syringe until pleural fluid is encountered.

The thoracentesis catheter is then inserted into the pleural space. An 18-gauge insertion needle on a 20-ml syringe is inserted, with the bevel directed inferiorly, into the pleural cavity in the same manner. The needle is slowly advanced superiorly over the edge of the rib, while constantly aspirating. Once pleural fluid is encountered, the syringe is removed and a finger placed over the needle to prevent air from entering the pleural cavity. Using the Seldinger technique, a guidewire is inserted through the needle into the chest, and then the needle is carefully removed leaving the wire. The catheter is inserted into the chest over the wire, and then the wire is removed. A finger is maintained over the end of the catheter to prevent air from entering the chest. The extension tubing and vacuum apparatus is attached, the stopcock opened, and fluid withdrawn. Slowly, the catheter is withdrawn to remove any pockets of fluid located proximal to the tip until the catheter is pulled out of the chest. About 1000 to 1500 ml of fluid removal is generally tolerated.

## VARIATIONS OF OPERATION

A lateral approach may be necessary when the patient is unable to sit upright. If this approach is selected, the patient is propped up with a rolled towel placed lengthwise beneath the back with the upper arm resting over the ear to open up the intercostal spaces. Likewise, when the pleural effusion is loculated, as evidenced by failure of the fluid to layer out on decubitus chest radiographs or chest CT scan, alternative areas are chosen to perform the thoracentesis and may warrant a change in patient positioning. Successful evacuation of loculated fluid may be aided by the use of fluoroscopy, ultrasonography, or less commonly, CT scan to localize the collection. When localization of the effusion is needed, however, it is important to be certain that it be done with the patient in the same position as he or she will be in for the thoracentesis to keep the surface landmarks constant.

## POSTPROCEDURE ORDERS

A stat chest x-ray is obtained to rule out pneumothorax and evaluate residual pleural fluid. Serum samples should be drawn at the same time for LDH, protein, and any other additional studies as the clinical situation applies.

Pleural fluid (about 50 to 100 ml, up to 250 ml for cytologic testing) should be sent off for the following, with test selection based on clinical differential diagnosis:

Lavender tube for cell count, with differential
Red top tube for total protein, LDH, glucose, triglycerides, creatinine
Syringe or vacuum bottle with 5000 to 10,000 U of heparin for cytologic examination
Gram's stain and cultures, acid-fast bacillus stains, fungal cultures/ KOH preparation

Anaerobic syringe on ice for pH
Amylase, lipase if warranted

## V. POTENTIAL COMPLICATIONS

Pneumothorax is the most common complication (10%) and is best
avoided by keeping air out of the system at all times. Tube thoracostomy
may be necessary if the pneumothorax is symptomatic or >10%. Intercostal vessel damage is minimized by positioning the needle directly over
the superior edge of the rib. If laceration occurs, the complication is monitored with serial chest x-rays with thoracostomy necessary for significant
hemothorax. Other complications include empyema and spleen or liver
puncture.

55

THORACENTESIS

# LUMBAR PUNCTURE

*Ali Chahlavi*

The brain and spinal cord are contained within the cerebrospinal fluid (CSF). By analyzing the CSF, the state of health or disease of the central nervous system is determined.

## I. PATHOPHYSIOLOGY

The CSF supports and cushions the central nervous system (CNS) against trauma, removes waste products, and serves as a medium for the transportation of hormones and ions within the brain. The CSF is a clear, colorless liquid containing all the substances normally found in blood plasma, but at different concentrations (see Table 56-1). Only one to five white blood cells (WBCs) may be considered to be within normal limits in any CSF sample; no red blood cells (RBCs) should be present.

The total volume of CSF is estimated to be 140 to 150 ml, of which 25 ml is in the ventricles. CSF is produced at about 0.35 ml/min, which is 450 to 500 ml/d (in newborns, there is **only 5 ml of total CSF** with a formation rate of 25 ml/d). Normal CSF pressure is 7 to 15 cm of $H_2O$ (greater than 18 is usually abnormal). In the pediatric population, normal CSF is <15.

## II. TYPICAL PRESENTATION

### INFECTIONS

The patient usually presents with severe headache, photophobia, and development of meningismus, with or without Kernig's or Brudzinski's sign. In the subacute presentation the patient can have drowsiness, lethargy, nausea, vomiting, and even coma. In infants less than 5 weeks old with a fever greater than 38.0°C, CSF analysis is mandated.

In bacterial meningitis, the CSF is under high pressure, has leukocytosis of 500 to 10,000 (predominately polymorphonuclear leukocytes in purulent infections and mostly lymphocytes in chronic infections), protein of 50 to 1000 mg/dl, and glucose less than 50 mg/dl. With turbid CSF and high γ-globulin, syphilis is likely to be the causative agent; whereas, "cobweb" clot (fibrinogen) in CSF suggests tuberculosis meningitis. In patients with brain abscess the CSF is high in pressure, leukocytosis, and protein about 65% of the time.

With fungal infection, leukocytosis occurs with predominately lymphocyte and in the case of cysticercosis, lymphocytes mixed with eosinophils; protein is usually high and glucose low. In cryptococcal meningitis, yeast from CSF can be seen with India ink or Wright stains. With *Candida,* cultures are required for diagnosis, but with *Blastomyces,* cultures are usually

**TABLE 56-1**

COMPOSITION OF LUMBAR CSF

Osmolarity = 295

Na = 138, K = 2.8, Ca = 2.1, Mg = 2.3, Cl = 119 mEq/dl

Glucose = 60 mg/dl, protein = 35 mg/dl, albumin = 15.5 mg/dl

IgG/IgA/IgM (mg/L) = 12.3/1.3/0.6

pH/$P_{CO_2}$/$P_{O_2}$ = 7.33/47/43

required. Leakage of echinococcal cyst can cause aseptic meningitic syndrome.

Viral infection causes an increase in CSF pressure 200 to 400 mm Hg, leukocytosis of 10 to 200/mm$^3$ (mostly lymphocytes), and mild increase in protein (50 to 80 mg/dl); glucose level is unaffected.

## CEREBROVASCULAR DISORDER

By definition, a single RBC in the CSF is technically a subarachnoid hemorrhage (SAH). These patients present with the "worst headache of their life." They have simultaneous onset of vertigo and vomiting with the onset of headache. They can also have nuchal rigidity. The CSF is uniformly bloodstained in most symptomatic patients (although up to 500 RBC/mm$^3$ can appear clear). Sometimes, the blood from intracranial bleeding can take 6 to 12 hours before reaching the lumbar subarachnoid space, and sometimes it may never reach it. The blood can persist for 7 to 14 days or may disappear within 24 hours. See Table 56-2 for differentiating traumatic lumbar puncture (LP) from SAH.

## MENINGEAL CARCINOMATOSIS

Half of the patients have high CSF pressure from the first LP. Malignant cells are found in ~60% (with repeated LP ~80%) of patients with leptomeningeal tumors, compared with ~2% of patients with tumors not involving the meninges. There is leukocytosis, usually less than 500/mm$^3$, and protein up to 1200 mg/dl. If the glucose is less than 50 mg/dl, diffuse meningeal involvement should be considered.

**TABLE 56-2**

DIFFERENCE BETWEEN TRAUMATIC LP AND SAH

| Traumatic LP | SAH |
|---|---|
| Blood streak/clot formation | Xantochromia (90% <12 h) (also present in |
| Clearing from tube 2 to 4 | intracerebral hemorrhage and subdural |
|  | hemorrhage if brain is lacerated) |
| 1 WBC per 700 RBCs | Leukocytosis in 24-48 h |
| 1 mg protein per 1000 RBCs | Increased protein in 24-48 h |

## PSEUDOTUMOR CEREBRI

The patients have elevated intracranial pressure (ICP) without evidence of cause (diagnosis of exclusion). They have symptoms of high ICP such as headache, dizziness, nausea, visual changes, and signs of papilledema, abducens nerve palsy, and scotoma. Otherwise, the neurologic examination can be normal with normal to small ventricles. The CSF cell count and glucose are normal, although the protein can be reduced.

## SEIZURE DISORDERS

Postictal pleocytosis and high protein (<100 mg/dl) can follow prolonged seizure or repetitive seizures.

## GUILLAIN-BARRÉ SYNDROME

Increased protein is found in the CSF for the first 2 to 3 weeks (up to 1000 mg/dl), with a characteristic albuminocytologic dissociation (leukocytosis only in 15%). The $\kappa/\lambda$ ratio is normal (~1.0).

## MULTIPLE SCLEROSIS

The CSF has a mild increase in lymphocytes (<50) 30% of the time with increased IgG and electrophoretic oligoclonal bands. The $\kappa/\lambda$ ratio is also high, >1.0. Increase in myelin basic protein occurs in acute episodes, although it is also present in generalized nervous tissue destruction.

## III. PREPROCEDURE WORKUP

Computed tomography (CT) or magnetic resonance imaging (MRI) should precede all LPs to rule out mass effect or noncommunicating hydrocephalus and to prevent herniation and death. LP should not be performed at an infected site. Severely infected tissue, from either bed sores, acne, or other causes, can result in contamination of the CSF and iatrogenic meningitis or epidural abscess. Other contraindications include coagulopathy or platelet count less than 50,000; therefore, a CBC with complete blood count with prothrombin time and partial thromboplastin time is needed before a LP in high-risk patients. High ICP or papilledema is not a contraindication.

Caution should be taken in aneurysmal SAH. Rapidly lowering the CSF pressure increases the transmural pressure across the aneurysmal wall and can cause rupture. Thus, a minimal amount of CSF should be removed slowly with a small-gauge needle.

## PREOPERATIVE ORDERS

Head CT or MRI
Check CBC, PT, PTT

## IV. SURGICAL ANATOMY

The conus of the spinal cord ends at the level of L1 and L2, and the thecal sac ends at S2. Thus, L3-4 interspace (at the level of the superior border of iliac crests) or one level lower is usually used to perform LP and withdraw CSF without penetrating the spinal cord. In children, the conus sits slightly lower at the level of L2-L3; consequently, in pediatric population, L4-L5 or L5-S1 is favorable for LP.

## V. CONDUCT OF OPERATION

The patient is placed in a relaxed horizontal knee-chest position on the edge of the bed for firm support. For a right-handed person, it is easier for the patient to lie on the left side. Sometimes for difficult or obese patients, the sitting position can be helpful. The puncture site of the spine is then marked. It is at the midline between the superior iliac crests. The back is prepped and draped in the usual sterile fashion, and the skin and the selected interspinous area is anesthetized with 1% to 2% lidocaine. A 20-gauge spinal needle is generally used for LP. A larger 18-gauge needle is useful in elderly patients with osteoarthritic backs. In patients suspected of high ICP, a 22-gauge needle should be used to prevent large dural holes and uncontrolled postoperative leakage.

The bevel should enter the dura parallel to the spinal cord and once inside the subarachnoid space should be turned to face superiorly. Before penetration, a slight resistance is felt, which is from the ligamentum flavum. The manometer is attached to the needle hub immediately after CSF flow is confirmed, and the opening pressure is measured (in millimeters of water). Drainage should be stopped immediately if CSF pressure exceeds 240 mm $H_2O$.

The CSF is collected in four tubes for diagnostic analysis. The first tube is for CSF culture and sensitivity of the organism. The following tube is used to measure the protein and glucose level, and the third one is for cell count. If the tap is traumatic or there is suspicion of SAH, the first and fourth tubes are used for cell count, and the second and the third tubes are used for culture and sensitivity and protein and glucose, respectively. In the traumatic tap the RBC count in tube 4 is much less than in tube 1; whereas in SAH the cell counts are similar (see Table 56-2.)

### POSTPROCEDURAL ORDERS

Send fluid for osmolality, Na, K, Mg, Ca, Cl, glucose, protein, albumin, immunoglobulins, pH, $Pco_2$, $Po_2$, cell count, cytologic study, bacteriology Gram's stain and cultures, and fungal if necessary.
Patients should remain flat for 1 hour after the procedure.
Puncture site should be checked for signs of hematoma.

## VI. POSSIBLE COMPLICATIONS

Herniation can be a grave consequence of lumbar puncture. A CT scan or MRI should always be done in an unconscious patient or when one suspects an intracerebral lesion such as a tumor, abscess, or empyema.

Epidermoid tumor can occur at the level of LP if the procedure is not properly performed. The physician must advance the LP needle with the stylet at all times; otherwise a core of epidermal tissue can be transplanted and increase the risk of epidermoid tumor.

Postlumbar headache occurs in 20% of patients. They usually last for 2 to 5 days. Bed rest, hydration, and mild analgesics or intravenous caffeine sodium benzoate is the treatment. If persistent, an epidural fibrin clot or blood patch is necessary.

Hematoma in subarachnoid, subdural, or epidural space may occur if the patient is anticoagulated after an LP. Other common complications are backache, intervertebral disk damage, nerve root or spinal cord injury, bleeding secondary to puncturing of epidural veins, and infection.

56

LUMBAR PUNCTURE

# INDEX

Note: Page numbers followed by t refer to tables.

## A

Abdominal hernia, umbilical, 183-186
Abdominal pain
  cholangiopancreatography in, 168
  mesenteric ischemia causing, 241, 243
Abdominal wall, peritoneal dialysis and, 251
Abdominal wound, 260-261
Abdominoperineal resection, 118-121
ABG Pro, 394-395
Abscess, perirectal, 105-110
  anatomy in, 107
  complications of, 110
  discharge orders for, 110
  pathophysiology of, 105-106
  preoperative workup for, 106
  presentation of, 106
  surgery for, 107-110
Accessories for personal digital assistant, 397-398
Achalasia, 47-52
  anatomy in, 49
  complications of, 52
  discharge orders for, 52
  evaluation of, 48-49
  pathophysiology of, 47
  presentation of, 47
  surgery for, 49-52
  treatment of, 47-48
Acral lentiginous melanoma, 270
Acute appendicitis, 75
Acute mesenteric ischemia, 241
Acute pancreatitis, 133-142. See also Pancreatitis.
Acute tubular necrosis, 350
Adenocarcinoma
  gastric, 67-68
  of lung, 307

Adenoma
  parathyroid, 198, 201
  salivary gland, 337
Adenomatous polyp
  colon cancer and, 85
  gastric cancer and, 67
  rectal cancer and, 115
Adhesion, intestinal, 38
  dialysis access and, 253
Adjuvant therapy
  for breast cancer, 231-232
  for skin or soft tissue tumor, 266
Adrenal disorder, 213-221
  anatomy in, 217-218
  complications of, 220
  discharge orders for, 221
  pathophysiology of, 213-214
  preoperative workup for, 215-217
  presentation of, 214-215
  surgery for, 218-220
Adrenergic-corticoid phase, 15-16
Adrenocorticotropic hormone, 213
Advancement flap, rectal, 103
Age, wound healing and, 258
Airway, tracheotomy for, 331-336
Alcoholism
  Mallory-Weiss tear in, 30
  pancreatitis and, 133
Aldosterone
  excess of, 215
  in Conn's syndrome, 216
Algorithm for pancreatic cancer, 161
Alimental formula, 20-21
Alkaline reflux gastritis, 72
Allograft. See Transplantation.
American Joint Committee of Cancer Staging System, 311
Amylase, 136
Anabolic phase, 16
Anal gland, 107

Analgesia
  hernia surgery and, 181
  in cirrhosis, 147
  in pancreatitis, 135
Anaplastic thyroid cancer, 191
Anastomosis
  ileorectal, 93
  ilial-pouch anal, 96
  in gastric cancer surgery, 70-71
  in pancreatic resection, 163
Anemia, 279-280, 279-283
Anesthesia, in cirrhosis, 147
Angina pectoris, 287
Angiodysplasia, bleeding in, 31
Angiography
  cardiac, 288
  for gastrointestinal bleeding
    lower, 32, 33
    upper, 28
  in liver cancer, 153
  in mesenteric ischemia, 243, 244
  in pancreatic neoplasm, 161, 208
Anorectal disorder
  fistula in ano, 99-104
  hemorrhoids, 111-114
  perirectal abscess, 105-110
  rectal cancer, 115-121
Anorectal space, 107
Antibody induction for renal
        transplantation, 349
Antigen, carcinoembryonic, in liver
        cancer, 152, 153
Antiinflammatory drugs in wound
        healing, 259
Antiplatelet drug
  cardiac valve disease and, 301
  in coronary artery bypass graft,
        289
Antireflux procedure, 51
Antithymocyte globulin for renal
        transplantation, 349
Antropometric measurement, 17
Aorta in coronary bypass, 291

Aortic insufficiency, 299
Aortic regurgitation, 305
Aortic stenosis, 298-299
  complications of, 304
Aortic valve repair or replacement,
        303
Appendectomy, 75-79
Arrhythmia after lung cancer surgery,
        315
Arterial graft, coronary, 287-295
Arterial secretin stimulation test, 208
Arterial stenosis, renal, 350
Arterial thrombosis
  hepatic, 368-369
  mesenteric, 241-242
Arterioportography, computed
        tomographic, 153
Artificial airway, 331-336
Ascites in cirrhosis
  assessment of, 145-146
  fluid therapy and, 147
Aspiration, 13-14
Aspiration biopsy
  in breast cancer, 227
  of salivary gland, 338
Atherosclerosis
  coronary artery bypass graft and,
        288
  in transplanted heart, 383-384
  mesenteric ischemia and, 241-
        243
  pathophysiology of, 235
Auricular nerve hypoesthesia, 341
Axillary lymph node dissection, 228-
        230

**B**
Bacterial meningitis, 411
Barium esophagraphy, 54
Barium study
  gastric cancer and, 68
  in ulcerative colitis, 95
Barium swallow, 48

Basal energy expenditure, 18-19
Basiliximab, 349
Battery life of personal digital
        assistant, 390
Bedside procedure
    chest tube insertion, 401-404
    lumbar puncture, 411-415
    thoracentesis, 405-409
Belsey Mark IV technique, 56-57
Benign tumor
    parathyroid adenoma, 198
    salivary gland, 337
Bile, 125
Bile duct leak, 369
Bile duct stone, 140
Biliary disorder
    liver transplantation and, 369
    pancreatitis with, 139
Biliary drainage, enteral feeding
        and, 9
Bilirubin in pancreatic cancer, 160
Biopsy
    in breast cancer, 227
    of melanoma, 270
    of salivary gland, 338
    thyroid, 192
Bjork flap, 334
Black pigment gallstone, 126
Bladder leak after pancreatic
        transplant, 359
Bleeding
    adrenalectomy and, 220
    carotid endarterectomy and, 239
    endoscopic retrograde
            cholangiopancreatography
            and, 171
    gastrointestinal, 27-30
        lower, 31-34
        upper, 27-30
    hemorrhoid surgery and, 114
    in cirrhosis, 158
    in esophageal surgery, 58
    nosebleed, 327-330

Bleeding—cont'd
    parotidectomy and, 342
    shock and, 41-43
    splenectomy and, 283
    thyroid surgery and, 195
    tracheotomy and, 335
    ulcer surgery and, 64
    variceal, 146
Blood
    coronary artery bypass graft and,
            289, 294
    in urine, after transplant
        pancreatic, 359
        renal, 350
    splenectomy and, 279-283
Blood cell count
    in appendicitis, 76
    in pancreatitis, 136
Blood chemistry
    in liver cancer, 153
    in pancreatitis, 135-136
Blood disorder, 279-283
    anemia, 279-280
    bypass graft and, 294
    cardiac valve disease and, 300-
            301
    myoproliferative, 280
    thrombocytopenia, 280
Blood gases in lung cancer, 308
Blood pressure, bypass graft and,
            293-294
Bone, hyperparathyroidism and, 198
Bowel ischemia, 141
Brain, digital peripheral, 389-398.
        See also Digital assistant,
        personal.
Breast cancer, 223-232
    anatomy in, 228
    carcinoma in situ, 223-224
    complications of, 230-231
    discharge instructions for, 231-
            232
    in pregnancy, 225

Breast cancer—cont'd
  inflammatory, 224-225
  invasive, 224
  male, 225-226
  Paget's disease and, 226
  preoperative workup for, 227
  presentation of, 226-227
  surgery for, 228-230
Bronchiolitis, obliterative, 376
Bronchopleural fistula, 315
Bronchopulmonary aspiration, 13-14
Bronchoscopy
  in lung cancer, 309, 310
  video-assisted thoracoscopic
    surgery and, 322
Brown pigment gallstone, 126
Budd-Chiari syndrome, 362
Bulge from umbilical hernia, 184
Bundle, intercostal neurovascular, 402
Bypass graft, coronary artery, 287-
    295

**C**
Cadaveric donor liver, 365
Calcitoninoma, 205
Calcium in hyperparathyroidism, 198
Calculus
  common bile duct, 140
  hyperparathyroidism and, 198
Calorie requirement, 18-19
Canal, inguinal, 177
Cancer. See Malignancy.
Carbohydrate requirement, 19
Carcinoembryonic antigen, 152, 153
Carcinoid, 152-153
Carcinoma in situ of breast, 223-224
Carcinomatosis, meningeal, 412
Cardiac arrhythmia after cancer
    surgery, 315
Cardiac output after bypass graft, 293
Cardiac transplantation, 379-385. See
    also Heart transplantation.
Cardiac valve disease, 297-305

Cardiogenic shock, 41
Cardioplegia, 291
Carotid artery
  cardiac valve disease and, 299
  mesenteric ischemia and, 241,
    244, 245-246
Carotid endarterectomy, 235-240
  anatomy in, 237
  complications of, 239
  discharge orders for, 240
  indications for, 235-236
  preoperative workup for, 236-237
  procedure for, 237-239
Cartilage in tracheotomy, 332
Case, personal digital assistant, 397
Catabolism, 15-16
Catecholamine, 214
Catheterization for peritoneal dialysis,
    249-253
Cell, islet, transplantation of, 357
Central nervous system infection,
    411-412
Central venous pressure, 7
Cerebrospinal fluid, 411-415
Cerebrovascular disorder
  carotid endarterectomy for, 235-
    240
  lumbar puncture for, 412
Chemically defined alimental formula,
    21
Chemotherapy for breast cancer, 231
Chest pain, 287
Chest tube, 401-404
Chest wall resection, 314
Chest x-ray
  chest tubes and, 401
  in achalasia, 48
  in lung cancer, 309
  video-assisted thoracoscopic
    surgery and, 322
Child
  appendectomy in, 78
  enteral feeding in, 9

Child—cont'd
  tracheotomy in, 333
  umbilical hernia in, 186
Child-Pugh score in cirrhosis, 145,
    145t, 149
Cholangiography
  intraoperative, 130
  percutaneous transhepatic, 167
Cholangiopancreatography,
        endoscopic retrograde, 167-
        172
  in pancreatic cancer, 160-161
  in pancreatitis, 139
Cholecystitis, 125-132
  anatomy in, 128-129
  complications of, 131
  discharge instructions for, 132
  pathophysiology of, 125-126
  preoperative workup for, 127-128
  presentation of, 126-127
  surgery for, 129-131
Cholescystostomy, 131
Cholestatic liver disease, 362
Cholesterol stone, 125-126
Chronic ambulatory peritoneal
    dialysis, 249-253
Chronic lymphocytic leukemia, 280
Chronic mesenteric ischemia, 242-
    243
Chronic obstructive pulmonary
    disease, 317-320
Chronic recurrent sialadenitis, 338
Cigarette smoking, wound healing
    and, 259
Circulation in cirrhosis, 143-144
Cirrhosis
  complications of, 148-149
  discharge instructions for, 149
  pathophysiology of, 143-144
  preoperative workup for, 144-147,
    145t
  presentation of, 144
  surgery for, 147-148

Clean-contaminated wound, 259
Clean wound, 259
Cleaning of wound, 261
Clip for wound closure, 263
Clotting factor, 294
Colectomy
  in Crohn's disease, 93
  in ulcerative colitis, 95
Colitis, ulcerative, 94-96
Collateral vessel in cirrhosis, 143-144
Collis gastroplasty, 57
Coloanal anastomosis, 118-121
Colon
  cancer of, 85-89
    hereditary nonpolyposis, 115
  diverticular disease of, 81-84
  obstruction of, 38
Colonoscopy, 33
Colorectal metastasis, 151
Common bile duct injury, 131
Common bile duct stone
  endoscopic retrograde
        cholangiopancreatography
        for, 168-169
  pancreatitis and, 140
Complete blood count
  in appendicitis, 76
  in pancreatitis, 136
Computed tomographic
    arterioportography, 153
Computed tomography
  carotid arterectomy and, 236
  gastrointestinal obstruction and, 36
  in cancer
    gastric, 68
    liver, 153
    lung, 309
    pancreatic, 208
    rectal, 116, 117
  in pancreatitis, 137
  thoracoscopic surgery and, 322
Computerization, 389-398. See also
        Digital peripheral brain.

Congenital adrenal hyperplasia, 213-214
Congestive heart failure, 379
Conn's syndrome, 215, 216
Contaminated wound, 259
Continent intraabdominal Kock pouch, 96
Continuous infusion for enteral nutrition, 21
Cord, spermatic, 177
Coronary artery bypass graft, 287-295
  complications of, 293-295
  discharge orders for, 295
  indications for, 287-288
  pathophysiology of, 287
  preoperative workup for, 288-290
  procedure for, 290-293
Coronary artery disease
  bypass graft for. *See* Coronary artery bypass graft.
  mesenteric ischemia and, 242
  transplantation for, 379
Corticoid-withdrawal phase, 16
Corticotropin, 214
Corticotropin-releasing hormone, 213
Cortisol, 216
Cranial nerve injury, 239
Cricoid membrane, 332
Cricothyroidotomy, 333
Crohn's disease, 91-94
Cullen's sign, 134
Cushing's syndrome
  preoperative workup for, 216-217
  presentation of, 214-215
Cyclic infusion for enteral nutrition, 22
Cyclosporine, 349
Cyst, 265-266
Cystic duct, gallstone in, 126
Cytomegalovirus, 351

**D**
DateBk4 software, 395-396
Death, umbilical hernia and, 186
Débridement
  of wound, 261
  pancreatic, 140-141
Deep postanal space, 107
  abscess of, 105-106
    surgery for, 108-109
Dehiscence, wound, 262-263
Dental evaluation in cardiac valve disease, 301
Dexamethasone, 216
Diabetes mellitus
  cardiac valve disease and, 301
  coronary artery bypass graft and, 290
  pancreatic transplant for, 353-359
Dialysis access, 249-253
  anatomy and, 251
  complications of, 252-253
  contraindications for, 250-251
  discharge instructions for, 253
  indications for, 249-250
  pathophysiology of, 249
  preoperative workup for, 251
  procedure for, 252
Diarrhea
  enteral nutrition and, 23
  ulcer surgery and, 65
Diet
  esophageal surgery and, 59
  gastric cancer and, 67
Dieulafoy's lesion, 30
Diffuse multinodular goiter, 189
Digital assistant, personal, 389-398
  accessories for, 397-398
  hardware manufacturers of, 391
  software for, 391-397
  system characteristics of, 389-390
Dilational tracheotomy, percutaneous, 333-334
Diphenhydramine, 349

Direct inguinal hernia, 175
Dirty wound, 259
Disease-specific alimental formula, 21
Distal splenorenal shunt, 146-147
Distributive shock, 41-42
Diverticular disease, 81-84
  anatomy in, 82
  bleeding in, 31
  complications of, 83-84
  discharge orders for, 84
  pathophysiology of, 81
  preoperative workup for, 81-82
  presentation of, 81
  surgery for, 82-83
Document viewer, 395
Donor
  heart, 381-382
  kidney, 346
  liver, 364
  lung, 372, 373-374
Dor operation, 57
Double-lung transplant, 374-375
Drainage
  biliary, enteral feeding and, 9
  of anorectal abscess, 110
  portal venous, 356
Dressing, wound, 262
Drug reference software, 392-394
Drug therapy, enteral feeding and, 9
Duct, parotid, 339
Ductal carcinoma in situ of breast, 223
Dumping syndrome
  gastric cancer surgery and, 72
  ulcer surgery and, 65
Duodenal segment leak after pancreatic transplant, 359
Duodenal ulcer, 61-65
Duplex scan
  carotid, 236
  in mesenteric ischemia, 244
Dyhydroepiandrosterone, 213

Dysphagia
  achalasia surgery and, 52
  reflux surgery and, 58
Dysrhythmia after lung cancer surgery, 315

E
Edema, pulmonary
  chest tube insertion and, 403
  postobstructive, 335-336
Effusion, pleural
  bypass graft and, 294
  thoracentesis for, 405-409
Electrolyte
  fluids and, 3-7
  in pancreatitis, 135
Embolism, mesenteric, 241-242
Empyema, chest tubes and, 404
End-stage disease, transplant for
  cardiac, 379
  lung, 371
Endarterectomy, carotid, 235-240
Endocavitary radiation, 120
Endocrine disorder
  adrenal, 213-221
  breast cancer, 223-232
  parathyroid, 197-204
  thyroid, 189-195
Endocrine tumor, pancreatic, 159
Endoscopic gastrostomy, percutaneous, 9-14
  complications of, 13-14
  discharge orders for, 14
  indications for, 9
  preoperative evaluation for, 10
  procedure for, 10-12
Endoscopic jejunostomy, percutaneous, 14
Endoscopic retrograde cholangio-pancreatography, 167-172
  anatomy in, 169-170
  complications of, 171-172
  discharge instructions for, 172

Endoscopic retrograde cholangio-
        pancreatography—cont'd
    for jaundice, 168-169
    in cholecystitis, 127
    in pancreatic cancer, 160-161
    in pancreatitis, 139
    pathophysiology of, 167-168
    procedure for, 170-171
    workup for, 169
Endoscopic ultrasonography,
        pancreatic, 208
Endoscopy
    anal fistula and, 101
    esophageal, 49
    gastric cancer and, 68
    gastrointestinal bleeding and, 33
    rectal cancer and, 116, 120
    ulcer and, 62
Enteral feeding, access for, 9-14
Enteral nutrition
    access for, 9-14
    surgical
        access for, 20
        assessment for, 17-18, 18t
        complications of, 21-22
        formula types for, 20-21
        indications for, 16-17, 20
        infusion methods in, 20-21
        nutritional requirements in,
            18-19
        protein-calorie malnutrition and,
            16
        stress-related metabolic
            changes and, 15-16
Enucleation for insulinoma, 210
Epidermal cyst, 265-266
Epidermoid tumor, 415
Epidural hematoma, 415
Epistaxis, 327-330
EPOC machine, 389
ePocrates qRx, 392
Esophageal leak, delayed, 52
Esophageal sphincter, lower, 47-48

Esophagogastroduodenoscopy
    for bleeding, 28
    for reflux, 54
    intraoperative, 210
Esophagogastropexy, 57
Esophagojejunal anastomosis, 71
Esophagojejunostomy, for gastric
        cancer, 70
Esophagraphy, barium, 54
Esophagus
    achalasia of, 47-52
    video-assisted thoracoscopy for,
        321
Exclusion criteria
    for heart transplant, 380
    for renal transplant, 345
Exercise testing in lung cancer, 308
External anal sphincter, 99-100
External hemorrhoid, 111
Extrapulmonary symptoms of lung
        cancer, 308
Extrasphincteric anal fistula, 100
Extubation, tracheotomy, 335
Exudative pleural effusion, 406-407

F
Facial nerve, parotidectomy and,
        341
Facial nerve in parotidectomy, 338
Familial adenomatous polyposis
    colon cancer and, 85
    rectal cancer and, 115
Fascia, abdominal, 260-261
Fasciitis, necrotizing, 13
Fasting, metabolic changes with, 15
Fat, requirement for, 19
Feeding, enteral, 9-14
Femoral hernia, 38
Fever in wound infection, 262
Fiberoptic bronchoscopy, 310
Fibrosis, idiopathic pulmonary, 371
Fine-needle aspiration biopsy
    in breast cancer, 227

Fine-needle aspiration biopsy—cont'd
  of salivary gland, 338
  thyroid, 192
  video-assisted thoracoscopic
    surgery and, 322
Fistula
  anal
    anatomy in, 101
    complications of, 104
    discharge orders for, 104
    pathophysiology of, 99-100
    preoperative workup for, 101
    presentation of, 100-101
    surgery for, 102-104
  bronchopleural, 315
  fluid and electrolyte loss from, 4-5
  gastrocolocutaneous, 13
  intestinal, 142
  tracheoesophageal, 335
  tracheoinnominate artery, 336
Flap
  advancement rectal, 103
  Bjork, 334
  parotidectomy and, 342
Fluid
  and electrolytes, 3-7
  cerebrospinal, 411-415
  cirrhosis and, 147
  in pancreatitis, 135
  pleural, 405-409
Fluid resuscitation
  for gastrointestinal obstruction, 36
  in shock, 42
Follicular thyroid cancer, 190
Foreign body in wound healing, 259
Formula, alimental, 20-21
Frey's syndrome, 342
Fundoplication
  for gastroesophageal reflux,
    55-56
  in achalasia, 51
  options for, 57
Fungal infection, 411

**G**
Gallbladder surgery, 125-132
Gallstone, pancreatitis and, 133-134, 139
Gas-bloat syndrome, 58
Gas exchange after bypass graft, 294
Gases, blood, in lung cancer, 308
Gastrectomy, for cancer, 69-72
Gastric cancer
  anatomy and, 69
  complications of, 72
  pathophysiology of, 67-68
  preoperative workup for, 68-69
  presentation of, 68
  surgery for, 69-71
Gastric decompression, 9
Gastric ulcer, 61-65
Gastric volvulus, 9
Gastrinoma, 152-153
  multiple endocrine neoplasia and, 205
  pathophysiology of, 204
  preoperative orders for, 208
  preoperative workup for, 207
  presentation of, 206
  surgery for, 209-211
  surgical anatomy and, 209
Gastritis
  bleeding in, 29
  gastric cancer surgery and, 72
Gastrocolocutaneous fistula, 13
Gastroesophageal reflux, 52, 53-59
  complications of, 58
  discharge instructions for, 59
  pathophysiology of, 53
  postoperative care for, 57-58
  preoperative workup for, 54-55
  presentation of, 53-54
  surgery for, 55-56
  surgical anatomy in, 55
Gastrointestinal disorder
  anorectal, 99-121. See also
    Anorectal disorder.

Gastrointestinal disorder—cont'd
  appendicitis, 75-79
  colon cancer, 85-89
  diverticular, 81-84
  enteral nutrition and, 23
  esophageal
    achalasia, 47-52
    reflux, 53-59
  fluid and electrolyte losses in, 4-5
  gastric cancer, 67-72
  Inflammatory bowel disease, 91-96
  intestinal obstruction, 35-39
  obstruction, 35-39
  pancreatic débridement and, 141, 142
  ulcer, 61-65
Gastrointestinal tract bleeding
  lower, 31-34
  upper, 27-30
Gastrojejunostomy, 70
Gastroplasty, Collis, 57
Gastrostomy, percutaneous endoscopic, 9-14
Gene, breast cancer, 223, 224, 225
Genetics
  of colon cancer, 85
  of rectal cancer, 115
Gland
  anal, 107
  parathyroid, 197-204
  salivary, 337-342
  thymus, 199
  thyroid
    disorder of, 189-195
    in tracheotomy, 332
Glucagon in pancreatic tumor, 204
Glucagonoma, 152-153
  preoperative workup for, 208
  surgery for, 209-211
Glucose intolerance, 21
Goiter, 189, 191
Goodsall rule, 101

Graft
  coronary artery bypass, 287-295
    complications of, 293-295
    discharge orders for, 295
    indications for, 287-288
    pathophysiology of, 287
    preoperative workup for, 288-290
    procedure for, 290-293
  in transplantation. See Transplantation.
Graft atherosclerosis, cardiac, 384-385
Graft rejection
  cardiac, 384
  liver, 369-370
  of pancreatic transplant, 358
  of renal transplant, 351
Graft thrombosis, pancreatic, 358
Graves' disease, 189-190, 191
Greater auricular nerve hypoesthesia, 341
Greater saphenous vein graft, 291
Grey-Turner's sign, 134
Groin, hernia in, 175-182
Groove, tracheoesophageal, 193
Guillain-Barré syndrome, 413
Gustatory sweating, 342
Gynecomastia, 224-225

## H

$H_2$ blocker, for ulcer, 61, 62
HandDBase software, 392
Hardware, digital, 391
Harris-Benedict equation, 18
Hartmann procedure for diverticulitis, 83
Harvest of cadaveric liver, 365
Hashimoto's thyroiditis, 189
Head of pancreas, cancer of, 162
Headache, postlumbar puncture, 415
Heart
  coronary artery bypass graft and, 287-295
  valvular disease of, 297-305

Heart failure, 379
Heart rate after bypass graft, 293
Heart transplantation, 379-385
    anatomy and, 381
    complications of, 384-385
    discharge instructions for, 385
    indications for, 379
    pathophysiology of, 379
    preoperative workup for, 379-381
    technique of, 381-384
*Helicobacter pylori,* 61, 62
Heller myotomy, 49-51
Hematologic disorder, 279-283
    anemia, 279-280
    bypass graft and, 294
    cardiac valve disease and, 300-301
    myoproliferative, 280
    thrombocytopenia, 280
Hematoma
    hernia surgery and, 182
    lumbar puncture and, 415
    parathyroid surgery and, 202-203
    parotidectomy and, 342
    thyroid surgery and, 195
Hematuria after transplantation
    pancreatic, 359
    renal, 350
Hemodialysis, 249-250
Hemodynamics, in cirrhosis, 144
Hemorrhage. *See* Bleeding.
Hemorrhagic shock, 41, 42
Hemorrhoid, 111-114
Hemothorax, 401
Hepatic artery thrombosis, 368-369
Hepatic failure, alimental formula for, 21
Hepatic transplantation, 361-370. *See also* Liver transplantation.
Hepaticojejunostomy, 163
Hepatobiliary disease
    cholecystectomy for, 125-132
    cirrhosis, 143-149
    liver cancer, 151-158

Hepatocellular disease
    carcinoma, 151-159
    liver transplant for, 362
Hereditary nonpolyposis colon cancer, 85
    rectal cancer in, 115
Hereditary spherocytosis, 279
Hernia, 38
    inguinal, 175-182
    paraesophageal, 53-59
    umbilical, 183-186
Herniation after lumbar puncture, 415
Hetertopic technique for heart transplant, 382-383
Hill esophagogastropexy, 57
Histamine-2 blocker, for ulcer, 61, 62
Hodgkin's lymphoma, 280
Hormonal therapy in breast cancer, 231
Hormone
    adrenocorticotropic, action of, 213
    corticotropin-releasing, 213
Horseshoe abscess, anorectal, 109
Hurthel cell cancer, 190
Hydrocortisone in renal transplantation, 349
Hydrolyzed alimental formula, 21
Hyperacute rejection of renal transplant, 351
Hyperaldosteronism
    preoperative workup for, 216-217
    presentation of, 215
Hyperamylasemia, 136
Hypercalcemia, 198
Hypergastrinemia, 207
Hyperglycemia, 136
Hyperlipasemia, 136
Hyperparathyroidism, 197-198
    complications of, 202-203
    discharge instructions for, 204
    persistent, 203
    preoperative workup for, 198-199

Hyperparathyroidism—cont'd
  presentation of, 198
  surgery for, 199-202
Hypertension
  bypass graft and, 294
  portal, in cirrhosis, 143, 146
  pulmonary, lung transplant for, 371
Hyperthyroidism, 189, 191-192
Hypocalcemia after parathyroid surgery, 203
Hypoesthesia, auricular nerve, 341
Hypoglycemia
  coronary artery bypass graft and, 290
  in pancreatitis, 136
Hypoparathyroidism, 195
Hypotension, bypass graft and, 293-294
Hypovolemic shock, 41

I
Iatrogenic injury
  nerve
    carotid endarterectomy and, 239
    parathyroid surgery and, 203
    parotidectomy and, 341
    thyroidectomy and, 195
  to common bile duct, 131
Idiopathic thrombocytopenic purpura, 280
Ileocecal resection, 93
Ileorectal anastomosis, 93
Ileostomy
  in Crohn's disease, 93
  in ulcerative colitis, 95, 96
Ilial-pouch anal anastomosis, 96
Ilioinguinal ligament, 177
Immunomodulatory alimental formula, 21
Immunosuppressive therapy
  for heart transplant, 383

Immunosuppressive therapy—cont'd
  for pancreatic transplantation, 358
  for renal transplantation, 349
  wound healing and, 259
Inborn error of metabolism, liver transplant for, 362
Incarcerated hernia, umbilical, 183
Incidental appendectomy, 75
Inclusion criteria for transplant
  pancreatic, 353-354
  renal, 346
Incontinence after anal fistulotomy, 104
Infarction, bowel, 141
Infected wound, 259
Infection
  cirrhosis and, 147
  coronary artery bypass graft and, 295
  cyst, 266
  dialysis access and, 253
  endoscopic retrograde cholangiopancreatography and, 171
  enteral nutrition and, 22
  hemorrhoid surgery and, 114
  hernia surgery and, 182
  liver transplant and, 369
  lumbar puncture for, 411-412
  lung transplant and, 376
  pancreatic, 139
  parotidectomy and, 342
  percutaneous endoscopic gastrostomy and, 13
  renal transplantation and, 350-351
  thyroiditis, 189
  wound, 262
Inferior mesenteric artery, ischemia of, 241, 242
Inflammation
  appendicitis, 75

Inflammation—cont'd
  cholecystitis, 125-127
  diverticular, 81
  pancreatic, 133-142. *See also*
      Pancreatitis.
  salivary gland, 338
  wound healing and, 257
Inflammatory bowel disease
  Crohn's, 91-94
  ulcerative colitis, 94-96
Inflammatory breast cancer, 224-225
Infusion, enteral nutrition, 21-22, 22t
Inguinal hernia, 38, 175-182
  anatomy in, 176-177
  complications of, 182
  discharge orders for, 181
  pathophysiology of, 175-176
  presentation of, 176
  surgery for, 177-181
Injury, iatrogenic. *See also* Trauma.
  nerve
      carotid endarterectomy and, 239
      parathyroid surgery and, 203
      parotidectomy and, 341
      thyroidectomy and, 195
  to common bile duct, 131
Insulin
  coronary artery bypass graft and,
      290
  pancreas transplant and, 290
Insulinoma, 152-153
  pathophysiology of, 204
  preoperative orders for, 208
  preoperative workup for, 207
  presentation of, 205, 206
  surgery for, 209-211
Intensive care unit, stress ulcers in,
      30
Intercostal neurovascular bundle, 402
Intermittent gastric volvulus, 9
Intermittent infusion for enteral
      nutrition, 22

Internal anal sphincteric, 99
Internal hemorrhoid, 111
Internal jugular vein, 237
Intersphincteric abscess, 108
Intersphincteric anal fistula, 99
Interval appendectomy, 75
Intestinal obstruction, 35-39
Intraabdominal Kock pouch, 96
Intraabdominal pressure, dialysis
      access and, 253
Intracerebral lesion, 415
Intraoperative choloangiography, 130
Intraoperative esophagogastroduo-
      denoscopy, 210
Intrathoracic pressure, 335-336
Intravascular space, third space fluid
      and, 5
Introducer endoscopic gastrostomy,
      11-12
Introducer percutaneous endoscopic
      gastrostomy, 11-12
Invasive breast cancer, 224
Iodine deficiency goiter, 191
Ischemia
  mesenteric, 241-247. *See also*
      Mesenteric ischemia.
  pancreatic débridement and, 141
Ischioanal abscess, 108
Ischioanal space, 107
Islet cell transplantation, 357
Islet cell tumor, 208

**J**
J-File, 392
Jaundice
  cholangiopancreatography for,
      167
  in pancreatic cancer, 160, 167
Jejunjejunostomy, 71
Jejunostomy, percutaneous
      endoscopic, 14
Jugular vein, internal, 237

## K

Keyboard for personal digital
    assistant, 397
Kock pouch, 96
Kwashiorkor, 16

## L

Laceration, tracheal, 335
Lag phase of wound healing, 257
Laparoscopy
    achalasia and, 49-51
    adrenalectomy, 218-219
    appendectomy and, 78
    cancer and
        gastric, 71
        pancreatic, 161-162
    cholescystectomy and, 129-130
    gastroesophageal reflux and,
        55-56
    hernia and, 180-181
        paraesophageal, 56
        umbilical, 185-186
    percutaneous endoscopic
        gastrostomy via, 12
    splenectomy and, 279, 281-282
Laparotomy, esophageal, 57
Large cell lung cancer, 307
Laryngeal nerve
    in thyroid surgery, 193, 195
    parathyroid surgery and, 203
Leak, bile duct, 369
Leakage
    after pancreatic transplantation,
        359
    esophageal, in achalasia, 52
    of dialysate, 253
    of percutaneous endoscopic
        gastrostomy, 13
Left adrenalectomy, 218, 219
Left colon cancer, 86
Lentigo maligna melanoma, 270
Leukemia, chronic lymphocytic, 280
Leukocytosis, 411-412

LexiDrugs software, 393
Ligament
    hepatic, 154
    ilioinguinal, 177
Ligation of hemorrhoid, 112, 113
Lipase in pancreatitis, 136
Lipid, 19
Lipoma, 266
Liver
    bile secretion by, 125-126
    cancer of, 151-158
    cirrhosis of, 143-149, 145t
    in pancreatic surgery, 210
Liver cancer
    anatomy in, 154-155
    complications of, 158
    discharge orders for, 158
    pathophysiology of, 151
    preoperative workup for, 153
    presentation of, 152-153
    surgery for, 155-158
Liver failure, alimental formula for, 21
Liver function
    cardiac valve disease and, 300
    coronary artery bypass graft and,
        289
    in cancer, 153
    in cirrhosis, 144, 145, 145t
Liver metastasis, 86
Liver transplantation, 361-370
    cholangiopancreatography after,
        168
    complications of, 368-370
    discharge instructions for, 370
    donor selection in, 364
    elective, 362-363
    urgent, 363-364
Liver tumor, transplant for, 362
Lobe
    liver, 154, 155
    salivary gland, 339
Lobectomy
    hepatic, 156

Lobectomy—cont'd
  lung, 313-314
Lobular carcinoma in situ of breast,
      223-224
Locally advanced breast cancer, 224
Loop ileostomy, 93
Low anterior resection, rectal, 118-
      121
Lower esophageal sphincter, 47-48
Lower gastrointestinal tract bleeding,
      31-34
Lumbar puncture, 411-415
Lumpectomy, 228, 230
Lung, chest tubes and, 401-404
Lung cancer, 307-315
  anatomy and, 313
  complications of, 315
  discharge orders for, 315
  pathophysiology of, 307
  preoperative workup for, 308-313
  presentation of, 308
  surgery for, 313-315
Lung reduction surgery, 317-320
Lung transplantation, 371-377
  complications of, 376
  discharge instructions for, 376-
      377
  indications for, 371-372
  pathophysiology of, 371
  preoperative workup for, 372-
      373
  technique of, 373-376
Lymph node
  in breast cancer, 228-230, 231
  in melanoma, 270
Lymphedema, 230-231
Lymphocele
  pancreatic transplant and, 359
  renal transplantation and, 350
Lymphocytic leukemia, 280
Lymphoma
  Hodgkin's, 280
  thyroid, 191

## M

Magnetic resonance imaging
  for carotid arterectomy, 236
  in liver cancer, 153
  in rectal cancer, 116
Maintenance fluids and electrolytes,
      3-4
Male breast cancer, 224-225
Malignancy. See Cancer.
  breast cancer, 223-232. See also
      Breast cancer.
  colon, 85-89
  esophageal, 321
  gastric, 67-72
  liver, 151-158
  liver transplant for, 362
  melanoma, 269-275
  meningeal carcinomatosis and,
      412
  pancreatic, 159-165, 205-212
  parathyroid, 198
  rectal, 115-121
  renal transplant and, 351
  retroperitoneal, 266
  salivary gland, 337
  skin, 265-268
  skin or soft tissue, 265-268
  thyroid, 190-191
Mallory-Weiss tear, 30
Malnutrition, wound healing and,
      259
Mammography, in male, 226
Manometry, esophageal, 49, 54
Marasmus, 16
Mass, inguinal hernia as, 175, 176
Mastectomy
  for breast carcinoma in situ, 223
  in male, 226
  modified radical, 228
Mathematics software, 393-395
Maturation, wound, 257
Mechanical complications of enteral
      nutrition, 22

Mechanical ventilation, 331
Med Calc software, 394
Mediastinal shift, 315
Mediastinal surgery, video-assisted, 321
Mediastinoscopy, 322
    in lung cancer, 309, 313
Medical mathematics software, 393-395
MedMath software, 393-394
Medullary thyroid cancer, 191
Melanoma, 269-275
    anatomy and, 271-272
    complications of, 275
    discharge orders for, 275
    pathophysiology of, 269
    preoperative workup for, 270-271
    presentation of, 269-270
    surgery for, 272-275
Membrane, cricoid, 332
Memory, computer, 389
Meningeal carcinomatosis, 412
Meningitis, 411-412
Mesenteric ischemia, 241-247
    anatomy and, 244-245
    complications of, 247
    pathophysiology of, 241-243
    preoperative workup for, 243-244
    presentation of, 243
    surgery for, 245-247
Mesenteric vessel in pancreatic cancer, 160, 162, 164
Metabolic disorder
    enteral nutrition and, 22
    liver transplant for, 362
Metastasis
    colon cancer, 86
    liver, 151-152
        pancreatic surgery and, 210
    lung cancer, 308
    retroperitoneal, 266
Methylprednisolone for renal transplantation, 349

Mitral regurgitation, 297
    complications of, 304
Mitral stenosis, 298
    complications of, 304
Mitral valve repair or replacement, 302-303
Modified radical mastectomy, 228
Modular alimental formula, 21
Moromonab for renal transplantation, 349
Mortality, umbilical hernia and, 186
Mucoepidermoid carcinoma of salivary gland, 337
Mucous plugging after tracheotomy, 335
Multinodular goiter, 189
Multiple endocrine neoplasia, 205
Multiple sclerosis, 413
Muscle
    abdominal, peritoneal dialysis and, 251
    perirectal abscess and, 107
Mycophenolate for renal transplantation, 349
Myeloproliferative disorder, 280
Myocardial infarction
    carotid endarterectomy and, 239
    risk for, 287
Myocardial perfusion, 287-288
Myocardial protection, 302
Myotomy, Heller, 49-51

N
Nasogastric suction in pancreatitis, 135
Nasogastric tube
    fluid and electrolyte loss from, 5
    for enteral feeding, 20
    for gastrointestinal obstruction, 37
Necrosis
    pancreatic, 133
    renal tubular, 350
    skin flap, in parotidectomy, 342

Necrotizing fasciitis, 13
Neoadjuvant therapy for skin or soft tissue tumor, 266
Neoplasm. *See* Cancer; Tumor.
Nerve disorder
  carotid endarterectomy and, 239
  Frey's syndrome and, 342
  parathyroid surgery and, 203
  parotidectomy and, 341
  recurrent laryngeal, 195
Neuroendocrine liver metastasis, 151
Neurogenic shock, 41-42
Neurologic deficit after carotid endarterectomy, 239
Neurovascular bundle, intercostal, 402
Nipple, Paget's disease of, 226
Nissen fundoplication, 55-56
Nitrogen balance, 17-18
Nodular melanoma, 270
Nodule, pulmonary, 310
Nonfunctional islet cell tumor, 208
Nonnodular goiter, 189-190, 191
Nonpolyposis colon cancer, hereditary, 115
Non–small-cell lung cancer, 307
  treatment of, 311-313
Nosebleed, 327-330
Nutrition
  enteral
    access for, 9-14
    surgical, 15-23
  esophageal surgery and, 59
  wound healing and, 259

**O**

Obesity, wound healing and, 259
Obliterative bronchiolitis, 376
Obstruction
  cystic duct, 126
  gastrointestinal, 35-39
    complications of, 39
    discharge instructions for, 39

Obstruction—cont'd
  gastrointestinal—cont'd
    pathophysiology of, 35
    preoperative evaluation of, 35-37
    presentation of, 35
    surgery for, 37-39
    tracheotomy for, 331
    umbilical hernia causing, 183
Obstructive pulmonary disease, chronic, lung reduction surgery for, 317-320
Occlusion
  coronary artery, 287
  renal transplantation and, 350
Octreotide, for ulcer, 65
Off-pump coronary artery bypass graft, 292
Omeprazole in pancreatic tumor, 212
Open cholecystectomy, 130
Operating system, Windows, 389-390
Opportunistic infection after renal transplant, 351
Orthotopic technique for heart transplant, 382

**P**

Packing
  for nosebleed, 329
  of wound, 262
Paget's disease of nipple, 226
Pain
  chest, 287
  in pancreatic cancer, 160
  in pancreatitis, 134, 135
  mesenteric ischemia causing, 241, 243
  postcholecystectomy, 167-168
  ulcer causing, 61
  umbilical hernia causing, 184
Palliative therapy
  in pancreatic tumor, 212
  splenectomy as, 280

Palm OS machine, 389, 390
PalmPrint, 396
Pancreatic cancer, 159-165
    complications of, 165
    discharge instructions in, 165
    pathophysiology of, 159
    preoperative workup for, 160-161
    presentation of, 160
    surgery for, 161-165
Pancreatic neoplasm, 205-212
    anatomy and, 209
    complications of, 212
    discharge instructions for, 212
    pathophysiology of, 205-206
    preoperative workup for, 207-209
    presentation of, 206-207
    surgery for, 209-212
Pancreatic transplantation, 353-359
    anatomy and, 355
    complications of, 358-359
    discharge orders for, 359
    inclusion crieteria for, 353-354
    pathophysiology of, 353
    preoperative workup for, 354-
        355
    technique for, 355-358
Pancreaticoduodenectomy, 210-211
Pancreatitis, 133-142
    anatomy in, 138
    complications of, 141-142
    discharge orders for, 142
    nonoperative management of,
        135
    pathophysiology of, 133-134
    post-ERCP, 171-172
    posttransplant, 358-359
    preoperative workup for, 135-138,
        137t
    presentation of, 134-135
    surgery for, 139-141
Papillary thyroid cancer, 190
Paraesophageal hernia, 53-59
    complications of, 58

Paraesophageal hernia—cont'd
    postoperative care for, 58
    preoperative workup for, 54-55
    presentation of, 53-54
    surgery for, 56-57
Parathyroid disorder, 197-204
    cancer, 198
    complications of, 202-203
    discharge instructions for, 204
    hyperparathyroidism, 197-198
    postoperative orders for, 202
    preoperative workup for, 198-199
    presentation of, 198
    surgery for, 199-202
Parathyroid gland, in thyroid surgery,
        193
Parotidectomy, 337-342
    anatomy and, 339
    complications of, 341-342
    discharge orders for, 342
    indications for, 337-338
    preoperative workup for, 338-
        339
    procedure for, 339-341
Patient keeper, 391
Patient tracking software, 391-392
PEG. See Percutaneous endoscopic
        gastrostomy.
Peptic ulcer disease, 61-65
    bleeding in, 29
Percutaneous dilational tracheotomy,
        333-334
Percutaneous endoscopic gastros-
        tomy, 9-14
Percutaneous endoscopic jejunos-
        tomy, 14
Percutaneous transhepatic cholangi-
        ography, 167
Perforation
    endoscopic retrograde cholangio-
        pancreatography and, 171
    esophageal or gastric, 58
    of appendix, 79

Perfusion
  myocardial, 287-288
  tissue, 261-262
Perianal abscess, 107-108
Peripheral vascular disease, 288
  cardiac valve disease and, 299
Perirectal abscess, 105-110
Peristomal infection, 13
Peritoneal dialysis, chronic
      ambulatory, 249-253
Peritonitis, 13
Personal computer, 389
Personal digital assistant, 389-398.
      See also Digital assistant,
      personal.
Pheochromocytoma
  complications of, 220
  preoperative workup for, 216-217
  presentation of, 215
Physicians Drug Handbook, 393
Pigmented gallstone, 126
Pleural effusion
  bypass graft and, 294
  thoracentesis for, 405-409
Pleural space, 401
Plug, mucous, 335
Plummer's syndrome, 189-190
Pneumomediastinum, 335
Pneumonectomy for lung cancer, 314
Pneumoperitoneum, 13
Pneumothorax
  bypass graft and, 294
  lung cancer and, 310
  thoracentesis and, 409
  tracheotomy and, 335
  trauma and, 401
Polymeric alimental formula, 20-21
Polyp
  gastric cancer and, 67
  rectal cancer and, 115
Portal hypertension, 143, 146
Portal vein thrombosis, liver
      transplant and, 361

Portal venous drainage, 356
Postanal space
  abscess of, 105-106
    surgery for, 108-109
  anatomy of, 107
Postcholecystectomy pain, 167-168
Postobstructive pulmonary edema,
      335-336
Postprandial pain, 243
Pouch
  ilial, 96
  Kock, 96
Prednisone for renal transplantation,
      349
Pregnancy, breast cancer during, 224
Pressure
  central venous, 7
  intraabdominal, dialysis access
      and, 253
  portal venous, 143
Printer for personal digital assistant,
      398
Proctocolectomy
  in Crohn's disease, 93
  in ulcerative colitis, 96
Proctoscopy, 101
Proliferative phase in wound healing,
      257
Protein-calorie malnutrition, types of,
      16
Protein requirement, 19
Pseudotumor cerebri, 413
Pull percutaneous endoscopic
      gastrostomy, 11
Pulmonary alimental formula, 21
Pulmonary disease, chronic
      obstructive, 317-320
Pulmonary edema
  chest tube insertion and, 403
  postobstructive, 335-336
Pulmonary function
  bypass graft and, 294
  in lung cancer, 308

Pulmonary function—cont'd
  video-assisted thoracoscopic
      surgery and, 322
Pulmonary hypertension, 371
Pulmonary insufficiency
  cardiac valve disease and, 300
  coronary artery bypass graft and,
      289
Pulmonary transplantation, 371-377
Puncture, lumbar, 411-415
Purpura, thrombocytopenic, 280
Push percutaneous endoscopic
      gastrostomy, 11

**R**
Radiation therapy
  in breast cancer, 231
  in rectal cancer, 120
  wound healing and, 259
Radical mastectomy, modified, 228
Radiographic evaluation
  anal fistula and, 101
  cholecystitis and, 127
  Crohn's disease and, 92
  gastrointestinal obstruction and, 36
  hyperparathyroidism and, 199
  liver cancer and, 153
  lung cancer and, 309
  pancreatic cancer and, 160
  pancreatitis and, 136-137
  percutaneous endoscopic
      gastrostomy and, 12
  renal transplant and, 346
  ulcerative colitis and, 95
Radionuclide scan in cholecystitis,
      128
Ranson's criterion in pancreatitis,
      138, 138t
Rectal bleeding, 31-34
Rectal cancer, 115-121
  anatomy in, 118
  complications of, 120-121
  discharge instructions for, 121

Rectal cancer—cont'd
  pathophysiology of, 115
  preoperative workup for, 116-118,
      117t
  presentation of, 116
  staging of, 117t
  surgery for, 118-120
Rectal flap, 103
Recurrence
  of anorectal abscess, 110
  of carotid stenosis, 239
  of hernia, 182
  of sialadenitis, 338
  of ulcer, 64-65
Recurrent laryngeal nerve
  in thyroid surgery, 193, 195
  parathyroid surgery and, 203
Reflux, gastroesophageal, 52, 53-59
Reflux gastritis, 72
Reflux pancreatitis, 358-359
Regurgitation, mitral, 297
  complications of, 304
Rejection of transplant
  heart, 383
  liver, 369-370
  lung, 376
  pancreatic, 358
  renal, 351
Remolding, wound, 263
Renal artery stenosis, 350
Renal failure
  alimental formula for, 21
  cardiac valve disease and, 300
  coronary artery bypass graft and,
      289
  dialysis access in, 249-253
  wound healing and, 259
Renal function
  coronary artery bypass graft and,
      295
  parathyroidectomy and, 197-198
Renal transplantation, 345-352
  anatomy and, 347

Renal transplantation—cont'd
  complications of, 350-351
  discharge orders for, 351-352
  indications for, 345
  pathophysiology of, 345
  preoperative workup for, 345-347
  technique of, 347-349
Respiratory system. *See also*
      Pulmonary *entries.*
  chest tubes and, 401-404
  lung transplant and, 371-377
Resting energy expenditure, 18-19
Restrictive lung disease, 371
Resuscitation, fluid, 36
Retrograde cholangiopancreatography,
      endoscopic, 167-172
  in pancreatic cancer, 160-161
  in pancreatitis, 139
Retroperitoneal tumor, 266
  surgery for, 267
Right adrenalectomy, 218-219
Right colon cancer, 86
Roux-en-Y esophagojejunostomy,
      70
Rubber band ligation of hemorrhoid,
      112, 113
Russell endoscopic gastrostomy,
      11-12

**S**
Sacks-Vine endoscopic gastrostomy,
      11
Salivary gland surgery, 337-342
Saphenous vein graft, 291
Sarcoma
  discharge orders for, 268
  pathophysiology of, 265
  surgery for, 267
Scan
  carotid duplex, 236
  in lung cancer, 309
  parathyroid, 199
Secretin stimulation test, 208

Secretion, tracheotomy and, 331
Seizure, 413
Selective arterial secretin stimulation
      test, 208
Sepsis
  hemorrhoid surgery and, 114
  metabolic changes with, 15
  splenectomy and, 283
Seroma
  hernia surgery and, 182
  tumor surgery and, 268
Serum amylase, 136
Serum lipase, 136
Setamibi scan, 199
Seton for anal fistula, 103-104
Shock, 41-43
Shunt, splenorenal, 146-147
Sigmoid cancer, 86
Sigmoid volvulus, 39
Single-lung transplant, 374
Skin
  melanoma of, 269-275
  wound healing and, 257-265. *See
      also* Wound healing.
Skin flap necrosis, 342
Skin tumor, 265-268
Sleeve lobectomy, 314
Small-cell lung cancer, 307, 313
Small intestine, obstruction of, 38
SmartDoc, 395
Smoking, wound healing and, 259
Soft tissue tumor, 265-268
Software
  drug reference, 392-394
  mathematics, 393-395
  patient tracking, 391-392
Solitary nodule, pulmonary, 310
Somatostatinoma
  pathophysiology of, 204-205
  preoperative workup for, 208
  presentation of, 206
  surgery for, 209-211
  surgical anatomy and, 209

Space
  anorectal, 105, 107
  pleural, 401
  third space fluid loss, 5-7
Spermatic cord, 177
Spherocytosis, hereditary, 279
Sphincter
  hemorrhoid surgery and, 114
  lower esophageal, 47-48
Splanchnic circulation in cirrhosis, 143-144
Splenectomy, 279-283
  anatomy and, 281
  complications of, 283
  discharge orders for, 283
  indications for, 279-281
  pathophysiology and, 279
  preoperative workup for, 281
  procedure for, 281-283
Splenorenal shunt, 146-147
Sputum in lung cancer, 309-310
Staging, cancer
  lung, 310-312
  melanoma, 270
  pancreatic, 159
  rectal, 117t
Staple, skin, 263
Starvation, 15
Stenosis
  aortic, 298-299
    complications of, 304
  carotid endarterectomy for, 235-240
  mitral, 298
    complications of, 304
  renal artery, 350
  tracheal, 336
Sternotomy
  cardiac valve disease and, 302
  coronary artery bypass graft and, 290
  lung volume reduction and, 319
Steroid
  cardiac valve disease and, 300

Steroid—cont'd
  coronary artery bypass graft and, 289
  wound healing and, 259
Stimulation test, secretin, 208
Stomach
  cancer of, 67-72. See also Gastric cancer.
  ulcer of, 61-65
Stone
  common bile duct
    cholangiopancreatography for, 168-169
    pancreatitis and, 140
  gallbladder, 125-126
  in hyperparathyroidism, 198
Storm, thyroid, 195
Strangulated hernia, umbilical, 183, 185
Stress gastritis, bleeding in, 29
Strictureplasty, 93
Stroke, carotid endarterectomy for, 235-240
Subarachnoid hematoma, 415
Subcutaneous tissue in wound closure, 261
Subdural hematoma, 415
Subtotal gastrectomy, 69-70
Suction, nasogastric, in pancreatitis, 135
Sulcus tumor, superior, 308, 314
Superficial spreading melanoma, 270
Superior mesenteric vessel, 244, 245-246
  in pancreatic cancer, 160, 162, 164
  ischemia of, 241
Superior sulcus tumor, lung, 314
Superior sulcus tumor of lung, 308
Superventricular dysrhythmia, 315
Supralevator abscess, 108
Supralevator space, 107
  abscess in, 105

Supralevator space—cont'd
  anatomy of, 107
Suprasphincteric anal fistula, 100
Surface area, peritoneal, 249
Surgery, for thyroid disorder, 193-
    195
Surgical wound, 259-263
Swallowing disorder, achalasia,
    47-52
Sweating, gustatory, 342
SynCalc software, 394

## T

99mTc-HMDP scan, in gastrointestinal
    bleeding, 32
TealDoc, 395
TealPhone, 396-397
Tear, Mallory-Weiss, 30
Thalassemia, 279-280
Third space fluid loss, 5-7
Thombolytic therapy for mesenteric
    ischemia, 244
Thoracentesis, 405-409
Thoracic surgery
  coronary artery bypass graft, 287-
    295
  for cardiac valve disease, 297-305
  for lung cancer, 307-315
Thoracoscopy
  in lung volume reduction, 318-
    319
  video-assisted, 321-324
Thrombocytopenia, 280
Thrombosis
  hepatic artery, 368-369
  mesenteric, 241-242
  pancreatic graft, 358
  portal vein, 361
Thrombotic thrombocytopenic
    purpura, 280
Thymoglobulin for renal
    transplantation, 349
Thymus gland, 199

Thyroid gland, 189-195
  cancer of, 190-191
  discharge instructions for, 195
  goiter and, 189, 191
  hyperthyroidism, 189, 191-192
  preoperative workup for, 192
  surgery of, 193-195
  surgical anatomy of, 193
  surgical complications of, 195
  tracheotomy and, 332
Thyroid storm, 195
Thyroiditis, 189
Thyrotoxicosis, 189-190, 191
Tissue perfusion, 261-262
TNM staging, of rectal cancer, 117
Total energy expenditure, 18-19
Total gastrectomy, for cancer, 70-71
Totally exptraperitoneal approach in
    hernia surgery, 180, 181
Toupet fundoplication, 57
Toxic nonnodular goiter, 189-190,
    191
Tracheoesophageal fistula, 335
Tracheoesophageal groove, 193
Tracheoinnominate artery fistula,
    336
Tracheotomy, 331-336
Transabdominal laparoscopic
    adrenalectomy, 218-219
Transabdominal preperitoneal
    approach in hernia surgery,
    180, 181
Transanal endoscopic microsurgery,
    120
Transhepatic cholangiography, 167
Transient ischemic attack, 235-240
Transplantation
  heart, 379-385
  liver, 361-370
  lung, 371-377
  pancreatic, 353-359
  renal, 345-352
Transsphincteric anal fistula, 99-100

Transthoracic surgery
  esophageal, 56-57
  for paraesophageal hernia, 58
Transudative pleural effusion, 406
Transverse colon cancer, 86
Trauma
  chest tubes and, 401
  facial nerve, 341
  metabolic changes with, 15
  nosebleed from, 327, 328
  splenectomy and, 281
  wound healing and, 260, 261
Triad, Whipple's, 205
Trismus, 342
Tube
  chest, 401-404
  nasogastric. See Nasogastric tube.
  tracheotomy, 335
Tubular necrosis, renal, 350
Tumor
  benign
    parathyroid adenoma, 198
    salivary gland, 337
  epidermoid, 415
  malignant. See Malignancy.
  pheochromocytoma
    complications of, 220
    preoperative workup for, 216-217
    presentation of, 215

**U**

Ulcer disease, 61-65
  bleeding in, 29
  complications of, 64-65, 65t
  discharge orders for, 65
  evaluation of, 61-62
  pathophysiology of, 61
  preoperative orders for, 62
  presentation of, 61
  surgery for, 63-64
  surgical anatomy in, 63
Ulcerative colitis, 94-96

Ultrasonography
  anal fistula and, 101
  appendicitis and, 76
  cholecystitis and, 127-128
  gastric cancer and, 69
  gastrointestinal obstruction and, 36
  pancreatic, 208, 210
  rectal cancer and, 116, 117
Umbilical hernia, 183-186
Uncinate process of pancreas, 162
Upper gastrointestinal tract bleeding, 27-30
Uremia, wound healing and, 259
Urologic complications of renal transplant, 350
Urologic evaluation for renal transplant, 346

**V**

Vagotomy for ulcer, 63-64
Valve disease, cardiac, 297-305
  complications of, 304-305
  discharge orders for, 305
  pathophysiology of, 297
  preoperative workup for, 299-302
  presentation of, 297-299
  surgery for, 302-304
Variceal bleeding, 29-30, 146
Vascular access for dialysis, 249-253
Vascular disorder
  cardiac valve disease and, 299
  carotid endarterectomy for, 235-240
  coronary, 287-293
  mesenteric ischemia, 241-247
  nosebleed and, 328-329
  peripheral, 288
  renal transplantation and, 350
Vascularity in wound healing, 259
Vasoactive intestinal polypeptide–secreting tumor. See VIPoma.
VATS, 321-324

Vein
  internal jugular, 237
  superior mesenteric, 160, 162, 164
Venous drainage, portal, 356
Venous pressure
  central, third space fluid and, 7
  portal, 143
Venous thrombosis
  mesenteric ischemia and, 242
  portal, liver transplant and, 361
Ventilation, tracheotomy and, 331
Ventricular filling, bypass graft and,
      293
Video-assisted thoracoscopic surgery,
      321-324
  in lung cancer, 309
Viewer, document, 395
VIPoma
  pathophysiology of, 204
  preoperative workup for, 207, 208
  presentation of, 206
  surgery for, 209-211
Viral infection, 412
Volume reduction surgery, lung, 317-
      320

Volume resuscitation, 43
Volvulus
  enteral feeding and, 9
  sigmoid, 39
Vomiting, Mallory-Weiss tear from, 30

W
Wedge resection, lung, 314
Whipple's triad, 205
White blood cells in appendicitis, 76
Whole protein alimental formula,
      20-21
Windows operating system, 389-390
WordComplete, 397
Wound healing, 257-264
  complications of, 262-263
  discharge orders for, 263
  factors affecting, 258-259
  pathophysiology of, 257-258
  postoperative orders for, 261-262
  preoperative workup for, 260
  surgical closure and, 260-261
  types of, 258
Wound infection after parotidectomy,
      342